ALLE·ZEIT·WACH
1842

Ad Aertsen Valentino Braitenberg (Eds.)

Information Processing in the Cortex

Experiments and Theory

With 102 Figures

Springer-Verlag
Berlin Heidelberg New York
London Paris Tokyo
Hong Kong Barcelona Budapest

Dr. Ad Aertsen
Universität Bochum
Institut für Neuroinformatik
Postfach 102148
Gebäude ND 04
W-4630 Bochum, FRG

Professor Dr. Valentino Braitenberg
Max-Planck-Institut
für biologische Kybernetik
Spemannstraße 38
W-7400 Tübingen, FRG

ISBN 3-540-55391-6 Springer-Verlag Berlin Heidelberg New York
ISBN 0-387-55391-6 Springer-Verlag New York Berlin Heidelberg

Library of Congress Cataloging-in-Publication Data.
Information processing in the cortex: experiments and theory / edited by Ad Aertsen and Valentino Braitenberg. p. cm. Includes bibliographical references and index.
ISBN 3-540-55391-6 – ISBN 0-387-55391-6 (U.S.)
1. Cerebral cortex. 2. Human information processing. 3. Cognitive neuroscience. I. Aertsen, Ad (Adrianus), 1948–. II. Braitenberg, Valentino. QP383.I54 1992 612.8′25–dc20 92-19742 CIP

Typesetting: Camera ready by Margarete Ghasroldashti, MPI, Tübingen
31/3145-5 4 3 2 1 0 – Printed on acid-free paper

Preface

There is a tradition of theoretical brain science which started in the forties (Wiener, McCulloch, Turing, Craik, Hebb). This was continued by a small number of people without interruption up to the present. It has definitely provided main guiding lines for brain science, the development of which has been spectacular in the last decades. However, within the bulk of experimental neuroscience, the theoreticians sometimes had a difficult stand, since it was felt that the times were not ripe yet and the methods not yet available for a development of a true theoretical speciality in this field. Thus theory remained in the hands of a fairly small club which recruited its members from theoretical physicists, mathematicians and some experimentalists with amateurish theoretical leanings. The boom of approaches which go by the name of 'computational neuroscience', 'neuronal networks', 'associative memory', 'spinglass theory', 'parallel processing' etc. should not blind one for the fact that the group of people professionally interested in realistic models of brain function up to the present date remains rather small and suffers from a lack of professional organization.

It was against this background that we decided to organize a meeting on Theoretical Brain Science. The meeting was held April 18 - 20, 1990 and took place at Schloss Ringberg, West-Germany, a facility sponsored by the Max-Planck-Society. There were of course precursors, notably a meeting in Ravello on Neural Networks in 1967, organized by E. Caianiello[1], a small meeting in 1972 and a more extensive one in 1978, both organized by Güttinger at the Center for Theoretical Physics in Trieste[2], a meeting in Tübingen (1977), organized by Heim and Palm[3], a meeting in Palo Alto (1983), organized by Gerstein and Perkel, and several informal meetings at the MPI Göttingen, organized by Christoph von der Malsburg, as well as several others in the U.S. and Europe.

The present meeting was the third in a row organized by a group who met for the first time in October 1984 at the International Center for Theoretical Physics in Trieste[4]. The same group with some variations met again in Bad Homburg[5] and, as an offshoot, a group partly overlapping with the first, organized a meeting in Nijmegen[6], and in Irvine (Shaw, 1988).

The group was held together by an interest in theoretical models that actively seek confrontation with experimental data from the functioning brain, and by a didactic effort aimed at experimentalists to present their data in a format that makes them more amenable to theory.

Since in the preceding meetings some more general questions of brain theory had been in the foreground it was decided this time to focus on a single topic, the cerebral cortex. There were three aspects which we wanted to highlight in the three days of the meeting. On the first day statistical aspects of cortical connectivity were discussed both from an anatomical and a physiological point of view. The second day was dedicated to the part of the cortex which has been studied most, the visual cortex. The third day concerned itself with the question at what level of resolution in space and time cortical activity makes sense.

Since this subdivision of items proved to be successful during the meeting, and since the sequence of presentations undoubtedly influenced contributions, even in their written version, in this book on the whole we followed the same pattern. Finally, in a fourth part we included two contributions not directly related to any of the three main topics.

Margarete Ghasroldashti not only had a crucial part in the organization of this meeting but equally in the preparation of this book. Hubert Preißl and Stefan Rotter provided valuable assistance, especially where it came to the layout of mathematical formulas.

The meeting at Schloss Ringberg was sponsored jointly by the Deutsche Forschungsgemeinschaft, the Reemtsma-Stiftung, and the European Commission. The facilities at Schloss Ringberg and financial support for members of Max-Planck-Institutes was provided by the Max-Planck-Society. The generous support by all these institutions is most gratefully acknowledged.

Ad Aertsen
Valentino Braitenberg

References

[1] Caianiello ER (ed): Neural Networks. Berlin: Springer, 1968

[2] Conrad M, Güttinger W, Dal Cin M (eds): Physics and Mathematics of the Nervous System. Berlin: Springer, 1974

[3] Heim R, Palm G (eds): Theoretical Approaches to Complex Systems. Berlin: Springer, 1978

[4] Palm G, Aertsen A (eds): Brain Theory. Berlin: Springer, 1986

[5] von Seelen W, Leinhos U, Shaw G (eds): Organization of Neural Networks: Structures and Models. Weinheim: VCH Verlag, 1987

[6] Johannesma PIM, Eggermont JJ, van Gisbergen JAM (eds): Activity patterns of neural populations. Brain and Behaviour Report Nr. 4. Nijmegen, The Netherlands, 1985

Contents

Part Three

Visual Cortex

Part Four

Outlook

Part One
Anatomical Connectivity

Randomness and Constraints in the Cortical Neuropil

Almut Schüz

Max-Planck-Institut für biologische Kybernetik, Spemannstrasse 38, 7400 Tübingen, Germany

Introduction

Among neuroanatomists working on the cerebral cortex there is a controversy about specificity of connections as opposed to randomness. I want to report on this topic here from the point of view of our research.

Most neuroanatomists nowadays would agree that the cerebral cortex is neither wired as precisely as an electronic device nor is it a network completely free of rules. Cortical neuroanatomists would, however, differ considerably with respect to the question as to which of the two extremes the cortex is closer to and on which of the two principles a cortical theory should be based. I want to discuss here to what extent the connectivity between neurons in the cortex is subject to rules and to what extent it can be considered as random.

In order to render the problem more explicit I shall start with some general considerations. One can imagine three basic kinds of networks (Fig. 1). Let us assume that each of them consists of neurons of two different types, type A and type B. The network of Fig. 1 a is characterized by specificity between cell types and between individual neurons. For example, the neurons A11 and A21 are connected to neuron B1 and never to neuron B2 which receives its input from the two neighbouring neurons A12 and A22. A prerequisite for this kind of connectivity is that the neurons can be individually labelled as is the case in some parts of invertebrate nervous systems in which the elements are arranged in strictly regular patterns.

In the network of Fig. 1 b the neurons have no regular arrangement nor any other marker which would allow them to be labelled in-

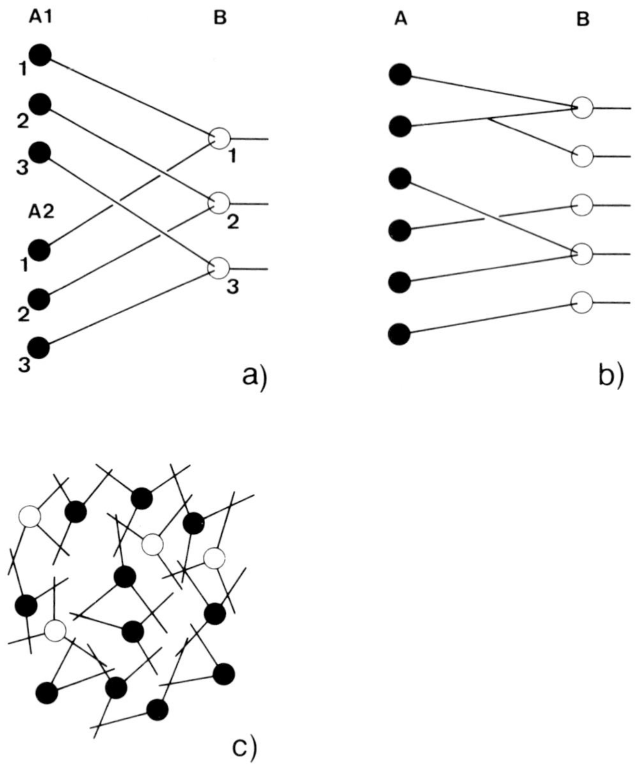

Fig. 1. Three kinds of networks. Network (**a**) is characterized by specificity of connections between different types of neurons (*A and B*) and between individual neurons. In network (**b**) there is specificity only between types. Network (**c**) has no specificity at all. (In c dendrites and axons are not distinguished)

dividually. Let us assume that this is not only the observer's problem but that it is impossible as a matter of principle. In such a network there can be no specificity between individual neurons but there may still be a specificity between different neuronal types. Such a network is probably realized in the cerebellum. Here, neurons of one type are always connected to neurons of a certain other type but there is probably no rule specifying whether a certain neuron of type A connects to an individual neuron of type B or rather to a neighbouring neuron.

One can, however, also imagine a network in which both specificity between individuals and between types is lacking (Fig. 1 c). The neurons of type A and type B are intermingled and make connections with everything which happens to be within their reach. What is within their reach depends on the shape of the dendritic and axonal arborizations, on the distance between neurons and on the proportion and distribution of the various types.

I shall use these schemes as a scaffold for the discussion of the structure of the cerebral cortex. For example, a strictly modular concept of the cortex based on the assumption of chip-like, identical subunits would be of the kind schematized in Fig. 1 a. An ever more detailed distinction of neuronal types may be based on a conception of the cortex as sketched in Fig. 1 b. Other concepts are based on the assumption that the cerebral cortex is better described as a network such as sketched in Fig. 1 c rather than as one of the other two kinds. Transitions between the schemes in Figs. 1 a and 1 b and between those of Figs. 1 b and 1 c can easily be imagined.

The question as to whether the cortical network is of one or the other kind is not only of fundamental interest for the understanding of the function of the cortex but also has implications for the approaches appropriate for cortical anatomy. For example, if a network is of the more specific kind as in Figs. 1 a or 1 b, it is essential to trace the wiring schemes which characterize this network in detail. In a network such as in Fig. 1 c, however, it does not make sense to seek for detailed connectivity. It is, though, appropriate to investigate global properties, such as the shapes of the dendritic and axonal arborizations, the number of neurons of each type and their spatial distribution.

For example, the number of neurons in each type has quite different implications in the case of a network of the type in Fig. 1 c as opposed to the other two cases. In the cerebellar cortex which is of type (b), there are about at least several hundred times more granular cells than Purkinje cells (Harvey and Napper, 1988) but one would not say that the Purkinje cells are less important for information processing in the cerebellum. Since the information is processed sequentially, all members in the chain are of equal importance. On the other hand, in the network (c) in which signals are dispersed onto all neighbours within reach, the character of the network may be decisively shaped by the frequency of neurons of each type.

In this kind of network it is also important to know to what extent it is homogeneous with respect to the shape, density and distribution of neurons and, if it is not, to ask for the rules according to which these properties vary. It is easy to imagine that by letting these properties vary in different regions, the network as a whole can be made into a network which is locally quite specialized in function in spite of a common scheme of random connections.

I shall now summarize some of the results of the histological investigations in our group and show how we came to the conclusion that a scheme such as in Fig. 1 c does more justice to the structure of the cortex than the other two schemes (Braitenberg 1978 a; Braitenberg 1986; Schüz and Palm 1989; Braitenberg and Schüz 1991). I will also show in what respects the cortex deviates from this simple scheme.

Basic properties of cortical structure

The neurons in the cerebral cortex can be divided into two main groups, the pyramidal and the non-pyramidal cells. Although most neuroanatomists would agree to this main distinction, they would draw the borderline between them at different levels and there is, indeed, at present no definition which would not imply some exceptions. The following definition seems to us the most correct one since it is not only based on cell shape but also on functional properties. It also entails the least number of exceptions:

Pyramidal cells have many dendritic spines; they make both local and long-range connections; they receive only Type II synapses on their cell bodies and their axon is presynaptic to Type I synapses (Colonnier 1968; LeVay 1973; Parnavelas et al. 1977; Peters and Fairén 1978; Somogyi 1978; Peters and Proskauer 1980)) which are supposed to be excitatory. The exceptions which we would still include into the group of pyramidal cells since they deviate only in one of these criteria, are certain large pyramidal cells which have few spines (Kaplan and Scheibel 1980; Hübener et al. 1990) and a certain population of spiny stellate cells the axon of which does not enter the white matter (Lund 1984).

The non-pyramidal cells are characterized by having few or no spines and by making no long-range connections via the white matter. They receive both Type I and Type II synapses on their cell bodies and the axons are presynaptically engaged in Type II synapses (Peters and

Fairén 1978; Peters and Proskauer 1980), implying that they are inhibitory.

A few individual cells have been described which seem out of place in this scheme (Peters and Kimerer 1981), and there are some cells of which it is not yet known with certainty if they are excitatory or inhibitory, such as the so-called Martinotti-cells. However, these do not seem to be numerically prevalent and shall not be considered further.

It is not easy to assess the percentage of pyramidal and non-pyramidal cells, but all attempts indicate that the pyramidal cells are in the majority (e.g. Werner et al. 1979; Winfield et al. 1980; Braak and Braak 1986). For our purposes, the figure of 85% pyramidal cells given by Peters and Kara (1985) seems most adequate since these authors use a classification similar to ours.

It is easier to quantify the number of connections each group contributes to the network. One can do this by counting the percentage of Type I and Type II synapses and the percentage of synapses on spines as opposed to synapses on dendritic shafts. Neglecting the few possible exceptions mentioned above and the relatively few synapses by afferent fibres from subcortical structures, one can assume that all Type I synapses belong presynaptically to pyramidal cells. Postsynaptically they belong either to dendritic spines (which means pyramidal cells) or to dendritic shafts (which can mean both pyramidal and non-pyramidal cells) or to cell bodies (which means non-pyramidal cells since pyramidal cells have only Type II synapses on their cell bodies). The Type II synapses come presynaptically from non-pyramidal cells and go postsynaptically mainly to the dendritic shafts or cell bodies of both pyramidal and non-pyramidal cells.

Our results for the neocortex of the mouse are the following: 75% of the synapses are situated on spines and thus on pyramidal cell dendrites (neglecting the few spines on non-pyramidal cells). 88% of the synapses are of Type I and thus belong presynaptically to pyramidal cell axons.

From this it is clear that pyramidal cells connect onto both pyramidal and non-pyramidal cells and non-pyramidal cells connect onto both groups as well. With respect to the sketches in Fig. 1, this excludes the type of specificity shown in Fig. 1 b, in which neurons of one type strictly connect to those of a certain other type, at least within the framework of the rough categorization given above.

These data also show that the two main groups do not play an equal role, but that the network is dominated by one type of cell, the pyramidal cells, not only as far as the number of these neurons is concerned but also with respect to the connectivity. Between 80 and 90% of the connections are between pyramidal cells. Since these connections are excitatory, it is also evident that the basic function of the cortex relies on excitatory interactions.

Divergence and convergence of connections between pyramidal cells

The next relevant question for the understanding of the network concerns the number of connections each neuron makes and the question as to how many different neighbours each neuron is connected to.

The average number of synapses each neuron makes can be calculated from the density of neurons and the density of synapses. For the mouse it is about 8000, for animals with larger brains it is even higher.

A clue as to how many different neighbours one neuron connects to is given by the shape of the axonal arborizations. Neurons which tend to stick to a certain target neuron can be recognized by the fact that their axon re-traces the shape of the dendritic tree or of the cell body of the postsynaptic cell. Well-known examples are the climbing fibres and the basket cells in the cerebellar cortex. The axonal trees of pyramidal cells do not show this kind of shape at all. Their axons show a far-reaching and very loose ramification and the individual branches tend to be straight without any indication that they would follow the outline of a special target. This makes it probable that the pyramidal cells tend to distribute their synapses onto many different postsynaptic neighbours. This may be less so in the case of various kinds of non-pyramidal cells which often have much denser axonal ramifications than the axons of pyramidal cells and which are known to make specific connections in some cases.

The number of postsynaptic neighbours of pyramidal cells has been quantified by Braitenberg (1978 b) on the basis of the geometry of the axonal and dendritic arborizations. One may ask how likely it is that overlapping dendritic and axonal trees touch each other, thus having the chance to make one or more synapses. For pyramidal cells it turned out that this probability is very low. Even if an axonal tree has a large overlap with a certain dendritic tree there is a considerable probability that they do not meet at all or that they meet only once or only few times. This makes it likely that the pyramidal cells distribute their synapses onto thousands of different neurons and that they receive their synapses from thousands of different neurons as well. This implies that the pyramidal cells are weakly connected to each other and are not likely to be able to drive each other individually.

Distribution of synapses along axons

One may argue that pure observation of the geometry of axons and dendrites is insufficient for a realistic picture of the connectivity. One could imagine that when a dendrite and an axon meet they often do not make a synapse, while at other places, when a cell has found an adequate postsynaptic neighbour, clusters of synapses are formed. It may also be that an axon makes its synapses according to certain rules, for example, that synapses are preferentially made on distal segments of the axonal tree. This would shift the statistics of connections in favour of more distant cells and would minimize connections between close neighbours. In order to answer such questions one should know the distribution of synapses along the cell processes.

The distribution of synapses on the postsynaptic side is rather well known in the case of pyramidal cells, since the dendritic spines which carry most of the synapses are well visible in the light microscope in Golgi-preparations. Apart from the portions of dendrites very close to the cell body, they are distributed throughout the dendritic tree, on average about two per micron.

The distribution of synapses on the presynaptic side is much more difficult to assess, but even more important for our purpose, since - as measurements on the mouse cortex show - the total axonal length of a pyramidal cell is about 10 times greater than the total dendritic length. Thus, supposing that there is about the same number of synapses on the dendrites and on the axons - which can hardly be otherwise - there is 10 times more space on axons than on dendrites for the synapses to be arranged.

The positioning of presynaptic sites can be deduced from various electron microscopic studies. However, electron microscopy is always restricted to relatively small samples, making it difficult to obtain a global impression. However, some of these studies have shown that the axonal swellings to be observed in the light microscope correspond quite well to the position of the presynaptic sites (Peters and Proskauer 1980; Somogyi and Cowey 1981; Schüz and Münster 1985). On the basis of this finding, a Golgi study was undertaken in our group (Hellwig 1990), the main results of which I shall summarize here.

The average distance between axonal swellings on pyramidal cell axons is between 4 and 5 μm, and they are distributed throughout the axonal tree as far as it can be traced in Golgi-preparations. Only on the descending segment of the axon is the density of swellings always lower than on the rest of the axonal tree.

Figure 2 shows some examples of primary collaterals of pyramidal cells and the position of their presynaptic boutons. There are no conspicuous patterns which would leap to the eye. In some cases there is a lower density near the origin of the collateral (2, 5) but this is by no means a general rule (6, 8). On some collaterals the swellings appear to have a tendency to cluster (6, 8, 11), on others one may suspect a certain periodicity in their arrangement (3). The question is whether these patterns go beyond what one would expect from a random distribution? To clarify this, we applied a statistical analysis (Hellwig et al. in preparation) which is commonly used for the detection of patterns in spike trains (e.g. Aertsen and Gerstein 1985). Figures 3 and 4 show examples of the results for some of the longest collaterals investigated, assuming that these give the most reliable statistics.

Figure 3 shows the interval histograms for four collaterals. For two of these, Figure 4 (top) presents a scatter diagram in which each interval is plotted against the neighbouring interval. Fig. 4 (bottom) shows the autocorrelograms for the same two collaterals. All three of these statistical tests speak clearly in favour of a random distribution. Fig. 3 speaks in favour of an exponential distribution, and there is no indication of any serial correlation in Fig. 4 (top), nor of any pattern, apart

---

Fig. 2. Examples for the distribution of axonal swellings on primary collaterals of pyramidal cells. For reasons of clarity, each collateral has been stretched to form a straight line, without changing the actual length. The brackets comprise collaterals which belong to the same neuron. The origin of the collaterals is at the leftmost side of the Figure (at the bottom of the page). (From Hellwig, 1990)

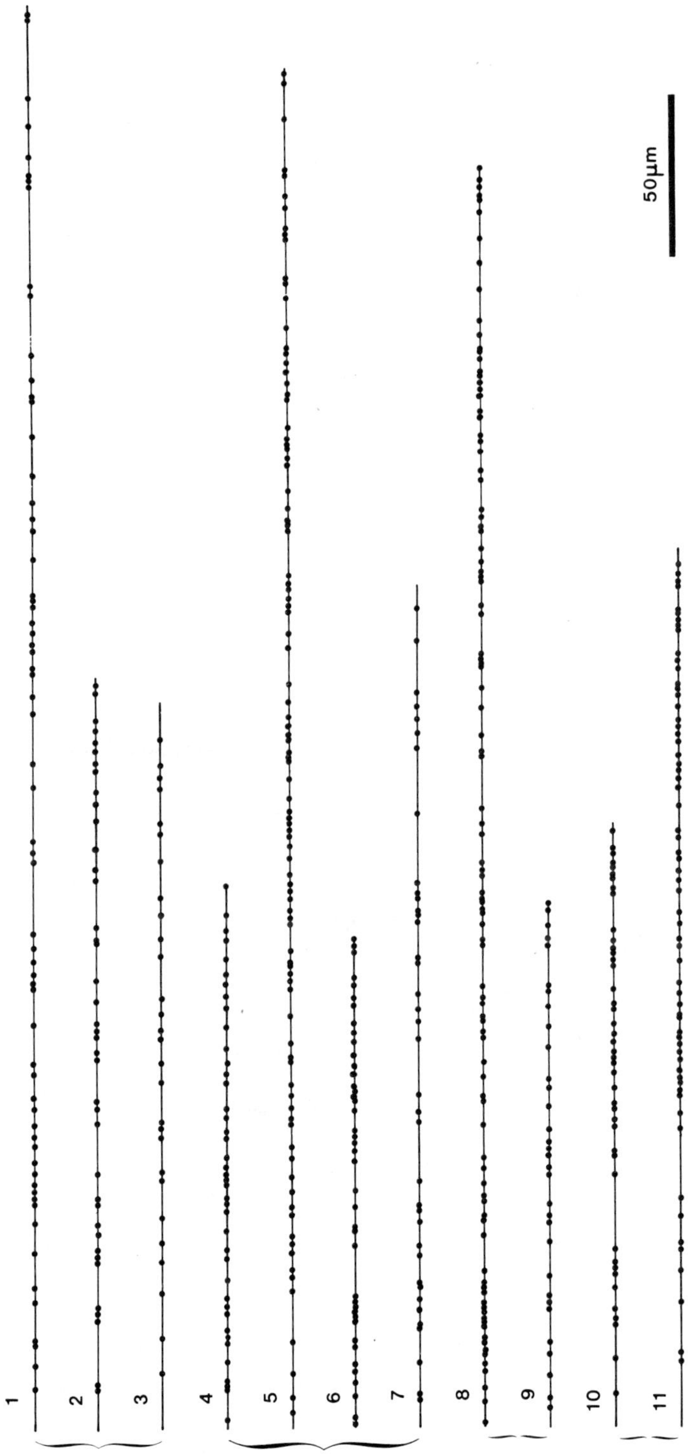
50µm
1
2
3
4
5
6
7
8
9
10
11

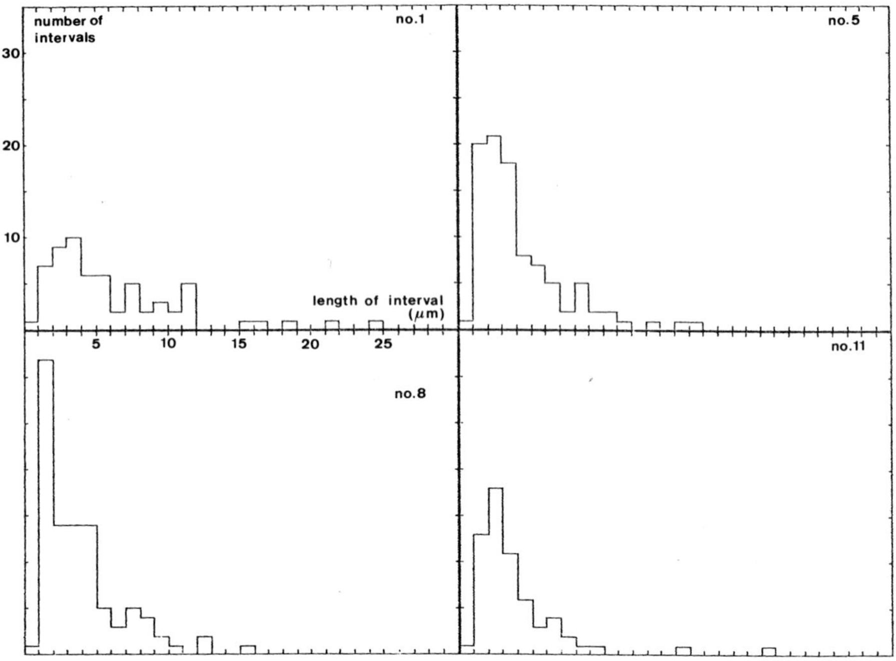

Fig. 3. Interval histograms of four of the longest collaterals. The numbers indicate which histogram belongs to which of the collaterals in Fig. 2. (From Hellwig et al., in preparation)

from the trivial peak at zero, in Fig. 4 (bottom). We conclude that the spatial distribution of presynaptic sites along the axon is adequately described by a Poisson distribution.

These results are compatible with the assumption that an axon makes a synapse wherever it happens to hit a dendrite during its course through the neuropil. The probability of connections between overlapping neurons, calculated on purely geometrical grounds, may therefore be quite realistic and one must indeed conclude that each pyramidal cell has thousands of different pre- and postsynaptic neighbours. In view of the fact that this concerns 10^7 neurons in the mouse and 10^{10} to 10^{11} neurons in large brains, the enormous complexity of the resulting network is incompatible with the idea of genetically determined precise wiring; a considerable amount of randomness must be assumed.

It may well be that such a lack of precision at the level of the individual synapse is not just a necessary evil due to the limited capacity

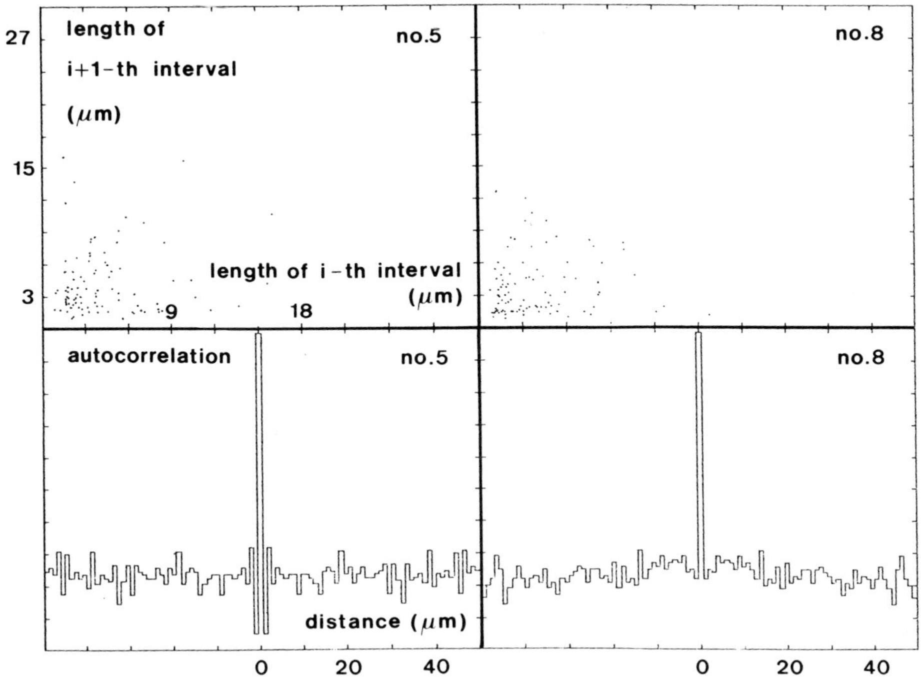

Fig. 4. Scatter plots (top) and autocorrelograms (bottom) for the collaterals nrs. 5 and 8. There is no indication of any pattern in either diagrams. (From Hellwig et al., in preparation)

of the genetic channel. It may even be a prerequisite for the realization of certain tasks. The structure of the cortex as presented here agrees well with the idea of learning by associations. A diffuse network connected at random guarantees a high degree of mixing of information which is an important condition for associative learning. Furthermore, the observation that the function of the cortex is mainly based on excitatory interactions, and additionally that the connections between pyramidal cells are weak, fit the interpretation of the cortex as a substrate for cell assemblies as envisaged by Hebb (1949) or for synfire chains as proposed by Abeles (1982). Both these theories imply that pyramidal cells ignite in a cooperative way rather than as a consequence of the action of individual neurons.

Randomness and constraints

I want to elaborate on the expression "considerable amount of randomness". It is clear that the cortex is not connected entirely at random. It is a prestructured network in which obviously the a-priori probability of a connection varies a great deal between different pairs of neurons. The most obvious condition for the establishment of a synapse between two neurons is that the axonal territory of one overlaps the dendritic territory of the other. This constraint is essentially given by the arrangement of the neurons and by the shapes of their arborizations, both of which are subject to rules. These rules are evident in the existence of different cell types, in the layering of the cortex, in its cyto- and myeloarchitectonics, in the pattern of cortico-cortical connections in the white matter, in the existence of blobs, of ocular dominance columns, etc. Thus, on a global level, the cortex is obviously far from random. However, the question remains open as to whether these morphological constraints are the only ones or if there are additional constraints which determine individual connections within groups of neurons whose processes overlap.

There are some obvious constraints referring to the locus on the neuron at which certain types of synapses can be made. This is evident in the distribution of Type I and Type II synapses and of spines on dendrites or cell bodies. For example, the cell body of pyramidal cells is not a target for synapses of other pyramidal cells. The distribution of synapses on axons mentioned above indicates that such internal constraints are mainly restricted to the postsynaptic side. It has also been shown that different postsynaptic loci on individual neurons select for axons originating from different sub-groups of non-pyramidal cells. The most extreme case is the chandelier cell which makes synapses exclusively on initial segments of axons (e.g. Somogyi 1979; Fairén and Valverde 1980; Peters et al. 1982). Other kinds of non-pyramidal cells have been found to avoid axon initial segments and cell bodies completely. Others again make synapses onto all kinds of loci but may be biased towards one of them (Somogyi 1989).

More relevant to the present discussion, however, are the findings which show a selectivity of connections between cell types. These findings have been extensively reviewed by White (1989).

There is clear evidence for target selectivity in some non-pyramidal cells: the chandelier cells which, as mentioned above, make their terminations on the initial segment of axons, connect exclusively with pyramidal cells and only onto their axon hillocks.

In some pyramidal cells a bias towards non-pyramidal cells was observed. In combined light and electron microscopic studies it is possible to determine whether the axon of an individual cell is presynaptic to spines (i.e. to pyramidal cells) or to dendritic shafts. In some of these studies the axons were found to make only 40 to 50% of their synapses on spines (Somogyi 1978; White and Hersch 1981; Winfield et al. 1981). In two other studies (mainly referring to intracortical collaterals of cortico-thalamic cells) it was even as low as 10% and 30% (McGuire et al. 1984; White and Keller 1987). If these neurons had distributed their synapses indiscriminately onto the targets within their reach, one would expect them to terminate on spines in 85% of the cases. (The argument is as follows: 75% of the synapses in the neocortex are localised on spines. Since all of the spines carry a Type I synapse and 88% of all synapses are of Type I, the spines carry 85% of all Type I synapses).

However, this is not true for all pyramidal cells. In about the same number of cases, the neurons were found to attach between 80 and 87% of their synapses onto spines (Kisvárday et al. 1986; Elhanany and White 1990; Gabbott et al. 1987), which corresponds very well to the expected figure.

Even within the class of non-pyramidal cells a strict target selectivity such as observed in the chandelier cells is likely to be the exception. Most other sub-types have been shown to project onto both pyramidal and non-pyramidal cells and onto various loci on these neurons (summarized in White 1989). But even if more specificities in the domain of non-pyramidal cells should be discovered, it would only concern a minority of connections in the cortex (10 to 15%).

The following simple calculation speaks in favour of the assumption that a strong selectivity between cell types is probably not the dominating principle (Braitenberg and Schüz 1991): If one assumes that 85% of the neurons are pyramidal cells and, in addition, that a non-pyramidal cell contributes on average as many synapses to the network as a pyramidal cell, one can calculate how many synapses there should be between pyramidal and pyramidal cells, between non-pyramidal and non-pyramidal cells and between pyramidal and non-pyramidal cells, under the assumption of a total lack of selectivity:

py to py: 85% x 85% = 72% Type I (most of them on spines),
py to non-py: 85% x 15% = 13% Type I (on dendritic shafts),
non-py to py: 15% x 85% = 13% Type II,
non-py to non-py: 15% x 15% = 2% Type II.

These numbers are remarkably close to the values one finds in the electron microscope. The number of spine synapses we counted in the cortex of the mouse was a few percent higher (75%) and that of Type II synapses slightly lower (12%) than the expected values. A deviation in this direction has to be expected since the subcortical afferents also contribute to the fraction of Type I synapses in the cortex.

On the other hand, it should be mentioned that the frequency of non-pyramidal neurons which we assumed in order to calculate the expected frequency of various kinds of synapses is at variance with some findings on the monkey and cat cortex (Hendry et al. 1987; Gabbott and Somogyi 1986). These authors find a proportion of about 25% to 20% GABAergic neurons, depending on the area. The discrepancy may be due to the different species examined, or our simple assumption that individual pyramidal and non-pyramidal cells are responsible for about the same number of synapses may be wrong. Cell types so radically different as pyramidal and non-pyramidal cells are, in fact, quite likely to carry different numbers of synapses.

There are statistical arguments against the assumption of a strong selectivity in the system of pyramidal cells. If one assumes for example that many pyramidal cells select for non-pyramidal cells as strongly as in the case of the corticothalamic cells, one is left with the question as to the source of input to the remaining spines. Subcortical afferents can hardly fill the gap. Although they account for about 20% of the synapses in layer IV in primary sensory areas (White 1978), they probably make up at most a few percent of all synapses in the cortex.

Another possibility which has to be examined is the following: the studies mentioned above have been restricted to the local axonal tree of pyramidal cells. It could be that the long-range connections via the white matter project more onto spines than does the local axonal tree. This is suggested by a study by Sloper and Powell (1979) on the monkey: in the motor cortex, callosal terminals made 96% of their synapses on spines. However, studies on other long-range systems (including callosal connections at the border of area 17/18 in monkey and cat) do not confirm such a rule (Fisken et al. 1975; Sloper and Powell 1979).

Another kind of target selectivity has also been observed in the callosal fibres: Pyramidal cells from the upper layers of the cortex have been found to receive from callosal fibres twice the number of synapses which pyramidal cells receive from deeper layers, when the different densities of dendrites of the two classes of pyramidal cells in the layer examined were taken into account (Porter and White 1986).

To summarize, a strict target selectivity as sketched in Fig. 1 b seems to be realized only in the system of non-pyramidal cells and may be the exception even there. As far as they have been investigated, all other populations of neurons were found to project onto all kinds of neurons within reach (Peters and Feldman 1976; White 1989). A number of findings are even compatible with a targeting which is completely unselective with respect to cell types. However, various results indicate that one must take a few constraints beyond those of overlap between neurons into consideration. Strong selectivities, as seen in the case of the non-pyramidal cells make one think of chemical specificity. Milder deviations from an unselective targeting could perhaps be explained by differences in maturation between populations of neurons. It is well-known that the various layers do not mature simultaneously. This is probably also true for the various fibre systems, and has been shown already for corticocortical as compared to thalamic input (Wise et al., 1977; Wise and Jones, 1978). Thus, even if an axonal tree indiscriminately makes synapses with every possible target, its connectivity may ultimately still deviate from the overall statistics of the neuropil. It may be that such statistical biases which concern large populations of neurons, and therefore require relatively little information from the genetic channel, prepare the network for its later tasks in an interesting way which yet has to be explained.

Although these constraints introduce unequal probabilities for the connections between certain neurons and thus reduce the degree of randomness, they do not invalidate the principle of an essentially probabilistic connectivity. They do not provide evidence for the cortex as a highly specific network of the kind sketched in Figs. 1 a and 1 b, nor do they justify a theory of the cortex in terms of electronic circuitry. Of course, there are all possible transitions between the extreme cases of Fig. 1 b and c. The data show that the cortex is somewhere in between, with traits of both. Our feeling is, however, that the connectivity of type 1 c belongs essentially to the cortical network, and is related to its basic function.

Learning and connectivity

In the preceding pages I have intentionally disregarded the phenomena of plasticity, although we believe that learning is the main function of the cortex and that it does affect its connectivity. There are reasons to believe that learning is mainly due strengthening of already existing connections rather than to the establishment of new ones (e.g. Schüz 1981; Merzenich et al. 1984; Jones 1990). However, weakening of inadequate connections up to the point of their elimination may also play a role (e.g. Apfelbach and Weiler 1985; Wallhäuser and Scheich 1987; Huttenlocher and de Courten 1987). But even if learning were responsible for the formation or consolidation of all synapses in the cortex, this would not free us from considerations of the above kind. Learning is assumed to play a role in both the cortex and the cerebellum and yet it certainly provides no reason for the fundamental differences in the connectivity of the two systems. Although learning does shape the final interaction between neurons (perhaps in an ever-changing way), the possibility for neurons to interact is decisively dependent on the basic construction of the network. A substrate such as network (c) certainly allows the incorporation of a much richer spectrum of correlations than the other two kinds of networks.

Acknowledgements

I am very grateful to Valentino Braitenberg for years of illuminating discussions, to Ad Aertsen for the statistical analysis in figs. 2-4, to Elisabeth Braitenberg and to Shirley Würth for linguistic support, and to Claudia Martin-Schubert for help with the pictures.

References

Aertsen A, Gerstein G (1985) Evaluation of neuronal connectivity: Sensitivity of cross-correlation. Brain Res 340:341-354

Abeles M (1982) Local Cortical Circuits. Springer, Berlin Heidelberg

Apfelbach R and Weiler E (1985) Olfactory deprivation enhances normal spine loss in the olfactory bulb of developing ferrets. Neurosci Lett 62:169-173

Braak H, Braak E (1986) Ratio of pyramidal cells versus non-pyramidal cells in the human frontal isocortex and changes in ratio with aging and Alzheimer's disease. In: Swaab DF, Fliers E, Mirmiran M, Van Gool WA, Van Haaren F (eds) Progress in Brain Research. Elsevier Science Publ. Amsterdam pp 185-212

Braitenberg V (1978 a) Cortical architectonics: general and areal. In: Brazier MAB, Petsche H (eds) Architectonics of the cerebral cortex. Raven Press, New York pp 443-465

Braitenberg V (1978 b) Cell assemblies in the cerebral cortex. In: Heim R, Palm G (eds) Lecture Notes in Biomathematics (21). Theoretical Approaches to Complex Systems. Springer, Berlin Heidelberg New York, pp 171-188

Braitenberg V (1986) Two views of the cerebral cortex. In: Palm G, Aertsen A (eds) Brain Theory. Springer, Berlin Heidelberg pp 81-96

Braitenberg V, Schüz A (1991) Anatomy of the Cortex. Statistics and Geometry. Springer, Berlin Heidelberg New York

Colonnier M (1968) Synaptic patterns on different cell types in the different laminae of the cat visual cortex. An electron microscope study. Brain Res 9:268-287

Elhanany E, White EL (1990) Intrinsic circuitry: synapses involving the local axon collaterals of corticocortical projection neurons in the mouse primary somatosensory cortex. J Comp Neurol 291:43-54

Fairén A, Valverde F (1980) A specialized type of neuron in the visual cortex of the cat: A Golgi and electron microscope study of chandelier cells. J Comp Neurol 194:761-779

Fisken RA, Garey LJ and Powell TPS (1975) The intrinsic, association and commissural connections of area 17 of the visual cortex. Phil Trans Roy Soc ser B 272:(919) 487-536

Gabbott PLA, Martin KAC, Whitteridge D (1987) Connections between pyramidal neurons in layer 5 of cat visual cortex (area 17). J Comp Neurol 259:364-381

Gabbott PLA, Somogyi P (1986) Quantitative distribution of GABA/immunoreactive neurons in the visual cortex (area 17) of the cat. Exp Brain Res 61:323-331

Harvey RJ, Napper RMA (1988) A quantitative study of Purkinje and granule cells in the cerebellar cortex of the rat. J Comp Neurol 274:151-157

Hebb DO (1949) Organization of Behavior. A neuropsychological Theory. 2nd edition (1961). Wiley & Sons Inc., New York

Hellwig B (1990) Dichte und Verteilung präsynaptischer Boutons. Ein Beitrag zur Synaptologie der Grosshirnrinde. Dissertation, Medizinische Fakultät, Universität Tübingen

Hellwig B, Schüz A, Aertsen A: Density and distribution of presynaptic boutons on Golgi stained axons in the cortex of the mouse. In preparation

Hendry SHC, Schwark HD, Jones EG, Yan J (1987) Numbers and proportions of GABA-immunoreactive neurons in different areas of monkey cerebral cortex. J Neuroci 7:1503-1519

Hübener M, Schwarz C, Bolz J (1990) Morphological types of projection neurons in layer 5 of cat visual cortex. J Comp Neurol 301:655-674

Huttenlocher PR, de Courten C (1987) The development of synapses in striate cortex of man. Human Neurobiol 6:1-9

Jones EG (1990) Modulatory events in the development and evolution of primate neocortex. In: Jones EG, Peters A (eds) Cerebral Cortex, Vol. 8A, Comparative Structure and Evolution of Cerebral Cortex, Part I. Plenum Press, New York London

Kaplan AS, Scheibel AB (1980) Giant spine-poor pyramidal cells in auditory cortex of young and aged cats. Soc Neurosci Abstr 6:557

Kisvárday ZF, Martin KAC, Freund TF, Magloczky ZF, Whitteridge D, Somogyi P (1986) Synaptic targets of HRP-filled layer III pyramidal cells in the cat striate cortex. Exp Brain Res 64:541-552

LeVay S (1973) Synaptic patterns in the visual cortex of the cat and monkey. Electron microscopy of Golgi preparations. J Comp Neurol 150:53-86

Lund JS (1984) Spiny stellate neurons. In: Peters A, Jones EG (eds) Cerebral Cortex Vol. 1,. Cellular components of the cerebral cortex. Plenum Press, New York London pp. 255-308

McGuire BA, Hornung J-P, Gilbert CD, Wiesel TN (1984) Patterns of synaptic input to layer 4 of cat striate cortex. J Neurosci 4:3021-3033

Merzenich MM, Nelson RJ, Stryker MP, Cynader, MS, Schoppmann A and Zook JM (1984) Somatosensory cortical map changes following digit amputation in adult monkeys. J Comp Neurol 224:591-605

Parnavelas JG, Sullivan K, Lieberman AR, Webster KE (1977) Neurons and their synaptic organization in the visual cortex of the rat. Cell Tiss Res 183:499-517

Peters A, Fairén A (1978) Smooth and sparsely spined stellate cells in the visual cortex of the rat. A study using a combined Golgi electron microscopic technique. J Comp Neurol 181:129-172

Peters A, Feldman ML (1976) The projection of the lateral geniculate nucleus to area 17 of the rat cerebral cortex. I. General description. J Neurocyt 5:63-84

Peters A, Kara DA (1985) The neuronal composition of area 17 of rat visual cortex. I. The pyramidal cells. J Comp Neurol 234:218-241

Peters A, Kimerer LM (1981) Bipolar neurons in rat visual cortex. A combined Golgi-electron microscopic study. J Neurocytol 10:921-946

Peters A, Proskauer CC (1980) Synaptic relationships between a multipolar stellate cell and a pyramidal neuron in the rat visual cortex. A combined Golgi-electron microscope study. J Neurocytol 9:163-183

Peters A, Proskauer CC, Ribak CE (1982) Chandelier cells in rat visual cortex. J Comp Neurol 206:397-416

Schüz A (1981) Prenatal formation of synapses and dendritic spines in Guinea pig cortex and their postnatal changes. In: Széleky G, Lábos E, Damjanovich S (eds) Adv. Physiol. Sci. Vol. 30. Neural Communication and Control. Pergamon Press

Schüz A, Münster A (1985) Synaptic density on the axonal tree of a pyramidal cell in the cortex of the mouse. Neuroscience 15:33-39

Schüz A, Palm G (1989) Density of neurons and synapses in the cerebral cortex of the mouse. J Comp Neurol 286:442-455

Somogyi P (1978) The study of Golgi stained cells and of experimental degeneration under the electron microscope: A direct method for the identification in the visual cortex of three successive links in a neuron chain. Neuroscience 3:167-180

Somogyi P (1979) An interneurone making synapses specificially on the axon initial segment of pyramidal cells in the cerebral cortex. J Physiol 296:18-19

Somogyi P, Cowey A (1981) Combined Golgi and electron microscopic study on the synapses formed by double bouquet cells in the visual cortex of the cat and monkey. J Comp Neurol 195:547-566

Sloper JJ, Powell TPS (1979) An experimental electron microscopic study of afferent connections to the primate motor and somatic sensory cortices. Phil Trans Roy Soc ser B 285:199-225

Wallhäuser E, Scheich H (1987) Auditory imprinting leads to differential 2-deoxyglucose uptake and dendritic spine loss in the chick rostral forebrain. Dev Brain Res 31:29-44

White EL (1978) Identified neurons in mouse SmI cortex which are postsynaptic to thalamocortical axon terminals: A combined Golgi-electron microscopic and degeneration study. J Comp Neurol 181:627-662.

White EL (1989) Cortical Circuits. Synaptic Organization of the Cerebral Cortex. Structure, Function, and Theory. Birkhäuser, Boston, Basel, Berlin

White EL, Hersch SM (1981) Thalamocortical synapses of pyramidal cells which project from Sml to Msl cortex in the mouse. J Comp Neurol 198:167-181

White EL, Keller A (1987) Intrinsic circuitry involving the local axon collaterals of corticothalamic projection cells in mouse SmI cortex. J Comp Neurol 262:13-26

Winfield DA, Brooke RNL, Sloper JJ, Powell TPS (1981) A combined Golgi-electron microscopic study of the synapses made by the proximal axon and recurrent collaterals of a pyramidal cell in the somatic sensory cortex of the monkey. Neuroscience 6:1217-1230

Winfield DA, Gatter KC, Powell TPS (1980) An electron microscopic study of the types and proportions of neurons in the cortex of the motor and visual areas of the cat and rat. Brain 103:245-258

Wise SP, Hendry SHC, Jones EG (1977) Prenatal development of sensorimotor cortical projections in cats. Brain Res 138:538-544

Wise SP, Jones EG (1978) Developmental studies of thalamocortical and commissural connections in the rat somatic sensory cortex. J Comp Neurol 178:187-208

An Example for Specific Connections in the Visual Cortex

Zoltán F. Kisvárday

Ruhr-University, Dept. of Neurophysiology, Universitätsstr. 150, MA 4/149, 4630 Bochum, Germany

Although the non-random origin and distribution of pyramidal and non-pyramidal cell axons has long been recognized from studies of Golgi impregnated neurons (Cajal 1899; Lorente de Nó 1922; Szentágothai 1973; Lund and Boothe 1975), and of intracellularly injected cells (Gilbert and Wiesel 1979, 1983; Martin and Whitteridge 1984), still there seems to be a disagreement between neuroscientists as to whether the cerebral cortex operates with random or specific neuronal connections.

To give an example for specific intracortical connections I deliberately chose a type of pyramidal cell in layer III which has been studied probably most thoroughly of all pyramidal cell types in the mammalian cerebral cortex. This type of pyramidal cell was first revealed in its full anatomical extent in cat visual cortex (area 17) using intracellular staining with horseradish peroxidase (Gilbert and Wiesel 1979, 1983). At the light microscopic level neither the somata nor the dendrites of these pyramidal cells do appreciably differ from those of other pyramidal cells in the same layer. However, their axons show a remarkable distinguishing feature; that is they span an overall longitudinal distance up to 4.9 mm parallel to the cortical surface (Fig. 1). Another characteristic feature of this cell type is that the axonal arbor is unevenly distributed, notably the main axon emits patches of fine collaterals within the dendritic field as well as in remote regions up to 2.8 mm from the parent somata. Each patch covers an area up to 400 μm in diameter (Fig. 1), though there can be considerable difference between individual patches of the same cell with respect to the density of fine collaterals and the overall area covered by the same axonal cluster. The unequal size and density of different patches provided by the same cell suggest different weighting functions at different target regions. This phenomenon is particularly evident for the patchy axonal system of

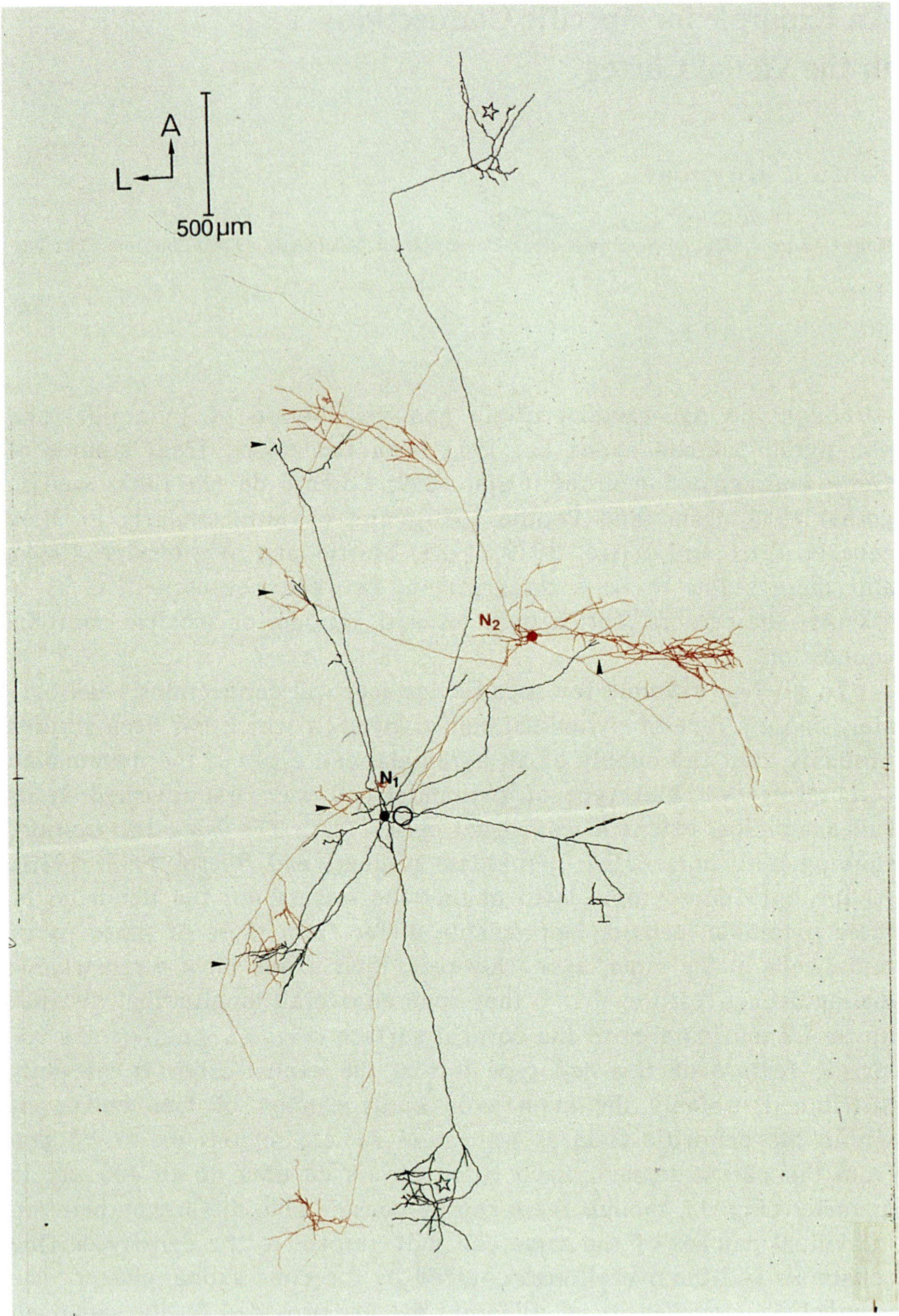
A
L
500µm
N2
N1

cell No 1 in Fig. 1 which establishes its densest patches (stars) at extreme distances up to 2.8 mm from the parent soma.

Recently we have started to analyze the spatial relationship between the patchy axons of pyramidal cells labelled after focal injection of a neuronal tracer. Namely, biocytin was applied with iontophoretic microinjection into layers II-III of cat visual cortical area 17 to reveal populations of cells in their entire morphology. It was then possible to reconstruct the patchy axons of several pyramidal cells labelled from the very same injected site. Three dimensional reconstruction of many of the labelled pyramidal cells revealed that their patchy axon termination fields apparently overlapped. This highly overlapping character is demonstrated in Fig. 1 for two cells, No 1 and 2 in black and in red, respectively. By superimposing the reconstructed axons it became evident that the two pyramidal cells shown in Fig. 1 shared their axonal patches at 5 distinct sites including the one at the injection site (circle in Fig. 1).

The patchy character and the laminar distribution of this pyramidal cell type suggest a high degree of target selectivity. Indeed, pyramidal neurons similar to the ones shown in Fig. 1 receive mainly axo-spinous contacts onto their apical dendrite from overlapping patchy axons of other remotely located pyramidal cells of the same long-range type (Kisvárday and Eysel, unpublished observation). The number of contacts from one cell to the other rarely exceeds 1 - 4, in most cases it is only 1, indicating that strong convergence of similar sources is required onto these cells.

Another line of evidence for the afore-mentioned specific pyramidal cell-pyramidal cell interactions derives from electron microscopic work on intracellularly horseradish peroxidase-labelled pyramidal cells. It was recently shown for the patchy axons of two intracellularly filled layer III pyramidal cells that the overwhelming majority of their tar-

---

Fig. 1. Composite drawing of the complete axonal distribution of two pyramidal cells (*N1* and *N2*) shown in black and in red, respectively, in layer III of cat visual cortex (area 17). Both pyramidal cells were labelled from the same small site following an iontophoretic microinjection of biocytin (circle) into layer III. Reconstruction of the axonal fields were made from large consecutive sections cut parallel to the cortical surface. Regions with overlapping axonal fields of the two pyramidal cells are indicated by arrowheads. The two densest axonal patches in extreme distance from the parent soma of cell No. 1 are marked by stars. The somata of pyramidal cells N_1 and N_2 are indicated by filled circles in black and in red, respectively. *A* = anterior, *L* = lateral

gets (85%) were dendritic spines, probably originating from other pyramidal cells in layer III (Kisvárday et al. 1986), and the remaining targets (15%) were dendritic shafts of small size, many of them of the spine bearing type with ultrastructural characteristics to identified pyramidal cell dendrites (Kisvárday et al. 1986). Taken together, the ultrastructural data suggest that pyramidal cells with patchy axons contact predominantly other pyramidal cells, most likely of the same type.

The highly specific anatomical properties of pyramidal cells of the above type, that is the large horizontal extent of the axons, their characteristic patchy distribution, and their target specificity (mainly dendritic spines) call for specific functional role(s). It has been supposed that patchy intrinsic connections directly connect far sites possessing certain orientation preferences (Mitchison and Crick 1982). Experimental evidence obtained so far, however, is somewhat contradictory as to whether long-range horizontal connections are made between cells of like orientation (Gilbert and Wiesel 1989; Ts'o et al. 1986) or of unlike orientation (Matsubara et al. 1985, 1987). Recent experiments, using physiological mapping for orientation preferences in large areas of cat area 17 and subsequent fine anatomical tracing of labelled horizontal axons of pyramidal cells suggest that regions with like orientation rather than with unlike orientation are interconnected by the patchy axonal system of pyramidal cells (Kisvárday and Eysel, unpublished observations). The above findings are in agreement with the results of Gilbert and Wiesel (1989) who used a combination of electrophysiological mapping, focal injection of fluorescent beads, and 2-deoxyglucose technique. It was found that retrogradely labelled cells appeared in remote patches possessing similar orientation preferences as shown with the alignment of physiologically determined sites or 2-deoxyglucose labelling in the same sections (Gilbert and Wiesel 1989). Further indication for the putative role of the specific patchy axonal system, supporting the "like orientation hypothesis", derives from cross-correlation experiments showing excitatory coupling between remotely spaced neurons only if their orientation preferences were similar (Nelson and Frost 1985; Ts'o et al. 1986).

The specific anatomical nature of long-range pyramidal cells and their specific character to interconnect cortical regions with like orientation preferences suggest that specific connections probably underlie specific functional tasks. Nevertheless, random-like axon arborization patterns of both pyramidal and non-pyramidal cells have been observed as well. However, it is conceivable that future studies using more advanced techniques than those available today may disclose that cortical cells that had been considered to have random-like connectivity patterns are highly specific, for example in the chemical composition of their postsynaptic targets.

References

Cajal R (1899) Estudios sobre la corteza cerebral humana. Corteza visual. Rev Trim Microgr 4:1-25

Gilbert CD, Wiesel TN (1979) Morphology and intracortical projections of functionally characterized neurons in the cat visual cortex. Nature 280:120-125

Gilbert CD, Wiesel TN (1983) Clustered intrinsic connections in cat visual cortex. J Neurosci 3:1116-1133

Gilbert CD, Wiesel TN (1989) Columnar specificity of intrinsic horizontal and corticocortical connections in cat visual cortex. J Neurosci 9:2432-2442

Kisvárday ZF, Martin KAC, Freund TF, Maglóczky, Zs, Whitteridge D, Somogyi P (1986) Synaptic targets of HRP-filled layer III pyramidal cells in the cat striate cortex. Exp Brain Res 64:541-552

Lorente de No, R (1922) La corteza cerebral del raton. I. La corteza acustica. Trab Lab Invest Biol Univ Madrid 20:41-78

Lund JS, Boothe R (1975) Interlaminar connections and pyramidal neuron organization in the visual cortex, area 17, of the macaque monkey. J Comp Neurol 159:305-334

Matsubara JA, Cynader M, Swindale NV, Stryker MP (1985) Intrinsic projections within visual cortex: evidence for orientation-specific local connections. Proc Natl Acad Sci USA 82:935-939

Matsubara JA, Cynader MS, Swindale NV (1987) Anatomical properties and physiological correlates of the intrinsic connections in cat area 18. J Neurosci 7:1428-1446

Martin KAC, Whitteridge D (1984) Form, function and intracortical projections of spiny neurones in the striate visual cortex of the cat. J Physiol 353:463-504

Mitchison G, Crick F (1982) Long axons within the striate cortex: their distribution, orientation, and patterns of connections. Proc Nat Acad Sci USA 79:3661-3665

Nelson JI, Frost BJ (1985) Intracortical facilitation among co-oriented, co-axially aligned simple cells in cat striate cortex. Exp Brain Res 61:54-61

Ts'o DY, Gilbert CD, Wiesel TN (1986) Relationships between horizontal interactions and functional architecture in cat striate cortex as revealed by cross-correlation analysis. J Neurosci 6:1160-1170

Szentágothai J (1973) Synaptology of the visual cortex. In: Jung R (ed) Handbook of Sensory Physiology, Vol VII. Springer, Berlin Heidelberg New York, pp 270-321

A Probabilistic Approach to the Analysis of Propagation Delays in Large Cortical Axonal Trees

Israel Nelken

Department of Physiology, Hebrew University Medical School, PO Box 1172, Jerusalem 91010, Israel

The most important means by which a neuron passes information to its postsynaptic partners is the propagation of action potentials from the soma to the synapses. Since the synapses are located at different distances from the soma, the action potential gets to them after different propagation delays. These propagation delays cause desynchronization in the computations performed by the cortical network. This paper presents an analysis of the propagation delays along a randomly branching axon. The model can describe propagation delays caused by both the randomness of the structure of the axon and by the changing electrical properties along its branches. The statistics of the branching axon are described by a subcritical branching process. It is shown that such a model does describe well some populations of axons. The propagation delays along the branching structure are random functions of the type of the branches. The main result is that the delays along the axon have an exponential or related distribution, which is wider than the Gaussian distribution with the same variance. Using some numerical estimates it follows that the coherence length in the cortex is in the order of magnitude of 1 mm. This result has implications concerning some current theories of brain function.

Introduction

An axon in the cerebral cortex is usually an extremely complex object, having between 10^3 and 10^4 synapses with other neurons in its vicinity or far off (Schüz and Palm 1989). Thus, in general, an action potential will activate different synapses on the axonal tree at slightly different times. The purpose of this paper is to analyze the distribution of these time delays.

Except for the intrinsic interest in this question, the main reason for this study of the propagation delays is to check the viability of some recently proposed models, which demand exact timing of spikes from several presynaptic sources converging onto one postsynaptic neuron. In all of those models, specific nonlinear effects are expected when such convergence occurs. These models include for example models for motion detection (Poggio et al. 1981), "shifter circuits" (Anderson and Van Essen 1987), and the synfire model (Abeles 1982). In the first two models, the converging post synaptic potentials (PSP's) are both excitatory and inhibitory. The nonlinear interaction is between the excitatory post synaptic potential (EPSP) and the inhibitory post synaptic potential (IPSP), which is assumed to have a reversal potential close to the resting potential. In such cases, there is a short time window around the time of occurrence of the EPSP during which the IPSP has to occur in order to effectively inhibit the excitation. The synfire model, in contrast, requires all PSP's to be excitatory, the nonlinear interaction being a result of the nonlinear transformation between membrane potential and firing probability. Nevertheless, the basic idea of nonlinear effects caused by synchronous convergence of several spikes is similar.

The delays along an axon are primarily caused by three mechanisms: the different distances between the cell body and the synapses, changes in the propagation velocity along the path from the soma to the synapses, caused by changing electrical properties, and delays introduced at branch points (Khodorov and Timin 1975).

Several studies attempted to clarify the relations between structural and electrical parameters on the one hand, and the propagation velocity on the other. Most of these used the cable equation and a Hodgkin-Huxley excitable membrane model (Khodorov and Timin 1975; Parnas 1979; Parnas and Segev 1979; Manor et al. 1991). There is also a quantitative understanding of the delays caused by branch points and by nonuniform axon properties (Parnas 1979, Parnas and Segev 1979). These studies begin at the micro level, and show how to compute the velocity of the action potential starting from "first principles". In this way, some specific geometrical forms can be analyzed: a single branch point, or specific changes in electrical properties along the axon. On the other hand, in order to understand what happens on a full axon in this approach, the set of equations describing the axonal tree has to be solved numerically. This is a lengthy task, and at the end one is left with a set of numbers which describe only the specific problem that was solved. Generalizing from the results of such simulations, without some theory to guide it, is problematic. Thus, a general theory, connecting this micro level with the macro level of propagation delays along a large branching structure is needed.

The approach taken in this paper is different from the analytical approach described above. Instead of trying to duplicate the details of one "typical" axon, then extracting global information from the solutions to the equations, the strategy here is to model some general picture of the axon, taking into account both the similarities between axons and the variance around that similarity (after all, no two axons are identical in the cerebral cortex), and then to find the distribution function of the delays on the whole axon at once. The price paid for this generality is, evidently, a loss of details, as compared to the previous approach.

The model has two components. The first is a probabilistic model of the structure of the axon. The second describes the delay along basic segments of the model axon. Integrating those two components, the result is a closed form expression for the distribution of the delays along the whole axon.

The main results of this paper are the analytical expressions for the distribution of the propagation delays. These expressions give quantitative information and enhance the qualitative understanding of the phenomenon and its consequences to various models of brain function. In addition, some examples of the applicability of the model to the description of axonal trees are given. A more thorough comparison of the model with cortical axons is in preparation (Nelken 1991).

Modelling the axon

To model the axon, the following assumptions are made (see Fig. 1 for a graphical illustration):

1. The axon is built from segments of constant properties. Such segments can be, for example, compartments in a compartmental model of the axon.

2. There may be several types of segments. Different parts of the axon that have different properties can thus be characterized by segments with different electrical and morphological attributes. The number of types is finite.
3. At the end of each segment, a probabilistic mechanism selects one of several possible combinations of descended segments. The parent segment may terminate (in which case it is called a terminal segment), or it may be continued by a segment of the same type, or it may be continued by a segment of a different type, or it may branch into segments of the same type or of different types.
4. The probabilities of these transitions depend only on the type of the parent segment, and not on anything else (like other segments in the neighborhood or previous transitions).

This set of assumptions describes, in general, a whole population of axons rather then a single specific axon. There is some "typical form" of the axons in the population, depending on the specification of the transition probabilities, and some "typical variance" around it. The major task in verifying the model, is to show that both the typical form and the typical variance can be deduced from it.

Assumptions 1, 2 and 3 describe the building blocks of the model, the segments, and the way these building blocks are connected to form a tree. They are natural in the sense that they fit any structure which can grow and branch. Although assumption 2 restricts somewhat the kind of changes the character of the axon might undergo, it does fit well with anatomical data. Indeed, as far as can be deduced from anatomical data, changes in the geometrical properties of axons are usually quite abrupt - at the transition from grey to white matter and vice versa, where the axon acquires or loses its myelin sheath (Feldman 1984; White 1989), or at a transition from one cortical layer to another, where the statistics of the branching may change suddenly (White 1989; Martin 1984). Assumption 3 is less restrictive than it seems, because the probabilistic mechanism is as yet not specified. Thus, any axon can be described exactly by it.

The crucial assumption for the analysis is assumption 4. By this assumption, any property of the subtree of descendants of a given parent segment depends on the type of the parent, and is statistically independent of anything else in the tree. This assumption does limit in an essential way the character of the axonal structures which can be described by the model. Its validity can be judged only by checking the predictions which can be derived from it against real data.

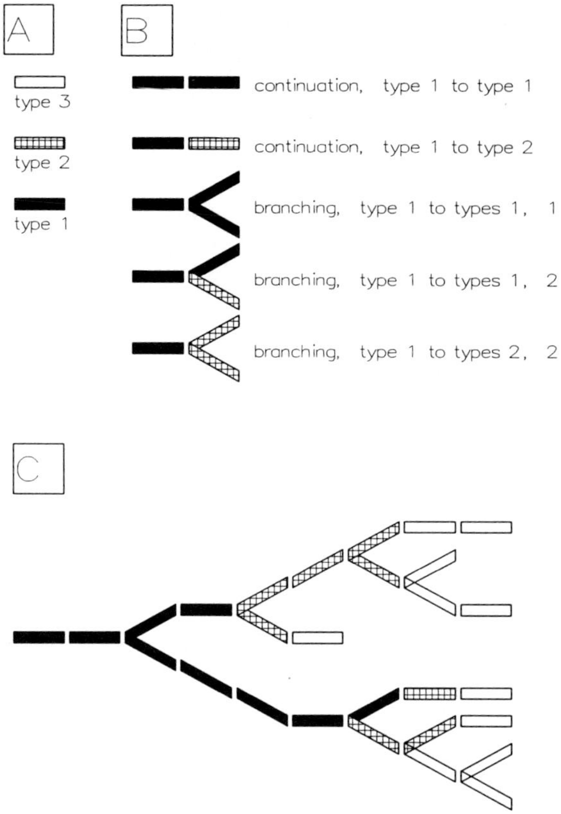

Fig. 1. A graphical illustration of the model. The axonal tree is modeled as a multitype branching process with constraints on the possible number of descendants and their types. **(A)** An illustration of 3 possible types of segments. **(B)** An illustration of all the possible transitions at the end of a segment of type 1. There may be a single descendant of type 1 (for elongation) or of type 2, or 2 descendants (and then there is a branch point). These may be of type 1 or of type 2. A segment of type 1 may not terminate (only the last type can terminate). **(C)** An axon fulfilling the assumptions of the model

Mathematically, these assumptions characterize a *multitype Markovian branching process* (Galton-Watson process, see Feller 1957). Usually, the analysis of such processes is aimed at obtaining the size of each generation of segments, but in the context of the axonal tree, the whole tree structure of the process is of interest. Thus, although these branching processes are well studied, their application to the description of axonal structure is new (for different approaches to the description of random branching patterns, see Triller and Korn 1986; Kliemann 1987; Verwer et al. 1987; van Pelt et al. 1989).

One additional assumption was made, to further simplify the analysis. This assumption is not crucial, but it agrees well with the anatomical knowledge.

5. The possible types of segments are numbered sequentially, and a branch of type i can be continued only by branches of types i and/or i+1. In addition, only binary branchings are allowed. Such a process will be called a *sequential* branching process.

Indeed, most branchings found on axons are binary (Triller and Korn 1986).

To describe a real axon, the structure generated from these assumptions should be finite. The process is then called "subcritical". A basic result for a sequential model is the following (proof in the appendix):

Lemma 1: For a sequential branching process with finite number of types, in order for the expected total number of segments to be finite, it is sufficient that for each type, the expected number of sons of the same type as their father is less than 1.

Given the assumptions above, the analysis of the statistics of the axonal tree is straightforward. The distributions and moments of quantities related to the tree, such as the number of terminal segments of the tree, the maximal length of a path along the tree, and so on, can be found easily. Some examples, which illustrate the general mathematical reasoning used, are given in the appendix.

The distribution of the propagation delays along the axon is intimately linked with the distribution of path lengths from the soma to the synapses. For the problem of computing propagation delays along the axonal tree, this is the most important distribution that has to be found. Intuitively, the reason is that in order to compute the expected delay from the soma to the synapses, one chooses first a "typical" path along the axon from the soma to a synapse, and then one computes the "typical" delay along such a path.

There is no unique way to specify this problem. The reason is that there are many ways to select a typical path along the axon, and different selection processes can result in different probabilities.

Two related questions can be naturally asked. The "forward" question concerns the length of the path traversed while following an action potential when it travels along the axon from the soma to a synapse. At each branch point, one of the two possible continuations is chosen, and this is done in a completely random fashion. In this case, synapses which are nearer to the soma are chosen with higher probability. For the "backward" question, first the whole axonal structure is examined, then one synapse is picked randomly, and the length of the path from the soma to that synapse is determined (this path is of course unique, because a tree does not contain any closed loop). In this case, given the structure of the axon, all synapses have equal probabilities to be selected.

The forward problem is the simpler one - it can be shown (see appendix) that if there are n possible types, then the length of the path is distributed like the sum of n geometrically distributed random variables, with parameters which are related to the branching probabilities of the types.

The backward problem is more complicated. A closed form solution was explicitly derived only for the single type model, and it is a mixture of negative binomial distributions (sums of geometrically distributed random variables). Although such a formula can also be written for the full model, it is complicated and not very illuminating. A full discussion is given in the appendix.

The common characteristic of these results is that all these distributions have tails decreasing, for large n, like p^n for some $p<1$. These become, in the continuous limit, exponential tails, decreasing like e^{-x}. The distributions are thus heavier-tailed than the Gaussian distribution. As an outcome, the probability of finding large deviations from the expected value are larger than for the Gaussian distribution with the same variance. The importance of this will be discussed later.

Before going on to describe the model of the delays along the tree, two examples illustrating the validity of the model for the description of cortical axons are presented. A fuller comparison between model predictions and actual statistics of axonal populations will be given elsewhere (Nelken 1991). The first example is taken from (Hellwig et al. 1991; see also Schüz, this volume). They analyzed the statistical characteristics of the distribution of boutons along axon collaterals in the mouse cortex. Their main findings may be summarized as follows: the distribution of the distances between boutons is essentially exponential, and successive intervals between boutons are statistically independent.

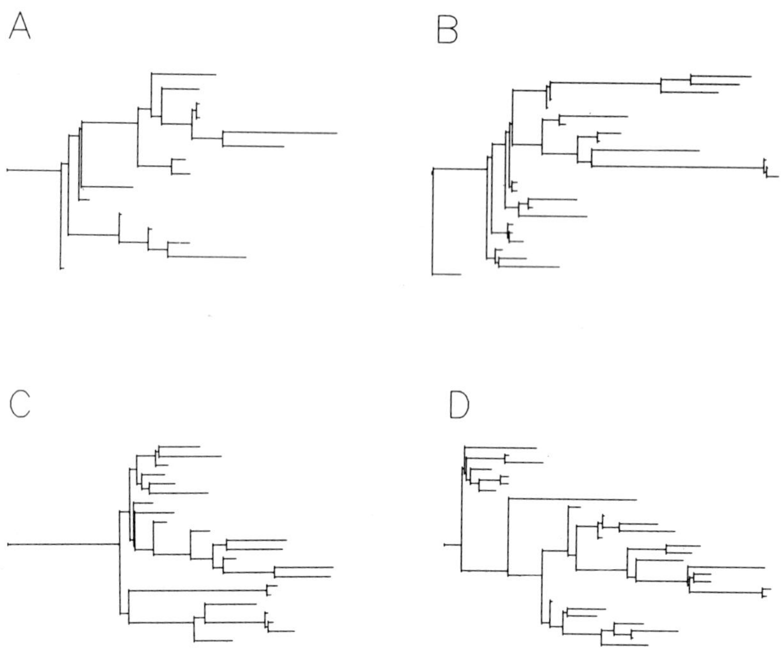

Fig. 2. Branching diagrams for 4 axons. The axons in **A**, **B** and **C** are from the somatosensory cortex of the mouse, from a data set collected by V. Braitenberg (with permission). The axon in **D** was generated from the model fitted for 9 cortical neurons, including the first three. The generation process was based on the prescription of the model - starting from the root segment, the segments were generated in a depth-first fashion, by choosing the continuations independently according to the estimated probabilities. Notice that the diagrams are essentially indistinguishable

A minimal branching model of these results has two types. One of them describes the collateral. The other, branching from it and terminating immediately, describes the occurrence of a bouton. The distribution of the length of the axon between successive branch points for a single type of segments is exponential, successive distances being independent. This model gives thus directly the main features of the distribution of boutons along cortical collaterals.

The second example is an informal comparison between a population of 9 axons from the somatosensory cortex of the mouse, chosen from a data set collected by Braitenberg (with permission), and one axon generated from a single-type model fitted to these axons. For details about the axons and the fitting procedure, see (Nelken 1991). In Fig. 2, branching diagrams of 4 axons are presented. One of them was generated by the model. It is not easy to distinguish between the true axons and the model axon.

To conclude this part of the paper, the morphological model describes quite well the phenomenology of the axonal structure. This of course does not prove in any way that the axon is built according to the model assumptions, although it strongly suggest that different parts of the axon do evolve relatively independently of each other.

Modelling the propagation delays

The propagation delays can now be modeled, based on the morphological model of the preceding section. The following assumptions are made about the electrical properties of a segment:

1. The segments are electrically homogenous.
2. Each segment has a list of parameters, describing its electrical properties. These parameters are chosen, according to some distribution, for each segment, but this distribution depends only on the type of the segment.
3. The delay along a segment is determined by its list of parameters.
4. The total delay to a terminal segment is the sum of the delays of all the segments on the path from the soma to the terminal segment.

Once the parameter list for each segment is given, the actual delay along the segment can be computed. It follows that the delays themselves are random variables. Knowing the distribution of the electrical characteristics of the segment fixes the distribution of that random variable uniquely. Thus, its distribution also depends only on the type of the segment.

This model apparently takes into account only delays along branches, and not delays caused by branch points. This problem can be remedied by postulating special types for the branching points themselves. In a model with such types, a branching occurs in two steps. First a transition to a segment of the branching point type is made. Then, with probability 1, the branching point segment branches into the two daughter branches. Branching point types do not have spatial attributes, and they are used only to carry the delays at the branch points.

In the preceding section, two ways to ask questions about the path along an axon were proposed. These can be translated immediately to questions about the delays along the axon. The forward problem consists now of following an action potential from the soma, taking randomly the left and right segments at branch points, and measuring the time it takes to get to a terminal segment. For the backward problem it is required to choose randomly a terminal segment, then to find the delay from the soma to that segment.

For general delay distributions along the segments, there is no closed form solution for the distribution of the delay along the whole tree, but the characteristic function (c.f. - the Fourier transform of the distribution function) of the total delay can nevertheless be given. This is based on a standard result for the c.f. of random sums (Feller 1957). As a reminder, for a probability distribution on the integers p_n, the probability generating function is given by

$$P(z) = \sum_{n=1}^{\infty} p_n z^n$$

Lemma 2: Let $f(t)$ be the c.f. of the delay along one segment. Let $G(z)$ be the probability generating function for the number of terms in the sum. Assume in addition that the number of terms in the sum is independent of their values. Then the c.f. of the sum is given by $G(f(t))$.

In the case of the single type axon, this result gives directly the c.f. of the delays for both the forward problem and the backward problem, because for both of those the corresponding G(z) is known explicitly (see preceding Section).

For a multitype model, there is an additional complication arising from the fact that the individual terms in the sum need not be identically distributed. A slight generalization of lemma 2 solves that problem:

Lemma 3: Let $f_i(t)$ be the c.f. of the delay along a segment of type i. Let $G(z_1,...z_n)$ be the n-dimensional probability generating function for the number of segments of each type along the path. Assume in addition that the number of terms in the sum is independent of their values. Then the c.f. of the sum is given by $G(f_1(t),...,f_n(t))$.

The proof of this lemma entirely parallels that of the simpler case, and is omitted.

For the forward problem model, the total length of the path from the soma to the terminal segment is a sum of independent geometrically distributed variables, one for each type. The n-dimensional probability generating function is then just the product of the individual terms, and the final result is

$$F(t) = \prod \frac{(1 - p(i))\, f_i(t)}{1 - p(i) f_i(t)}$$

where p(i) is the probability of transition from type i to itself along the path.

For the backward problem of the single type model, the corresponding formula is more complicated:

$$F(t) = \sum_{n=0}^{\infty} E\left(\frac{R_1}{K + K^{(n)}}\right) (2p_2)^n \left(\frac{f(t)}{1 - p_1 f(t)}\right)^{n+1}$$

where R_1 is the number of terminal segments at depth 1, K is the total number of terminal segments in the same tree, and $K^{(n)}$ is a sum of another n independent copies of K. p_1 and p_2 are the elongation and branching probabilities of the model respectively. This equation is somewhat obscure, and its intuitive meaning will become clearer when its asymptotic form is derived.

The backward problem for a multitype model is amenable to analysis, but the resulting formulas are even more complicated and will not be given here.

The two equations, as given above, are exact and can actually be used to compute the distribution of the delays for the two problems, by computing the c.f. and then inverting the Fourier transform to get the distribution function. Unfortunately, it is difficult to deduce general properties of the solution from them. To get more transparent equations, but without losing too much generality, an asymptotic analysis of these equations was made.

First, the relevant limit has to be specified. The most obvious limit is to make the length of each segment shorter and shorter, thus increasing the number of segments, but keeping the total length between two branch points equal. In terms of the parameters of the model, the elongation probability of each type becomes larger and larger, converging to 1, while the other probabilities decrease to zero. To keep the form of the tree, those other probabilities must keep the same ratios between themselves. For example, in the single type model there are 3 probabilities: p_0, the termination probability, p_1, the elongation probability and p_2, the branching probability. The limit will have then one parameter, the ratio p_2/p_0. To have a finite tree, it must be less than 1, and the nearer it is to 1, the more "bushy" the tree is.

Now the limiting forms of the distributions can be given. The basic term in the two equations above has the form of

$$\frac{f(t)}{1 - p_1 f(t)}$$

and its limiting form is given by the following lemma (proof in the appendix):

Lemma 4: Let T be the random variable whose value is the sum of N independent r.v. with c.f. f(t), where N is distributed geometrically and is independent of the individual terms. If the expected value of each term is greater than 0, then the limiting distribution of T/E(N) is exponential.

Thus, for the forward problem the limiting distribution is a sum of exponential distributions, while for the backward problem the limiting distribution is a mixture of sums of exponential distributions.

The importance of the results stems from the fact that these distributions are skewed to the right and have a heavier tail than the Gaussian with the same variance. Thus, it is expected that the range of random samples from such a distribution will be larger than for random samples from a Gaussian distribution.

Discussion

The model presented here is, like many models, only a caricature of the real world, but statistical analysis of real axons shows that it gives a relatively good description of at least some of the axons in real brains (Nelken 1991). Thus, the results concerning the distributions of the propagation delays may give a reasonable feeling for what happens in reality.

The model assumes relatively little about the structure of the axon. To summarize, the most important assumption about the structure of the axon is the "Markovian" assumption (assumption 4). This assumption is crucial for the mathematical simplicity of the model. Although there is no direct biological reason to make it, in some sense it is the "simplest possible" assumption, so that any other assumption about the growth of the axonal tree has to be justified based on biophysical data. Since theoretical distributions calculated from the model agree fairly well with the statistics of populations of axons (as described in the foregoing, or in Nelken 1991), and since the derivation of the theoretical distributions in all the examples relies quite heavily on the Markovian structure of the model, it is quite improbable that other, essentially different, sets of assumptions will give the same results (of course, the same mathematical model may result from more than one set of assumptions!). Thus, it may be concluded that assumption 4 does hold, at least approximately, for the axons in those examples. It has to be stressed that both examples are from central nervous systems of vertebrates. It may be that for other parts of the nervous system or for other animals the rules are different.

The general model has complete freedom in the number of types, and the large number of parameters poses problems for the parameter estimation procedures. In the examples discussed, the number of types was selected based on a general impression, and then the parameters of the model were estimated by manually assigning a type to each segment, then computing the mean length and branching probabilities. Such a manual procedure was possible because the database was small. For a large thalamocortical axon, with its thousands of terminal segments (Martin 1984; White 1989), a manual procedure is of course practically impossible. One direction of further work is to find a simple parameter estimation procedure. Some work on parameter estimation using hidden Markov chain models and the related estimation algorithms (Dempster et al. 1977) was already started.

The main result of the paper is the asymptotic form for the distribution of the path length and the propagation delays along the axon. It is, under the assumptions of this model, an exponential or a related distribution. The important characteristic of this family is its being overdispersed with respect to the Gaussian distribution. As a result, the range of the delays on a single axonal tree is larger than expected from the Gaussian assumption. To illustrate this point, for a single type model, the delay propagation distribution is a simple exponential. In this case, the standard deviation is equal to the mean of the distribution. As a result, a fit by a Gaussian will have a large negative tail, and this is an inconvenience for a quantity which is always positive. Secondly, the 1% critical point for a Gaussian distribution is approximately 2.236 standard deviations above the expected value, but the cumulative probability beyond this point for the exponential distribution is approximately 3.6%, that is, there is 3.6 as much probability of getting a longer delay, and this factor is even bigger for larger deviations from the expected value. Although for small axons this is not an appreciable factor, for large cortical axons this probability represent an appreciable number of endings.

To translate these numbers into absolute delays, some knowledge of the propagation velocity of action potentials in the cortex is needed. In (Manor 1990) it was assumed that the velocity is about 30 cm/sec, which is a reasonable guess for non-myelinated axons, as they are in the cortex. For a small axon, with mean branch length of 300 μm, this gives a mean delay of 1 msec, and this is also the standard deviation. In such a case, two action potentials starting at the same location will get to their target with a dispersion of less then 5 msec with probability of almost 1. On the other hand, for the longer branches, with a typical branch length of 3000 μm (Martin 1984), the mean delay will be 10 msec, and with standard deviation of 10 msec a dispersion of less then 5 msec is not likely any more.

This rough computation gives a tentative answer to the problem raised in the introduction - the "coherence length" (that is, the distance in the cortex for which small dispersion is expected) for propagation delays in the cortex seems to be on the order of magnitude of 1 mm (as in the rough estimate above), which is the size of a hypercolumn. For such distances, coherent activity is possible, with dispersion on the order of magnitude of 1 msec. Thus, models requiring good local timing are possible in the cortex. These are for example the Poggio and Koch models for direction selectivity (where the excitation and inhibition are generated at the same location), or the synfire chain. On the other hand, it is improbable to expect the required timing between hypercolumns or between cortical areas. Indeed, because of the large dispersion in the delays, it is expected that activity which starts as a coherent burst of spikes will desynchronize to a continuous distribution of excitations at different distances from the cell body. Thus, a model like the shifter circuits of Anderson and van Essen (Anderson and van Essen 1987) looks implausible, unless further mechanisms are postulated. It follows that if such long-range coincidence models are indeed verified experimentally, there must be some synchronizing mechanisms at work. Such mechanisms do exist in nature, but it is not clear whether they are important in the cortex. They include for example ephaptic interactions between neighboring axons, or "time filtering" by a group of neurons which are active in the synchronized mode (Abeles 1991).

On the other hand, this dispersion opens the door to other families of models. For example, it may be possible to transform a short, intense burst of spikes into a relatively long, constant excitation of a cortical region. This can serve for example for the transition from a coincidence code, like the synfire model predicts, to a rate code used in the periphery.

Another use of such blurring of time details may be in the interpretation of Hopfield-type neural network models: it may be used to make the active state of the single neuron effectively longer than the duration of the action potential. In such a version of the neural network, the random update needed for the sequential model may be interpreted in terms of the delays in the propagation of the action potentials.

Another question which is raised by this model is the interpretation of its success in the morphological description of the axonal trees. The fact that the statistics of populations of axons can be described by a Markovian model like the present one suggests that axonal growth may follow such rules. This is not so far fetched - it is known that the axon grows from its growth cones, which behave according to environmental cues. In a relatively homogeneous medium, where there are mostly random fluctuations, two growth cones may see environments which are essentially uncorrelated, and thus behave in an independent way. The different types are then explained by the different environments through which the axon is passing. Such a speculation may lead to a solution to the problem of the specification of the form of the axons from their genes. Indeed, the genes are responsible for the specification of the "transition probabilities", that is, the rules of what a growth cone should do at any given constellation of external influences. This is combined with the Markovian global generation mechanism to give the final form of the axon.

Appendix

In the appendix, the proofs omitted from the main text are given.

Proof of Lemma 1: first the single type model will be discussed. For the finiteness of the tree it is necessary that the branching process becomes extinct with probability 1 (Feller 1957). Thus, it must be a critical or subcritical branching process. Although a critical branching process becomes extinct with probability 1, its expected size is infinite (Feller 1957). Thus, to get a tree with finite expected size, the process must be subcritical. For a simple, one-type model, the condition for subcriticality is that the equation P(s)=s, where P(s) is the probability generating function for the number of descendants, has a root which is smaller than 1. Under assumption 5, of binary branchings only, the equation takes the form

$$p_0 - (p_0 + p_2)s + p_2 s^2 = 0$$

and its solutions are easily found to be 1 and p_2/p_0. Thus, the condition for subcriticality is $p_2/p_0<1$ or $p_2<p_0$. Now, since $p_0+p_1+p_2=1$, it follows that $p_1+2p_2<1$. But the left side of this inequality is exactly the expected number of descendants of any segment.

For the sequential model, it is easily found that the condition for having a tree with finite expected size is that all the subtrees built from segments of one single type have finite expected size. This follows from the fact that the expected number of subtrees of any type whose roots are direct descendants of a given segment is always finite (because of assumption 5), and thus a tree cannot become large because one segment has "too many" direct descendants. Thus, the only way for a sequential tree to become large is that one of the types composing it generates large subtrees. But then the previous discussion applies, and the lemma follows.

For the rest of the appendix, let $p^i_{(j,k)}$ denote the probability of a segment of type i to give rise to j segments of type i and k segments of type i+1. Under assumption 5, j+k can be 0, 1 or 2.

Distribution of path length for the forward problem: if the path is currently on a segment of type i, then the probability of the next segment on the path to be of the same type is, according to the assumption of the forward problem, $p^i_{(1,0)}+p^i_{(2,0)}+0.5p^i_{(1,1)}$. The probability of transition to the next type of segments is the complement of this. It follows that the number of segments that the path stays on any given type is distributed geometrically with the parameter above. The whole path is formed of successive parts, passing through all the types sequentially. Thus, the whole length of the path is a sum of such random variables. The independence follows from the Markovian assumption.

Distribution of path length for the backward problem, single type model: let R_n be the number of terminal segments of the tree whose distance from the root is n segments. Let K be the total number of terminal segments. On a tree with a given structure, the probability of choosing randomly a terminal segment with path of length n is then R_n/K. The unconditional probability for such a segment is then $E(R_n/K)$. To compute this expression, a recursion on n is developed, by conditioning on the first transition and using the Markovian assumption:

$$E\left(\frac{R_n}{K}\right) = E\left(\frac{R_1}{K}\right)\delta_{n1} + p_1 E\left(\frac{R_{n-1}}{K}\right) + 2p_2 E\left(\frac{R_{n-1}}{K+K^{(1)}}\right)$$

where $K^{(1)}$ is an independent copy of K. The last term in the sum needs then a separate recursion on n, and the general recursion is:

$$E\left(\frac{R_n}{K+K^{(m)}}\right) = E\left(\frac{R_1}{K+K^{(m)}}\right)\delta_{n1} + p_1 E\left(\frac{R_{n-1}}{K+K^{(m)}}\right) + 2p_2 E\left(\frac{R_{n-1}}{K+K^{(m+1)}}\right)$$

where $K^{(m)}$ is the sum of m independent copies of K. Define now the generating function

$$G_m(z) = \sum_{n=0}^{\infty} E\left(\frac{R_n}{K+K^{(m)}}\right) z^n$$

and from the recursion above it is found that

$$G_m(z) = \frac{z}{1-p_1 z} E\left(\frac{R_1}{K+K^{(m)}}\right) + \frac{2p_2 z}{1-p_1 z} G_{m+1}(z)$$

Since $K>0$, it follows that $G_m(z)$ tends to 0 with m, for every z. Iterating the formula, the final result is

$$G_0(z) = \sum_{n=0}^{\infty} \frac{z}{1-p_1 z} E\left(\frac{R_1}{K+K^{(n)}}\right)\left(\frac{2p_2 z}{1-p_1 z}\right)^n$$

As is easily seen, this is the generating function of a mixture of negative binomial distributions (sums of geometrically distributed variables).

Distribution of number of terminal segments of the axon: let $p^i(n)$ be the probability of a subtree whose root is a segment of type i to have n terminal segments. Then, by conditioning on the first transition, the following recursion holds:

$$\begin{aligned} p^i(n) =& p^i{}_{(0,0)}\delta_{n1} + p^i{}_{(1,0)}p^i(n) + p^i{}_{(0,1)}p^{i+1}(n) + p^i{}_{(1,1)}\sum_{k=1}^{n} p^i(k)p^{i+1}(n-k) \\ &+ p^i{}_{(2,0)}\sum_{k=1}^{n} p^i(k)p^i(n-k) + p^i{}_{(0,2)}\sum_{k=1}^{n} p^{i+1}(k)p^{i+1}(n-k) \end{aligned}$$

where each term comes from one of the possible transitions from a segment of type i.

Passing to generating functions, the recursion gives the following equation:

$$\begin{aligned} P^i(z) =& p^i{}_{(0,0)}z + p^i{}_{(1,0)}P^i(z) + p^i{}_{(0,1)}P^{i+1}(z) + p^i{}_{(1,1)}P^i(z)P^{i+1}(z) \\ &+ p^i{}_{(2,0)}\left(P^i(z)\right)^2 + p^i{}_{(0,2)}\left(P^{i+1}(z)\right)^2 \end{aligned}$$

which is a recursion for $P^i(z)$. Starting from the last type, for which the equation is just a quadratic equation, the transform can be computed, and then inverted to find the actual distribution.

Conditional expectation of number of endings given the maximum depth of the tree: this is done for a single type model only. The derivation starts with a recursion for p(n,k), the probability of having a tree with k endings and maximal depth of n. Conditioning on the first transition, the following formula is found:

$$p(n,k) = p_0\delta_{n1}\delta_{k1} + p_1 p(n-1,k) + p_2 \sum_{l=1}^{n-1}\sum_{k'=1}^{k-1}(2-\delta_{ln-1})p(n-1,k')p(l,k-k')$$

The second term comes from the fact that if the first transition is a simple continuation, then to have a tree with k endings and maximal length n, the subtree based on the first segment must also have k endings but maximal depth of n-1. The third term comes from enumerating all the possibilities for the case of branching: one of the subtrees has to have maximal depth of n-1, the other can have any maximal depth less than or equal to n-1, and the k endings are distributed between the two.

Passing to the generating function on k, with n as parameter, the following recursion on n is found:

$$P_n(z) = p_0 z \delta_{n1} + p_1 P_{n-1}(z) + p_2 P_{n-1}(z) \sum_{l=1}^{n-1} (2 - \delta_{ln-1}) P_l(z)$$

Finally, the conditional expectation E(K|n) is given by E(K|n) = E(K;n)/$P_n(1)$, and

$$E(K|n) = \frac{d}{dz} P_n(z)|_{z=1}$$

so that there are two recursions to be computed - $P_n(1)$ which is computed directly from the recursions for the generating functions, and $P'_n(1)$ which is easily derived from that recursion.

Asymptotic distribution of delays for geometric path length (Lemma 4): let N be the random variable giving the path length, Θ the delay along a single segment and T the total delay along the path. Let f(t) be the c.f. (characteristic function) of the distribution of Θ and F(t) the c.f. of T. The probability of having path length n is then

$$g(n) = (1-p)p^{n-1}$$

where p is the geometrical parameter. The generating function is

$$G(z) = \sum_{n-1}^{\infty} (1-p)p^{n-1} z^n$$

and the c.f. of the distribution of the delays is given by

$$F(t) = \frac{(1-p)f(t)}{1-pf(t)}$$

Now, EN = 1/(1-p), and the characteristic function of T/EN is given by F((1-p)t). In addition, f(t) can be written as f(t)=1-imt+o(t) where m=EΘ, and so

$$F((1-p)t) \approx \frac{(1-p)(1-i(1-p)mt)}{1-p(1-i(1-p)mt)} = \frac{(1-i(1-p)mt)}{1+pimt} \rightarrow \frac{1}{1+imt}$$

when p increases to 1. But the last function is the c.f. of an exponential distribution with parameter m, as was to be shown.

References

Abeles M (1982) Local cortical circuits. Springer, Berlin Heidelberg New York

Anderson CH, van Essen DC (1987) Shifter circuits: a computational strategy for dynamic aspects of visual processing. Proc Nat Acad Sci 84:6297-6301

Abeles M (1991) Corticonics: neural networks of the cerebral cortex. Cambridge University Press, Cambridge

Dempster AP, Laird NM, Rubin DB (1977) Maximum likelihood from incomplete data via the EM algorithm. J R Stat Soc B 39:1-38

Feldman ML (1984) Morphology of the Neocortical Pyramidal Neuron. In: Peters A, Jones EG (ed) Cerebral Cortex vol 1. Plenum Press

Feller W (1957) An Introduction to Probability Theory and its Applications. John Wiley & Sons, New York London

Hellwig B, Schüz A, Aertsen AMHJ (1991) In preparation

Khodorov BI, Timin YN (1975) Nerve impulse propagation along nonuniform fibers (investigation using mathematical models). Prog Biophys Molec Biol 30:145-184

Kliemann W (1987) A stochastic dynamical model for the characterizations of the geometrical structure of dendritic processes. Bull Math Bio 49:135-152

Manor Y (1990) Theoretical analysis of the propagation of action potentials in branching axon by computerized simulation. M.Sc. Thesis (in Hebrew)

Manor Y, Koch C, Segev I (1991) The effect of geometrical irregularities on propagation delay in axonal trees. Biophys J (in press)

Martin KAC (1984) Neuronal Circuits in Cat Striate Cortex. In: Peters A, Jones EG (ed) Cerebral Cortex vol 2. Plenum Press

Nelken I (1991) In preparation

Parnas I (1979) Propagation in nonuniform neurites: form and function in axons. In: Schmidt FO, Worden FG (ed) The Neurosciences, Fourth Study Section. M.I.T. press

Parnas I, Segev I (1979) A mathematical model for conduction of action potentials along bifurcating axons. J Physiol (Lond.) 295:323-343

Poggio T, Koch C, Torre V (1981) Microelectronics of nerve cells: dendritic morphology and information processing. M.I.T. A.I. memo no. 650, October 1981

Schüz A, Palm G (1989) Density of Neurons and Synapses in the Cerebral Cortex of the Mouse. J Comp Neurol 286:442-455

Schüz A (this volume)

Triller A, Korn H (1986) Variability of Axonal Arborizations Hides Simples Rules of Construction: a Topological Study From HRP Intracellular Injections. J Comp Neurol 253:500-513

van Pelt J, Verwer RWH, Uylings HBM (1989) Centrifugal-order distributions in binary topological trees. Bull Math Biol 51:511-536

Verwer RWH, van Pelt J, Noest AJ (1987) Parameter estimation in topological analysis of binary tree structures. Bull Math Biol 49:363-378

White EL (1989) Cortical Circuits: Synaptic Organization of the Cerebral Cortex, Structure, Function and Theory. Birkhauser, Boston Basel

Part Two

Cortical Activity at Different Levels of Resolution in Space and Time

The Biological Role of Neocortex

Horace B. Barlow

Physiological Laboratory, Cambridge, CB2 3EG, UK

The neocortex is the part of the brain that enlarged progressively during the evolution of mammals reaching its greatest development in the great apes and man. But the known properties of the neurons of the neocortex hardly begin to explain the behaviour they bring about, so we need some crucial new insight.

The types of behaviour mediated by neocortex all require good knowledge and understanding of the environment in which the animal lives, a point first emphasised by Herrick. Craik and Tolman extended this with their ideas about working models and cognitive maps, which enable an animal to predict what will happen next, and the probable results of its active interference with the environment.

These models and maps must be built up by observing the associative structure in sensory messages. The essential operation is to detect that two sensory messages occur together more often than expected from their individual probabilities, based on previous experience; ie they constitute a cliché or suspicious coincidence. These are important because they are indicators of new causal factors in the environment. Hitherto, perception has been thought to provide a simple representation of "what is where", but this is not enough for efficient detection of suspicious coincidences: one also needs to know how unexpected are the objects and events signalled. Without such knowledge of prior probabilities one could never distinguish reliably between accidental coincidences and those that betray genuine new causal factors at work.

But knowing the unexpectedness of the individual items in perception is still not sufficient. A versatile learning system should be sensitive to conjunctions of elementary signals, and finding the prior probabilities of conjunctions is very much easier if it is justifiable to assume that the individual items are independent. Thus a worthwhile computational goal for neocortex would be to categorise experience into elements that occur independently and with known prior probability in the normal environment, and to represent the current scene by the occurrence of these elements.

If the neocortex elaborates a representation of the world that makes available the prior probabilities of what is happening, this would greatly improve the efficiency and versatility of associative learning; it would explain the evolutionary advantage of neocortex and why it developed explosively in mammals. The computational task postulated is horrendously complex, but it can be modelled and I shall show some preliminary efforts.

The biological role of neocortex

This is an amazing problem, for neocortex contains the secret of mankind's place in nature. As Herrick (1926) said, it is "the organ of civilisation". How should we approach it?

Obviously we should first look at the comparative anatomy of the brain, and then at the new range of behaviour that evolved with the neocortex; though this is old-fashioned, old-established knowledge, I think it contains important lessons that have been overshadowed by the glamorous advances made over the past few decades in neurophysiology and neuroanatomy.

After that I shall describe some ideas about visual perception since I think these suggest a computational goal for the whole neocortex. This may guide us in interpreting the neurophysiology, and may also enable us to design a network to achieve that goal.

Defining the problem

In "The Descent of Man" Darwin (1871) gave a lengthy catalogue of the differences in behavioural capacities that separate Man from the great apes, but he added that these differences were ones of degree rather than of kind. Furthermore he thought that these capacities could be traced back to much lower forms.

In the half century that followed, comparative anatomists defined the anatomical correlate of this striking growth in behavioural capacities, and to cut a long story short, the *neocortex* is the answer. It is not the only part of the brain that is unusually large in man and primates, for so are the *thalamus* and the lateral lobes of the cerebellum, but these are closely associated with neocortex. The *hippocampus* too is relatively large. But neocortex is thought to be the most important new structure that developed, and its vast expansion during the evolution of the mammals is sufficiently striking for Elliot Smith (1924) to have coined the phrase "neopallial explosion" to describe it. So I think one can accept that relative enlargement of neocortex is what distinguishes the brains of great apes from those of primitive mammals and our own brains from those of the great apes. Data showing that man's brain is larger (though not very much) than might be expected from his body size can be found in Jerison (1973, 1983), and the location of the part that enlarged, the neocortex, is described in textbooks of comparative neuroanatomy such as Sarnat and Netsky (1981).

Behaviour and neurophysiology appear to have no connection

Table 1 shows some aspects of behaviour that are thought to be mediated by neocortex, but they are not much use to a neurophysiologist who wants to find out how nerve cells *explain* this behaviour. How are they connected with the properties of cortical neurons that neurophysiologists are concerned with? What on earth does *consciousness* have to do with a train of action potentials? How is *reason* related to receptive fields? What do *free-will* and the *moral senses* tell us about feature detection, columns, mapping, or long-term potentiation?

Perhaps one should not expect to see a connection between behavioural capacities and the hardware that underlies them, because even a clearly stated computational problem can be solved in many possible ways. But one *should* be able to see how nerve cells produce behaviour, while in fact the gulf looks no smaller from this point of view. What do the things neurophysiologists are currently discovering tell us about the way the organ they are investigating brings about the remarkable things we do with our brains? Many neurophysiologists and neuroanatomists doubtless chose to work on cortex because of its role in making human-kind pre-eminent, but their detailed results seem to make no contact with the issue that presumably aroused their interest.

Cortical columns, modules, multiple sensory areas, synchrony of firing, and other such developments are of great interest in the field of physiology and anatomy, but they seem to have precious little bearing on the behaviour the neocortex is thought to be responsible for.

Whole Animal	Neocortical Neurons
Consciousness	Action potentials
Free will	Receptive fields
Intelligence	Feature detection
Adaptability	Maps of sensory surfaces
Voluntary movements	Columns
Perception	Synchronisation
Moral sense	40 Hz oscillations
Insight	Long term potentiation

Table 1. Some aspects of the behaviour of the whole animal thought to be mediated by neocortex, and some properties of the neurons that should bring about this behaviour. Can you see any connection? How can this gap be filled?

This chasm between current work in the neurophysiology of the cerebral cortex and what is needed to account for it being the "organ of civilisation" makes me very uneasy. I feel it is as if, in studying the heart, we had become involved in a detailed examination of the ionic currents and membrane channels of the Purkinje fibres *before* making the all-important discovery that the heart pumps blood around the body. There is something crucial missing; we desperately lack understanding at levels intermediate between the detailed physiology and anatomy of neurons and the behaviour the brain is responsible for.

Filling the gap

To bridge these intermediate levels I think we must first try to find the common requirement of cortically mediated types of behaviour, for this is what the cellular neurophysiology should explain. Of course it is absurdly ambitious to attempt this, but we shall be lost without the answer.

Knowledge as prerequisite for neocortical behaviour

Philosophers, psychologists, theologians and computer scientists could argue indefinitely about the common requirements for the behavioural capacities especially characteristic of humankind, but at the end of the day I'm not confident that they would agree about anything except this: everything neocortex makes possible, from consciousness to the moral senses, requires knowledge and understanding of the animal's environment, and effective use of this knowledge and understanding. This is self-evidently important for intelligence and for the effective use of reason, and without such knowledge the exercise of free will would be quite aimless. With regard to the social and moral senses, knowledge and understanding of other members of one's own species are obviously crucial.

It must be agreed that this knowledge is *necessary* for the diverse and adaptable forms of behaviour that neocortex makes possible, though it may not be *sufficient* for this purpose; however we can leave the philosophers and theologians arguing about what else may be needed, for the necessity of knowledge of the world already gives a pointer to what neocortical neurons must do.

Herrick, Craik, and Tolman

To Herrick (1928) it seemed obvious that neocortex stores detailed knowledge of the environment, and he summarised this by stating that the neocortex constitutes the "filing system of the central executive". At the time he was saying this psychologists were becoming obsessed by the behaviourists' idea that learning only occurs following re-inforcement, and this may have prevented them from appreciating the vast amount of background information that has to be acquired, stored, and accessed in order to produce intelligent behaviour. Craik and Tolman, however, saw Herrick's point clearly.

Craik (1943) argued that the construction of "working models" is the essential operation underlying the most interesting things we do with our brains. He was not interested in models that just *looked* like the real thing; they had to *work* like the real thing too. Such a model must embody the principles which enable the object modelled to carry out its characteristic functions, and it must react the same way to outside interference or intervention. Thus his idea was certainly not restricted to the representation of things that might have been modelled mechanically, but is perhaps more generally stated in terms of the need to represent the *causes* that make the world work the way it does.

Tolman's contribution (1948) was to show by ingenious experiments that some embodiment of the geography of the environment (a cognitive map) is used in the control of behaviour and must therefore be incorporated in the brain. The essential feature of a map is the representation of spatial relations or associations, while we have seen that working models represent causal relations, so the two ideas can be combined by saying *the brain must work out and represent the causal and associative structure of the environment.*

What all cortical behaviour requires	**A computational goal for neocortex**
Knowledge and understanding of the environment incorporated in working models based on the associative structure of sensory messages.	Categorise and represent sensory scenes by features of known prior probability that occur almost independently in the normal environment.

Table 2. The common requirements of cortically mediated behaviour, and a computational goal that would lead to their fulfillment. The resulting improvements in the versatility and efficiency of associative learning may have provided the energy for the neopallial explosion

I think this is the common requirement for the behavioural capacities that evolved in mammals and reached their highest point in primates, so I think this is what neocortex must do. Neither Craik nor Tolman actually specified the anatomical locus of their models or maps, but their idea goes a good deal further than Herrick's "filing system" and in fact incorporates what he (Herrick 1928) alluded to in another quotable remark: "the essence of cortical function is correlation". The idea will be carried forward (see table 2), but first we shall consider the possible role of the neocortex in vision in order to gain further insight.

A new role for neocortex in vision

The usual account of the biological role of vision is that it tells you *what* is *where* in the world around you. This definition, with which Marr (1982) started his book, has been fruitful, especially for computer scientists who wish to emulate seeing, but we actually use our eyes for more than object recognition and discovering the spatial positions of objects: we acquire almost all our knowledge and understanding of the environment through perception, so we *learn* from what we see. One cannot ignore the fact that perception both uses stored information, and continually adds to this store.

A photograph or TV image can be analysed fairly well to give an account of the objects in it and where they are, but the result will not give anything approaching the depth of understanding that we obtain when we actually perceive a scene. The objects in it instantly recall for us previous experience with similar objects, and it is this stored information that enables us to predict what will happen if we intervene and do something to these objects. Furthermore it is the continual additions to this store that make our visual system so useful. Therefore the problem is: What kind of representation might contain the richness of associative knowledge that our perceptions give us, and how can this associative knowledge be continuously updated in such a representation?

That is not an easy question, and to simplify it still further let us concentrate on the requirement for keeping the representation up to date. This demands the ability to detect new associations when they arise, and can perhaps be epitomised as the ability to spot suspicious coincidences with the greatest possible reliability and efficiency. Admirers of Sherlock Holmes, Hercule Poirot, and Miss Marple will not need to be told that this ability is the cornerstone of intelligence, and hence the key function of cerebral cortex.

Detecting suspicious coincidences

We all have a pretty good intuitive understanding of the factors that make a coincidence suspicious, and therefore important, but it is worth spelling them out. The evidence for a new association is provided by the occurrence of some sequence or conjunction of two events - the cause and its effect - more often than would be expected if the association did not exist. To be good at spotting such conjunctions you must of course detect them and estimate how often they occur, but you must also be able to assess the expected frequency with which they *would* occur if the two events were *not* associated. Without the evidence on which such an expectation can be based there would be no way to distinguish between a random conjunction and a coincidence that betrays a genuine causal relation.

Importance of prior probabilities

What this really boils down to is that a representation to be used for learning must not only be an adequate image (as a photograph or a tv picture is), but it must also include information about the prior probabilities of the items represented. *What* and *Where* are not enough: you also need to know *How Unexpected*.

To show how important this is consider the formation of a conditioned reflex. When an important event occurs, such as an unanticipated reward or punishment, you must look for possible predictors of the important event among the other recent events that have low prior probabilities on the hypothesis that the causal nexus in the environment is unchanged; events of high prior probability are obviously likely to happen anyway, without there being any relation with the reward or punishment. Hence a representation to be used effectively in learning must indicate the unexpectedness of the features and events being signalled.

Note that this is a statement about what is logically required to detect new associations, and its truth is independent of empirical support. But well known experiments in learning (Kamin 1969; Rescorla and Wagner 1972; Mackintosh 1974) confirm that prior probability is crucially important: previous familiarisation with a conditional stimulus makes conditioning more difficult, an effect called "latent inhibition", and familiarisation means that the prior probability of the stimulus is increased. An efficient learning system *must* show such an effect, but of course without the experimental evidence we would never have known that learning actually is efficient in this way.

Having access to prior probabilities is also intuitively plausible: we all have an eye for the unexpected, and perception certainly seems to draw attention automatically to the improbable. Artists know this, so they use the visually surprising to attract attention in the same sort of way that a writer will use a rare word or an unusual word order. To me it is eminently plausible that the intensive element of our perceptions corresponds (but only approximately of course) to novelty or unexpectedness - some inverse measure of prior probability. For higher level perceptual attributes, surprisingness takes the place of brightness, brilliance, loudness, or other correlates of low level sensory intensity.

Definitions

Talking about probabilities needs care. By the probability of an event or occurrence I mean what is estimated in any one epoch by taking the ratio: *Actual number counted : Maximum possible number in that epoch*. The true probability would be obtained from an infinitely long epoch, and it is obvious that the epoch one is considering should be stated. Probabilities measured over any period from under a minute to a lifetime may be important to us, and the relevant epoch may not even be the most recent period of the specified duration.

The duration of the epoch determines the numbers of events and hence how accurately probabilities can be estimated, and if the epoch is short it may be necessary to categorise the sensory input coarsely in order to obtain sufficient samples for reasonable probability estimates to be obtained. These important issues cannot be further considered here, but one must realise that the brain often has to deal with very poor estimates of probabilities based on small numbers.

Associations

The above qualitative discussion implied that there is evidence for an association between C and U when

$$N(C.U) > E(C.U)$$

where N is the actual number of counts, (C.U) is a compound occurrence such as "the conditional stimulus C followed by the unconditional stimulus U", and E is the expected number of occurrences according to the null hypothesis of "no association". This needs clarifying both with regard to the direction of the inequality, and with regard to its magnitude.

The sign of the inequality given above corresponds to the customary thought that suspicious coincidences are significant *positive* associations, but is there any valid reason for confining one's attention to positive and neglecting negative associations? I think there is, for the following reason.

In everyday talk about coincidences one is usually referring to the co-occurrence of events that are themselves infrequent. The expected rate of co-occurrence is therefore very low and under these circumstances it is a difficult or impossible task to prove that the actual rate of occurrence is significantly below this expected rate; for instance if the two events each had an estimated probability of .001, the expected co-occurrences would have an expected rate of 10^{-6}, and one would have to wait for many million possible co-occurrences before gaining much evidence for a negative association. The situation is quite different with positive associations, for a very small number of co-occurrences is sufficient to make one doubt a null hypothesis that predicts nearly zero, and a significant result of this sort could be obtained after a few thousand trials. This asymmetry is clear and obvious, and Palm (1981) has drawn attention to related problems.

With regard to magnitude, the expression should be elaborated to

$$N(C.U) > E(C.U) + K\sigma\{E(C.U)\}$$

where $\sigma(E)$ is the standard deviation of the estimate of E and K is a constant setting the degree of confidence required before the existence of an association is accepted. Obviously the right hand side can be expanded in terms of the estimated prior probabilities of C and U, and the number of possible occurrences under consideration. There is no need for the probabilities to have been estimated over the same epochs as each other, or as that over which (C.U) is counted, but if they are not the same then stationarity as well as independence must be assumed for the null hypothesis.

Probability matching

In the qualitative discussion it was claimed that one should look for conditional stimuli among the *unexpected* occurrences and events preceding unconditional stimuli, because the expected ones were more likely to occur anyway and thus be of no significance. That is correct, but only because it is plausible to assume that rewards and punishments - the unconditional stimuli - are themselves of low prior probability. The more general statement is that one should search for associations between events of *equal* prior probability. It is obvious that the most useful associations are the complete ones for which C always and only occurs just before U, and where that is so the prior probabilities of C and U must of course be equal. But one can put this more generally.

The gain in knowledge that results from finding an association can be expressed as the reduction of entropy that is obtainable from knowing about the association; it is simply the redundancy that results from it. Thus if C and U are not known to be associated, the upper bound of the entropy is the sum of the individual entropies:

$$- [P_C \ln P_C + Q_C \ln Q_C + P_U \ln P_U + Q_U \ln Q_U]$$

where Q=1-P. But if it is known how they are associated the entropy can be calculated from the probabilities of the four compound events U.C, U.~C, etc., and this gives a reduced upper bound:

$$- [P_{C.U} \ln P_{C.U} + P_{C.\sim U} \ln P_{C.\sim U} + P_{\sim C.U} \ln P_{\sim C.U} + P_{\sim C.\sim U} \ln P_{\sim C.\sim U}]$$

Figure 1 shows contour maps of the maximum reduction of entropy of two binary messages that can be obtained from knowing how they are associated. When both P_C and P_U are less than 1/2 this maximum occurs when $P_{C.U}$ is equal to the lesser of P_C and P_U, so the contours are only drawn up to P=1/2. The left half represents in bits the reduction of entropy, or gain in knowledge, that occurs when the association is established; it peaks at one bit and has a ridge along the line of equal probabilities. In the right figure log scales of probabilities are used and the percentage reduction of entropy rather than the absolute reduction is plotted; this is constant at 50% along the ridge at 45°, falling off sharply on either side. Searching for associations among events of equal prior probability is advisable because it brings greater rewards when they are found.

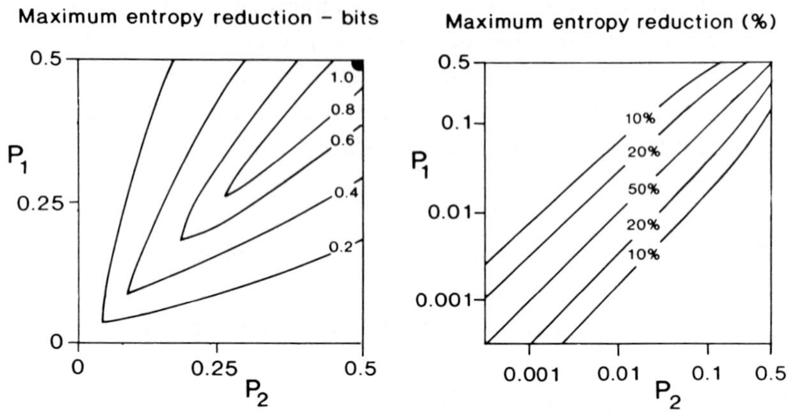

Fig. 1. This shows the difference between the entropy calculated from the probabilities P_1 and P_2 of two binary variables, and that calculated from the 4 input state probabilities. This represents the maximum benefit obtainable from knowledge of the association between two binary variables. The benefit is greatest when the two probabilities are equal, illustrating the merit of seeking associations between events of equal prior probability

I cannot decide whether the following additional argument for probability matching is valid or not. For every other variable one can think of, events that share the same value of the variable are more likely to be associated than events that do not. Proximity in time or space are the classic bases for induction in J. S. Mill's philosophy, and it can be argued that similarity in direction of motion, orientation, texture, colour, and disparity are the Gestalt qualities that cause segregation for precisely the reason that similarity in these variables indicates a likely association.

Is the same true for the variable *probability*? Is an event occurring on average, say, once a day more likely to be associated with another event occurring once a day than with an event that occurs, say, once a week? Or is one prompted to search for such associations solely because one gains more from them when they are identified?

Importance of independence

There is another desirable feature of a representation to be used for learning that follows directly from the importance of prior probabilities. I have talked so far as if detectable predictors of rewards and punishments are simple sensory events, but often they are compound events, that is conjunctions of simpler sensory stimuli. A learning system should be able to discriminate red circles both from red squares, and from green circles, and advanced animals can of course learn to do this.

Now you cannot calculate the prior probability of the conjunction of two elements in a representation if you only know their separate prior probabilities; you must either know about their degree of association, or you must assume something about it. If a complete matrix of the correlations between all elements of a representation was separately stored, it would have to be accessed for each pair of elements in a scene - a horrendously complex task. A much simpler way of solving the problem is to devise a representation in which separate elements occur approximately independently of each other under normal circumstances. Joint probabilities can then be calculated as simple products of the separate prior probabilities, or the sum of their logarithms.

There are possible alternatives: the degree of correlation might be constant so that it can be allowed for, or it might be coded by some other property of two neurons, such as their spatial distance apart in the cortex. Such possibilities are worth thinking about, but coding for independence seems to me the simplest solution, and that is the possibility I shall develop.

You may object that the degree of dependence follows directly from the environmental experience. For instance in the above example the independence of "form of a circle" and "red" might appear to depend solely upon the animal's previous experience. But "form of a circle" and "red" were categories my brain invented, and there are an infinity of other possible categorisations of the sensory information pertaining to forms and colours, some of which would provide categories that were more nearly independent than others. Thus the desirability of independence has implications for the way experience should be categorised.

Limitations on attainability of independence

The perceptual system surely has choice in how it categorises sensory messages, but is it always possible to devise a representation in which the elements are independent? The answer is "No", for the following easily seen reason (see also Barlow et al. 1989).

Each input stimulus causes a particular combination of representative elements to be active, and each of these combinations might occur with an arbitrary prior probability. If the elements were independent, this probability would be the product of the probabilities of the state (0 or 1) of each individual element; but since there are far fewer elements than combinations of elements, there are obviously too few variables for this to be possible, in general. There are, however, two reasons why this limitation may not greatly diminish the importance of coding aimed at independence.

The first is that the probabilities of the simple events will often not be known precisely because they were estimated from small numbers of events, and no advantage is to be gained by seeking a code that would predict the probability of compound events more precisely than is allowed by the errors of the probability estimates for simple events. The second is that there are vast differences in the amounts of dependence in different categorisation schemes, and it will usually be possible to improve independence by applying the appropriate categorisation. My argument is simply that the brain should select a categorisation scheme where the dependencies are low, even if they cannot be zero, for then the assumption of independence will not lead to enormously incorrect estimates of the prior probabilities of compound events.

The importance of theoretical limits

You may object that real brains cannot be expected to follow these theoretical needs, and I am sure they will not do so perfectly. But if they were flagrantly violated an animal would either fail to detect genuine new causal factors in its environment, or it would accept random coincidences as spurious evidence for causal factors that do not exist. If it did the former it would fail to exploit opportunities that were open to it, while if it did the latter it would execute the unadaptive behaviour appropriate if the causal factor had been genuine.

Hence there is strong selection in favour of the mechanisms I have proposed.

The objection that theoretical limitations are irrelevant in biology was often raised when people started talking about the fundamental physical limits in vision. It was assumed by some that eyes had such poor optics, and photoreceptors such poor sensitivity, that the *physical* factors limiting performance, such as diffraction at the pupil and quantum fluctuations in the photoreceptors, would be insignificant compared with the biological imperfections. We now understand that this is not the case at all, and that vision performs close to the physical limit at many tasks (Rose 1942; Barlow 1986); paying attention to these physical limits has enormously increased our understanding of the physiology.

Limiting factor	Importance
Optical Diffraction	
	Limiting resolution of simple eyes (e.g. human)
	Ommatidial size and spacing in compound eyes
Quantum Fluctuations and Thermal Isomerisation	
	Threshold of vision in humans, toads, insects, etc.
Statistical Efficiency of Discriminatory Mechanisms	
	Central detection of various targets
	Detecting mirror symmetry
	Do the statistical limits on detecting suspicious coincidences also belong here?

Table 3. Theoretical limiting factors of proven importance

The same change has taken place with regard to statistical factors that limit the ability of the brain to interpret images. One can measure the ability to detect psychophysical test targets on an absolute scale, and for suitably chosen tests the performance is astonishingly high, even if one takes a rather abstract task such as detecting bilateral symmetry (Barlow and Reeves 1979). Therefore the visual system is not only fed by physical instruments whose performance approaches absolute physical limits, but it also employs efficient statistical programs to interpret certain types of information it receives.

We do not yet have results from any absolute measures of brains performing the task of detecting new associations, but it is easy to see that, in a competitive environment, efficiency at this task would confer great selective advantage. Although proving that an association exists may be a more difficult task than detecting symmetry, the enormous importance of learning leads one to expect that the absolute performance at appropriate learning tasks will be high.

Signalling unexpectedness may power the neopallial explosion

This new outlook suggests that the representation provided by neocortex signals the novelty or unexpectedness of features and events, and that it categorises the sensory input into features and events that occur as nearly as possible independently in the environment the animal knows and understands. From this would follow more efficient and versatile learning, and the survival value of such an improvement may explain the energy of the neopallial explosion that culminated in mankind's brain.

This may seem too simple an answer to the big question we started with, and I do not claim it is the complete answer. But I hope I have correctly identified a task that might be responsible for some of the remarkable things the neocortex does for us. The 19 words on the right of Table 2 are deceptive, for the task they describe is not easy.

But how might the cortex undertake the categorisation of sensory inputs that would make such high efficiencies possible?

Networks for detecting independent coincidences

It is easiest to answer this by explaining our current concept of a network element that might achieve the computational goal that has been postulated above as the primary neocortical function. The element has been developed mainly by Földiák (1989; 1991) and has three stages.

Hebbian detection of common coincidences

The first step, that of detecting commonly occurring associations of sensory stimuli, is done by forming the weighted sum of a set of sensory inputs making synapses on to an output cell (fig. 2, left). This weighted sum will be highest for the input pattern that matches the weights, and if we now suppose that the weights are adjusted according to a simple linear Hebbian rule, this simple unit will adjust its input weights so that its response vector is aligned with the principle component of the variance of the inputs (Kohonen and Oja 1976). It will then respond best to this input vector.

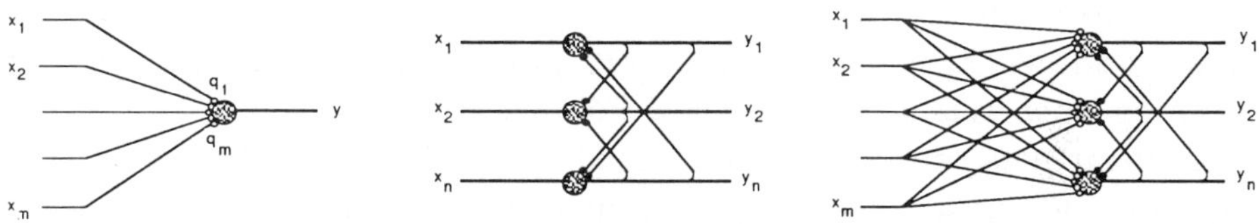

Fig. 2. The unit on the left forms the weighted sum of its inputs and fires when a threshold is exceeded; the weights are adjusted according to a Hebbian rule, so the the unit becomes selectively responsive to the commonly occurring patterns in its input - the clichés or suspicious coincidences. The middle group of units have modifiable feedback connections that follow an anti-Hebbian rule; these decorrelate the units and ensure that they respond to different clichés. At the right the two sets of connections are combined. The thresholds of the units are adjusted so that each has a pre-determined probability of firing, so *a priori* probabilities are propagated through the network. A network made up of such units tries to categorise the input into patterns that have known prior probability and are approximately independent (from Földiák 1989; 1991)

The above is true if the Hebbian adjustments depend on the correlation between the input along each channel and the linear weighted sum collected by the unit. But suppose the unit has a threshold, and the Hebbian adjustment only occurs when this threshold is exceeded and the unit fires. The behaviour then becomes much more complicated: the initial values of the weights can have lasting effects, and there may be no unique solutions, but one can see that the weights will tend to be adjusted to match those inputs which actually fire the neuron. With appropriate choice of threshold, this will approximate to the most commonly occurring input pattern.

If more than one such unit is connected to the same inputs, there will be a tendency for them to adjust their input weights in the same way, and hence to respond to the same input pattern. This is avoided as follows.

Decorrelation by anti-Hebbian lateral connections

Suppose that the outputs of a set of such units make inhibitory connections to other members of the set, as indicated in fig. 2 (middle). One can see at once that this will discourage two or more of them responding to the same input pattern, because if they did they would mutually inhibit each other. One can improve on this by postulating that the strength of the inhibition is increased when the two fire together, and we have shown that this ultimately leads to the outputs becoming uncorrelated (Barlow and Földiák 1989).

A linear network of this sort would provide outputs that define the same subspace as a true principle component analysis, but here we are interested in the non-linear system obtained by imposing thresholds on the outputs. By varying this threshold, the probability of firing of each output neuron can be adjusted to a predetermined value, so that when it does fire the prior probability of the feature or event it signals is known. Thus the output of such a network categorises the inputs into groups, which may overlap, each with an approximately known prior probability of occurring in the normal environment

Parenthetically it is worth noting that the same anti-Hebbian effect as that provided by variable synapses for lateral inhibition could be obtained with lateral *excitatory* synapses that follow an anti-Hebbian rule, i.e. they become weaker when they fire together with the output neuron. This may be more a realistic model, because excitatory interconnections between cortical neurons are a prominent (and hitherto unexplained) feature of the cortex. But it is also more complicated and would require additional inhibitory negative feedback to prevent an explosive chain reaction from uncontrolled positive feedback.

Joint action of the Hebbian and anti-Hebbian connections

It may not initially be obvious how elegantly the anti-Hebbian decorrelator modifies the action of the positive Hebbian coincidence detector. The inhibition (or anti-Hebbian excitation) helps to determine what makes an output neuron fire, and whether it fires or not determines which of the Hebbian synapses from the input are strengthened. Thus, because of the threshold, the decorrelator ensures that the Hebbian process causes each neuron to become selectively sensitive to an input pattern that is almost uncorrelated with the others.

Does it actually work?

Many features have not been specified in this cursory account, such as the overlap between adjacent cells, the numbers of them, the initial pattern of connectivity, and so forth, but the following example may give the flavour of what the network sketched above can do.

Each of 16 output units had an 8 x 15 pixel input, and the weights from each pixel can be represented as its receptive field. The input population to which it was exposed consisted of 82 alphanumeric characters, each presented with the frequency at which it occurs in normal English prose. Figure 3 shows how the input weights adjust themselves from their initially random values, and you can see that the 'receptive fields' which develop become vaguely letter-like. But of course there are not enough of them to resolve all the characters by each signalling one character, as in a grandmother cell representation. Instead most letters are quite good fits to two or more receptive fields and are therefore represented by the firing of two or more units, with the commoner letters on the whole requiring fewer active units.

The output is not completely unambiguous, so the coding loses some information, but because the ambiguities occur with infrequent letters this loss is small and 97% of the information is successfully transmitted.

The possibility of hierarchical networks

There is a slight inconsistency between the model and the argument I used to justify it. It was suggested that knowledge of prior probabilities was necessary for the efficient detection of non-random coincidences, yet it was the output of Foldiak's coincidence detecting element that gave an indication of prior probability by virtue of the

0
4 000
8 000
16 000

adjustment of its threshold: How about the inputs to these units, amongst which coincidences are to be detected?

I have suggested (Barlow 1969, 1972) that the output of a retinal ganglion cells can be regarded as signalling the unexpectedness of the current pattern of light on the hypothesis that there has been no change, and this argument could reasonably be extended to other sensory modalities. Hence I don't think this is a serious difficulty, but it does draw attention to the fact that elements that are used in a hierarchical manner must communicate the unexpectedness of the features being signalled as well as their occurrence. For this reason Földiák elements are ideal for building into hierarchies.

There are at least two reasons why the suitability for use in a hierarchy is extremely important. The first is practical, for a single element cannot and does not access directly all the sensory information that is required in pattern recognition and learning, so a hierarchical arrangement seems the only way of achieving wide access of individual elements to the input.

The second is more theoretical and concerns the actual possibility of determining the probabilistic structure of a complex input. If this is large the number of possible input states would be so vast that it would be impossible to estimate their relative frequencies in an epoch of reasonable duration. The only way that I can see of solving this problem is to combine signals in small groups hierarchically: the lowest level detects non-random coincidences of a limited number of inputs from the sensory input, and signals upward the non-random coincidences among those inputs; the next level elements do the same for the subsets of inputs each receives, and so on. Each element deals with a limited subset, but the higher elements have access to a wide input through a series of lower elements.

Incidentally the same argument must surely apply to temporal aspects of the categorisation process, where it would seem necessary to start with the probabilistic structure of short duration epochs, and

---

Fig. 3. A network like the rightmost in Fig. 2 was used to categorise alphanumeric characters presented with the frequency with which they occur in normal English. Each of the 16 units had an 8 x 15 pixel input, and the weights were initially random, as in the top row. After 16000 samples the weights formed receptive fields that had become somewhat letter-like. Each letter activated two or more, the rarer characters being represented by more active units. 97% of the information in the input was effectively transmitted (from Földiák 1989; 1991)

when that categorisation has been fixed, to combine elements over longer epochs, and so on.

Is this what's actually done?

I have argued here that neocortex must adapt the animal to its environment by using information derived from its experience of that environment. There are two areas where one might look for confirmation or disproof of these ideas. One is in the developments of learning theory that have taken place since it has been appreciated that the prior probabilities, based on past experience, of the various stimuli play a crucial role in the ease with which they are learnt. The other is in the developmental neurophysiology of the visual cortex. Since this tests the ideas at a cellular level I shall start with it, returning for a few brief words about learning at the end. How are cortical neurons influenced by what has happened to them, and do these effects fit our model?

Rapid desensitization due to decorrelation

I think there is good experimental evidence for two types of plasticity in the physiological mechanisms of perception, the rapid habituation-like process revealed by pattern adaptation, and the slower, more permanent, effects revealed by deprivation in the sensitive period. There may well be many other forms of plasticity, but let us confine ourselves to these for the moment.

Rapid adaptation or habituation leads to well known illusions. I have recently reviewed these (Barlow 1990) with the idea that the changes during exposure do not correspond simply to fatigue or exhaustion of pattern selective neurons as is commonly assumed, but correspond instead to an active attempt by the neurons to decorrelate their responses - i.e. it is the operation of the anti-Hebbian part of Földiák's network (Barlow and Földiák 1989). For instance, during adaptation to a vertical grating we think all the cortical units tuned to that orientation and periodicity will be strongly co-activated; this correlated activity will increase the strength of the mutual inhibition between them (or decreases the mutual excitation) so that population of units becomes less sensitive than normal.

This explanation is also capable of explaining tilt and size after-effects. Notice that it differs from the usual explanation which says that the units exposed to the adapting grating are simply fatigued or adapted, for it is the *correlated firing* of neurons, not the fatigue of each individual one, that is thought to lead to desensitization. There is plenty of evidence that the effects occur at neuronal level, and some evidence that this is not a matter of a particular class of neurons simply decreasing in sensitivity (Movshon and Lennie 1979). It would be possible to devise experiments that would distinguish between the two hypotheses, but current results do not provide a clear answer.

There are innumerable forms of this effect and I shall not enumerate them here. They characteristically show up either when you impose massive new correlations during an adaptation period, or in a situation where two aspects of sensory stimulation that are associated in normal life become dissociated. I suspect that whenever neurons in the cortex lying within easy communicating distance of each other (i.e. about 1 or 2 mm) are co-activated, they will develop mutual repulsion - that is they will mutually inhibit each other more strongly, or mutually reinforce each other less strongly, and that this change will persist over a period of minutes.

This has not yet been directly tested, but the measurements of correlations between neuronal firings reported elsewhere in this volume provide some supporting evidence: although the positive effects naturally attract most attention, one of the striking findings is that many neurons do *not* show correlations, even when they pick up from strongly overlapping populations of inputs. There must surely be a mechanism for producing this striking independence, and that postulated here is an obvious candidate which should be readily testable.

Long term sensitization

The other form of plasticity is that, long known to ophthalmologists, whose physiological basis was revealed by Hubel and Wiesel (1970) in their celebrated experiments on visual deprivation in kittens. In contrast with the first form of plasticity this requires a longer period to induce, it occurs mainly during a restricted sensitive period early in life, and the results tend to persist indefinitely. Note in particular that plasticity in the sensitive period *increases* (or preserves) sensitivity to the inducing experience, whereas the other process actively *desensitises* the system to the adapting stimulus. The properties of these two forms of plasticity are summarised in Table 4.

	Forward connections	*Lateral connections*
Synapse type	Hebbian	Anti-Hebbian
When modifiable	Post-natal period only	Throughout life
Experimental demonstration	Deprivation in sensitive period	Pattern adaptation
Functional role	Detecting clichés or suspicious coincidences	Decorrelation - making units detect different coincidences

Table 4. Two types of neural plasticity that may be mediated by Hebbian forward connections and anti-Hebbian lateral connections.

We attribute the increase or preservation of sensitivity in the sensitive period to the Hebbian part of Földiák's network, and the idea that there is such a process at work is quite widely supported (Rauschecker and Singer 1981). But the synergistic action with the anti-Hebbian decorrelating mechanism is new, and it offers an interpretation of the functional role of the sensitive period, in the following manner.

During the sensitive period pathways that cause excitation become permanently connected, but the decorrelating mechanism influences which pathways result in activity and thereby helps to determine the permanent pattern of connections that is established. If the animal is deprived of experience during the sensitive period the Hebbian process presumably still takes place, but any correlations present in the spontaneous maintained activity are quite different from those that normally result from patterns in the outside world, so the network adjusts itself inappropriately. The consequence will be a disordered pattern of connectivity unadapted to the statistical characteristics of the normal sensory input.

It is an intriguing feature of the model that a mechanism with a rapid time constant at a later stage in the network can have permanent effects on connections at a previous level. But having said that, I must admit that I cannot see why the probabilities that form the basis for the Hebbian coincidence detecting process should be estimated over a fixed epoch early in life, while those for the anti-Hebbian decorrelation should be continuously estimated over a relatively short epoch of the recent past. In spite of many such uncertainties I hope the model may reconcile the conflicting views about mechanisms, consequences, and purpose of the sensitive period (Movshon and Van Sluyters 1981). Miller, Keller and Stryker (1989) describe a satisfactory quantitative model for the effects of deprivation in the sensitive period, but it is descriptive and gives no understanding of the rationale for these mechanisms. We think our model provides this, and because it explains the useful consequences of the process, it could be an informative model for the influence of experience on connectivity elsewhere in the brain.

Learning and concept formation

I can only briefly indicate two possible applications of such mechanisms at higher levels.

First, the way we have suggested that the sensory input is categorised and represented would form an ideal preparation for learning what sensory stimuli are associated with reinforcement. We are thus proposing that perception is the prologue to associative learning that makes it versatile and efficient, and we specify the computational goal of this prologue. We think the mechanisms that try to attain this goal might explain such phenomena as blocking, latent inhibition, latent learning and perceptual learning.

Second, the intellectual discovery of high level explanatory concepts seems to have much in common with the process of low level categorisation that we have proposed. Coincidences that are unexpected according to what is already known must first be noted, and this is analogous to the Hebbian coincidence detection stage of the model. But such coincidences must not be explainable in terms of other "concepts" that have arisen in response to other past or present co-occurrences, so an anti-Hebbian decorrelation process is also required. Thus these high level processes may simply be a continuation of the low level ones; instead of explaining Helmholtzian unconscious induction by analogy with conscious inference, we may come to regard the latter as an extension of the former.

It is too early to say how well a hierarchical recoding network of the type suggested will work on realistic tasks that are much more complex, but we are rather encouraged. We feel that we are on the right track with regard to the use of unexpectedness and the probabilistic structure of the input, though we are well aware that some big problems, especially concerning the temporal structure of sensory messages, have not yet been included in our approach.

Summary

I have been speculating on the relation between the neurophysiology of cortical neurons and the almost magical things they do for us. Because we know a good deal about them, and are in a position to model what they do, it seems foolish not to try to bridge the gulf between neurons and the behaviour they mediate, so these are my suggestions:

1) An efficient mechanism for associative learning needs to receive signals showing "How Unexpected" are the objects and events signalled, as well as "What is Where".
2) Unexpectedness must be based on knowledge and understanding of the environment, and therefore requires the filing, modelling, and mapping postulated by Herrick, Craik and Tolman.
3) To promote efficient learning, the sensory input should be categorised in such a way that the representational elements occur independently and with known prior probability in the normal environment.
4) The achievement of this computational goal might provide sufficient selective advantage to explain the "neopallial explosion" that blew up our neocortex from oppossum-size to human-size in the period of evolution of the mammals.
5) These thoughts define a computational goal that is by no means simple or easy to achieve, but one can begin modelling it.

References

Barlow, HB (1969) Pattern recognition and the responses of sensory neurones. Annals of the New York Academy of Sciences 156:872-881

Barlow HB (1972) Single units and sensation: a neuron doctrine for perceptual psychology? Perception 1:371-394

Barlow HB (1986) Why can't the eye see better? In: Pettigrew JD, Sanderson KJ, Levick WR (eds) Visual Neuroscience. The Festschrift for P.O. Bishop. Cambridge University Press, Cambridge, UK

Barlow HB (1990) A theory about the functional role and synaptic mechanism of visual after-effects. In: Blakemore CB (ed) Vision: coding and efficiency. Cambridge University Press, Cambridge, UK

Barlow HB, Földiák P (1989) Adaptation and decorrelation in the cortex. In: Durbin R, Miall C, Mitchison G (eds) The Computing Neuron. Addison-Wesley, Wokingham, England

Barlow HB, Kaushal TP, Mitchison GJ (1989) Finding minimum entropy codes. Neural Computation 1:406-416

Barlow HB, Reeves HB (1979) The versatility and absolute efficiency of detecting mirror symmetry in random dot displays. Vision Res 19:783-793

Craik KJW (1943) The Nature of Explanation. Cambridge University Press, Cambridge

Darwin C (1871) The Descent of Man. John Murray, London

Elliot Smith, G (1924). The Evolution of Man. Oxford University Press, Oxford

Földiák P (1989) Adaptive network for optimal linear feature extraction. IEEE/INNS International Joint Conference on Neural Networks, Washington D.C. 1:401-405

Földiák P (1991) Forming sparse representations by local anti-Hebbian learning. Biol Cybern: *in press*

Herrick CJ (1926) Brains of rats and men. University of Chicago Press, Chicago

Herrick CJ (1928) An Introduction to Neurology. W.B. Saunders Co., Philadelphia

Hubel DH, Wiesel TN (1970) The period of susceptibility to the physiological effects of unilateral eye closure in kittens. J Physiol 206:419-436

Jerison HJ (1973) Evolution of the Brain and Intelligence. Academic Press, New York

Jerison HJ (1983) The evolution of the brain as an information-processing system. Advances in the study of Mammalian Behavior. pp 113-146. Special Publication 7 of the American Society of Mammologists

Kamin LJ (1969) Predictability, surprise, attention and conditioning. In: Campbell BA, Church RM (eds) Punishment and aversive behavior. Appleton-Century-Crofts, New York

Kohonen T, Oja E (1976) Fast adaptive formation of orthogonalizing filters and associative memory in recurrent networks of neuron-like elements. Biol Cybern 21:85-95

Mackintosh NJ (1974) The Psychology of Animal Learning. Academic Press, London

Marr D (1982) Vision. W H Freeman, San Francisco,

Miller KD, Keller JB, Stryker MP (1989) Ocular dominance column development: analysis and simulation. Science 245:605-615

Movshon JA, Lennie P (1979) Pattern selective adaptation in visual cortical neurones. Nature 278:850-852

Movshon JA, Van Sluyters RC (1981) Visual Neural Development. Annual Review of Psychology 32: 477-522

Palm G (1981) Evidence, information, surprise. Biol Cybern 42:57-68

Rauschecker JP, Singer W (1981) The effect of early visual experience on the cat's visual cortex and their possible explanation by Hebb synapses. J Physiol 310:215-239

Rescorla RA, Wagner AR (1972) A theory of Pavlovian conditioning: Variations in effectiveness of reinforcement and non-reinforcement. In: Black AH, Prokasy WF (eds) Classical conditioning II: Current Research and Theory. Appleton-Century-Crofts, New York

Rose A (1942) The relative sensitivities of television pick-up tubes, photographic film, and the human eye. Proceedings of the Institute of Radio Engineers 30:293-300

Sarnat HB, Netsky MG (1981) Evolution of the Nervous System. Oxford University Press, New York

Tolman EC (1948) Cognitive maps in rats and men. Psychol Rev 55:189-208

Coding and Computation in the Cortex: Single-Neuron Activity and Cooperative Phenomena

Eilon Vaadia[1] and Ad Aertsen[1,2,3]

[1] Dept. of Physiology, Hadassah Medical School, P.O. Box 1172, Hebrew University, Jerusalem, Israel
[2] Max-Planck-Institut für biologische Kybernetik, Spemannstrasse 38, 7400 Tübingen, Germany

Introduction

There is widespread consensus among neurophysiologists and neuropsychologists that neurons are involved in information processing and computations carried out by the brain. Yet there is still remarkably little understanding of the mechanisms underlying these processes. Similarly, also the nature of the neural code (or codes) being used by the brain is still very much open for discussion. In view of this, it is essential to consider different alternatives. Not only does each of them dictate a way of thinking about brain mechanisms, they also suggest different experimental approaches toward experimental studies of these mechanisms.

A common view among many neurobiologists suggests that the basic element of the neural code resides in the spike activity of a single neuron. A different view was first presented by Hebb (1949), who suggested that the coherent activity within groups of neurons ('cell-assemblies') is the basis of the neural code. In this paper we will present results from an ongoing electrophysiological study of cortical function, focussing on different aspects of coding and processing revealed by recordings of single and multiple neuron activity. We will illustrate our considerations by experimental results from different cortical areas in anaesthetized, as well as in awake, behaving monkeys.

---

[3] present address: Institut für Neuroinformatik, Ruhr-Universität, P.O. Box 102 148, 4630 Bochum, Germany

Cortical activity at the level of single-neuron spike trains

Single-neuron firing rate as a neural code

It is generally assumed, at least implicitly, that the most relevant parameter to be extracted from the spike train is the rate of spike occurrence, the single-neuron firing rate. Barlow (1972) suggested that, "The frequency of neural impulses codes subjective certainty: a high impulse frequency in a given neuron corresponds to a high degree of confidence that the cause of the percept is present in the external world." (See also Barlow's contributions to this Volume.) Thus, according to this view, the neural code is the firing rate of a single neuron and the appropriate experimental tool is a microelectrode that can isolate and record the activity of a single neuron ('single-unit activity').

Indeed, single-unit studies in many cortical and sub-cortical areas have clearly demonstrated highly specific changes of firing rates that were related to sensory and/or motor processing. Amongst others, this culminated in a wealth of data on 'receptive field' properties of neurons in various parts of the sensory system, exemplified in the work of Mountcastle (1957, 1977) and Hubel and Wiesel (1968, 1977). In addition, however, this approach also turned out to be fruitful in the study of cognitive and other higher brain functions, such as perceptual analysis of sensory input, selective attention, short-term memory, etc. (Fuster 1973, 1989; Evarts et al. 1984; Perrett et al. 1982; Goldberg and Segraves 1987; Goldman-Rakic 1987; Niki and Watanabe 1976, 1979; Gottlieb et al. 1989).

An example which illustrates how specific aspects of higher cortical function may be expressed in the firing rate of a single neuron is presented in Figure 1 (from Vaadia et al. 1986). It shows the responses of a neuron in the frontal cortex of a monkey which was trained to respond to acoustic or visual stimuli, presented at one of 5 possible locations. In one paradigm the monkey had to touch a key at the location of the stimulus. There were two such 'localizing' tasks: *auditory localization (AL)* and *visual localization (VL)*. In addition, the same monkey was also trained to perform an *auditory detection (AD)* paradigm. In this 'detection' task, one of the 5 keys was randomly designated as a 'detect key' and the monkey had to touch this key, irrespective of the stimulus location, until a new 'detect key' was designated. The VL, AL, and AD conditions were alternated in blocks of 20 trials. In each block of AD trials, a different key was designated as the 'detect key'. This latter task was designed to produce hand and eye movements during the detect task that were similar to those employed by the monkey in the AL and VL conditions (for details on the task and additional control conditions, see Vaadia et al. 1986). Five groups of five histograms each are shown. The first row shows that the neuron did not respond to auditory stimuli when the monkey was not performing any behavioral task (non-performing condition: NP). The second (AD(S)) and third (AD(R)) rows show that the neuron did not respond to stimuli (AD(S)) in the 'auditory detect' condition, nor was it

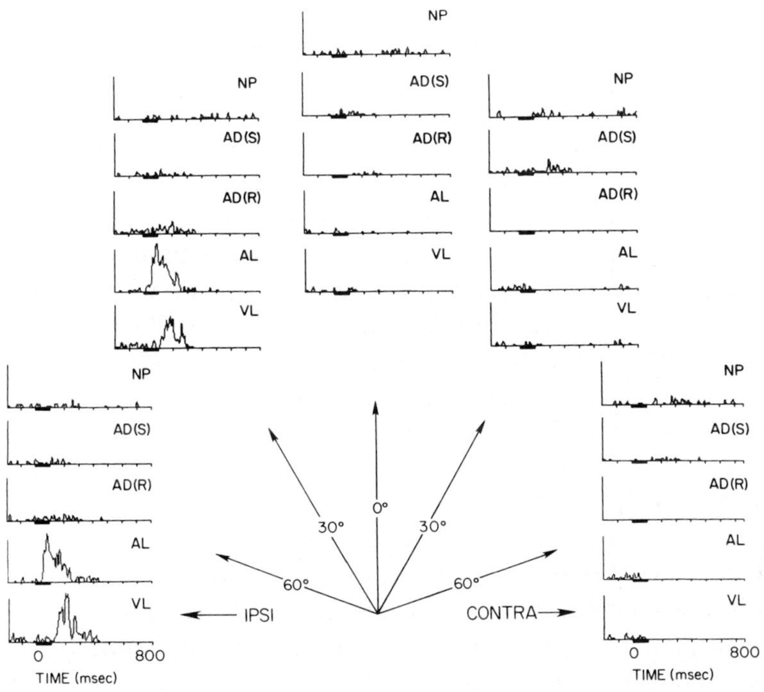

Fig. 1. PST histograms showing the activity of one neuron as a function of stimulus location in 5 behavioral conditions. *NP*: non-performing conditions (stimuli: noise bursts of 100 ms). *AD*: responses during performance of the auditory detection task, with *AD(S)*: histograms of the responses, sorted according to the location of the stimulus, *AD(R)*: histograms of the responses sorted according to the directional location of the arm movement. *AL*: responses of the unit when the monkey had to localize auditory stimuli. *VL*: responses of the neuron when the monkey had to localize visual stimuli. (From Vaadia et al. 1986)

activated in relation to arm movements that were made towards the targets (AD(R)). However, the last two rows reveal that a clear response to stimuli from 60 and 30 degrees at the ipsilateral side (irrespective of their modality) was evoked when the monkey had to localize the stimuli (AL, VL).

The responses of the neuron demonstrated in this Figure were not related strictly to auditory or visual stimuli, nor were they related to movements per se. The neuron was activated only when the location of the stimulus, irrespective of its modality, served as a cue for the appropriate behavioral response. It was therefore suggested that this neuron was involved in a mechanism that extracts spatial cues from at least two modalities.

Under appropriate behavioral conditions, prolonged slow waves of activity, marking distinct perceptual, cognitive and linguistic processes, and lasting hundreds of milliseconds to several seconds, can be recorded in a single cortical area (Donchin 1984; Deeke et al. 1985; see also the contributions by Elbert and by Arieli in this Volume). Signs of such long processing could also be found in the activity of single neurons recorded from sensory, association, premotor and motor cortices of behaving monkeys during some specified stages of behavior (Fuster 1989; Wise and Mauritz 1985; Gottlieb et al. 1989; Vaadia et al. 1989). An example from such studies is shown in Figure 2 (from Gottlieb et al. 1989). This Figure illustrates the behavior of the firing rate of a single neuron in the auditory cortex of a monkey, trained to perform an auditory short-term memory task. Two tone bursts (S1 and S2), separated by a silent inter-stimulus interval of 1 second, were presented in each trial. The monkey had to touch one key if the tones were identical, and another one if they were different. The firing rate of the unit while the monkey was performing correctly is shown as the solid line. The broken line shows the activity of the same single unit when the water spout was removed and the monkey did not perform the task.

Though it is not possible to tell from such an experiment how this particular unit was engaged in forming the short-term memory of pitch, it is clear that the neuron did not end its role when the stimulus was turned off. On the contrary, Figure 2 clearly shows that the neuron took part in, or was affected by, a prolonged process that took place in the primary auditory cortex during the inter-stimulus interval, persisting long after the information was presumably transmitted to other cortical areas. Approximately 60% of the recorded neurons in

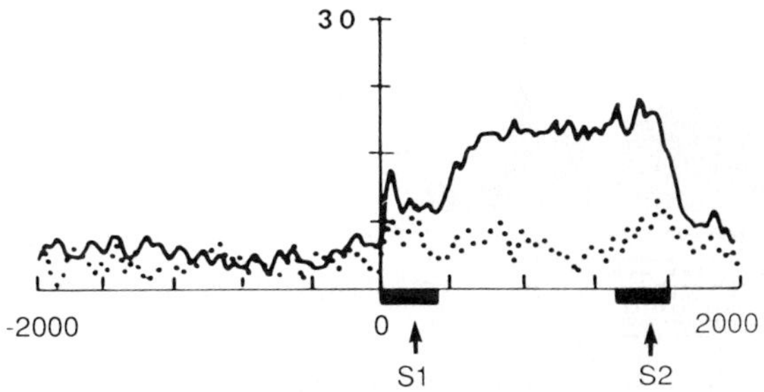

Fig. 2. Activity of a single neuron in the auditory cortex of the Rhesus monkey. The solid line shows a PST-histogram, collected during performance of the short-term memory task. The broken line shows the PST-histogram, collected when the stimuli were presented but the monkey did not perform the task. The abscissa describes the time from 2.0 sec before onset of the first stimulus (*S1*) until 0.45 sec after the second stimulus (*S2*) ended. The ordinate describes the firing rate in spikes/sec. (Adapted from Gottlieb et al. 1989)

this study showed such prolonged changes in their firing rates during the interval between the two tones (Gottlieb et al. 1989).

The activity of a single neuron may be quite complex. An example of this is given in Figure 3. It shows a raster-display and PST-histogram, illustrating the activity of a neuron in the premotor cortex of a monkey, recorded during performance of a stimulus-guided reaching task (after Vaadia et al. 1988). The monkey initiated a trial ('INIT') by touching a key (located in front of him in a mid-sagital location) and waited for 6 seconds. Then, one of two keys (either on the left or on the right) was illuminated (the 'cue', marked as 'Q' in Fig. 3). The monkey had to maintain contact with the center key for an additional 500 msec and then touch the illuminated key. Three components of activity can be seen in the PST-histogram. First, the unit was activated during the waiting period (from INIT to CUE, starting about 3 sec before cue onset). EMG recordings of superficial muscles indicated that the monkey did not attempt to make movements during the pre-cue interval. This and other considerations led to the suggestion that this activity was not related to the preparation or execution of the movements, but rather to other aspects of task performance, such as expectation or timing of events (Vaadia et al. 1988). Subsequently, the spike discharge of the unit was suppressed in response to the directional-cue onset and, finally, it was activated again later at the time of

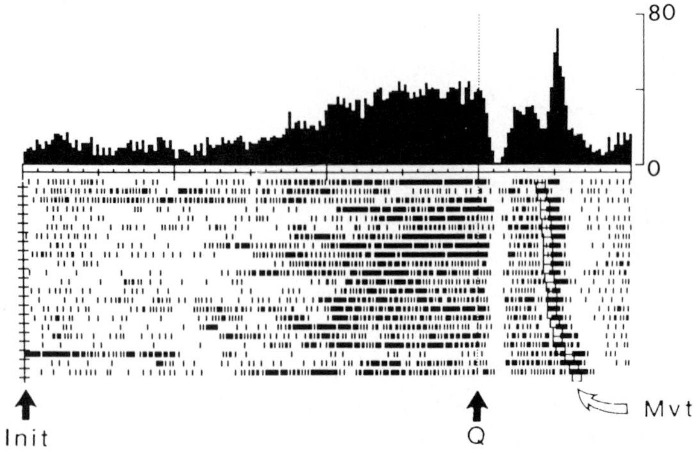

Fig. 3. Activity of a single neuron in the premotor cortex of the Rhesus monkey. The raster display and PST-histogram show 8 sec of activity centered around the onset time of the spatial cue (*Q*). Trial initiation (*INIT*) is marked by a plus sign on each raster. The beginning of the limb movement (*MVT*) is marked by an empty square. (From Vaadia et al. 1988)

movement onset (marked by an empty square on each line of the raster display). This last component of activity was direction-specific and could be easily matched with some of the EMG records, suggesting that it was related to motor function. As this result illustrates, this type of complex activation pattern strongly suggests a single neuron is not dedicated to the processing of just one single function.

Summarizing, the notion that the rate of single-neuron firing may serve as a neural code is supported by the above findings. Nevertheless, these findings do no tell us what the mechanism is by which the bi-modal responses (cf. Fig. 1) or the prolonged (cf. Fig. 2) and complex (cf. Fig. 3) rate modulation patterns were generated. Moreover, these findings do not rule out the possibility that increased firing rate may not be the sole encoding mechanism, or may even be a by-product of other mechanisms. Finally, there is a conceptual problem. If we accept the notion of firing rate as the sole basis of neural encoding, this implies that a neuron carries information only whenever its rate is elevated, but that all other spikes, the so-called 'background' activity, do not. It turns out, however, that the probability of finding a cortical neuron with an elevated firing rate is extremely low: the average cortical neuron spends over 99.8% of its time being idle (Abeles et al.

1990). This, evidently, makes it rather unlikely that single-neuron firing rate serves as the sole mechanism for neural encoding in the cortex. We conclude that it is important to also examine alternative codes.

Single-neuron firing patterns as a neural code

It is quite conceivable that a neuron may be coding for something (be it as a 'grandmother' neuron, or as a member of a functional group) without any observable change in its firing rate. One such possibility of an alternative code resides in the temporal firing pattern of the neuron. We present here two examples to demonstrate the feasibility of such a single-neuron firing pattern code, one taken from the somatosensory cortex, the other from the auditory cortex. For other examples of single-unit firing patterns as a potential neural code we refer to Dayhoff and Gerstein 1983a,b; Abeles 1983; and Abeles al. 1983.

An example which demonstrates the effect of stimuli on the firing pattern of single cortical neurons is shown in Figure 4. This result was taken from a study by Ahissar and Vaadia (1990), who examined properties of oscillatory neurons in the upper bank of the lateral sulcus (a polisensory area, were many neurons responded to tactile stimuli) of an awake, behaving monkey. The Figure shows the effect of two different tactile stimuli on the firing patterns of two simultaneously recorded neurons. Both neurons (4 and 6) showed clear oscillatory patterns when no stimuli were applied ('spontaneous activity' (SP1-3)), which could be suppressed by tactile stimuli (STIM1: soft strokes of the contralateral small toes at 1 stimulus/second, and STIM2: soft strokes of the contralateral big toe at 1 stimulus/second). The Figure further illustrates that tactile stimuli had different effects on the mean firing rates and on the temporal firing patterns of the two neurons. For example, the oscillatory firing pattern of unit 4 was suppressed by both STIM1 and STIM2, whereas only STIM1 affected the firing rate, which was enhanced in this case. For unit 6, on the other hand, again both STIM1 and STIM2 suppressed the oscillatory firing pattern, but now the firing rate was only affected (i.e. enhanced) by STIM2. It was further reported that in most of the cases no consistent relations were found between the effects of stimuli on a neuron's firing rate and their effects on its oscillatory firing pattern. In none of the cases could a significant cross-correlation be observed between any of the pairs of

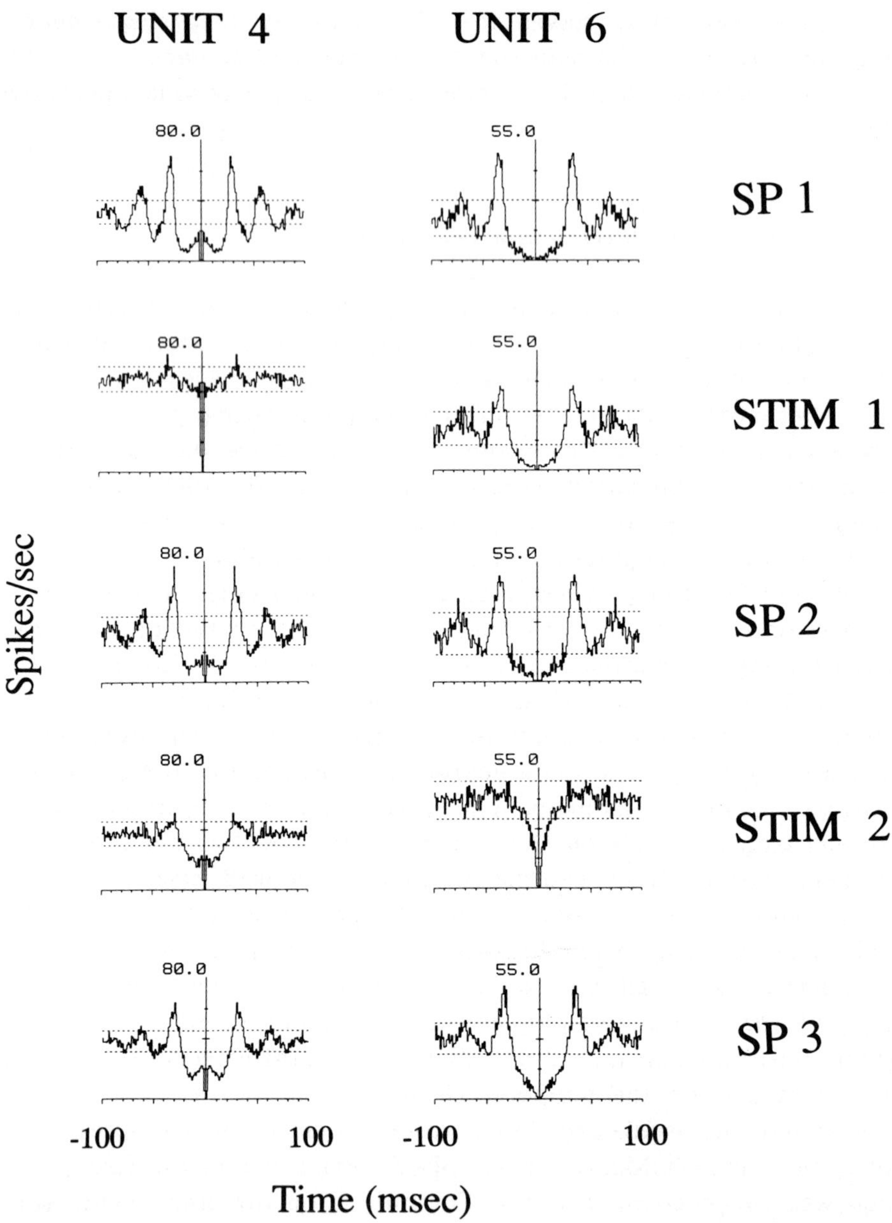

Fig. 4. Suppression of oscillatory activity in the somatosensory cortex of a monkey by tactile stimuli. (Left) Neuron 4 (33 Hz, full scale: 80 spikes/s). (Right) Neuron 6 (27 Hz, full scale: 55 spikes/s). Five consecutive periods are shown. SP-1, 131 s of spontaneous activity; the oscillatory activity is clearly seen. STIM-1, 147 s of soft strokes (1/s) to the contralateral small toes; the oscillations of unit 4 were suppressed and its averaged firing rate was elevated from 32 to 62 spikes/s; the firing rate of unit 6

oscillating neurons, not even when they were recorded on a single microelectrode.

In contrast to the oscillatory firing patterns in the upper banks of the lateral sulcus, the most striking feature of firing patterns of single neurons in the auditory cortex of monkeys and cats was the absence of periodicities (e.g. Abeles 1982a; Vaadia and Abeles 1987; Gottlieb et al. 1989; Ahissar et al. 1992). Nevertheless, in some cases it was found that the firing pattern was clearly affected by the behavioral state, even though the average firing rate remained almost the same. An example of this is given in Figure 5, which shows two 'snowflake' displays, mapping the timing of triplets of spikes. Each triplet is defined by two intervals T_B-T_A and T_C-T_B, where T_A, T_B and T_C are the times of occurrence of the spikes A, B and C. A triangular coordinate system is used to map the triplets into unique points in a hexagon. For example, a bin which maps the cases where the spike C occurred 100 msec after spike B, and the spike B occurred 50 msec after spike A, lies at the point where the vertical line, perpendicular to the upper-left axis (T_B-T_A) at +50 msec meets the line perpendicular to the lower-left axis (T_C-T_B) at +100 msec. (For more details on 'snowflake' display see Perkel et al. 1975 and Abeles 1982a). In this particular example, all spikes were taken from a single spike train. Therefore, the snowflakes represent the three-spike auto-correlation of the neuron: each triplet of spikes is represented in three bins, and the displays are symmetric in a triangular fashion.

By computing such 'snowflake' displays for different sections of recorded activity, we can observe changes in the neuronal activity and, in particular, extract the temporal patterns of spike triplets which dominated during each of these sections. The two snowflakes in Figure 5 represent the activity of a single neuron in the auditory cortex of a monkey, recorded during each of two behavioral paradigms in an

---

was not affected and its oscillations were affected only very slightly. SP-2, 90 s of spontaneous activity; note the recovery of unit 4's oscillations. STIM-2, 117 s of soft strokes (1/s) to the contralateral big toe; the oscillations of the two neurons were suppressed; while the firing rate of unit 6 increased from 22 to 40 spikes/s, the firing rate of unit 4 was not affected. SP-3, 136 s of spontaneous activity; the oscillations recovered again. Recording of the two neurons lasted while the procedure (SP-1, STIM-1, SP-2, STIM-2, SP-3) was repeated seven times with similar results. In three sets, the procedure was carried out under ketalar anesthesia. (From Ahissar and Vaadia 1990)

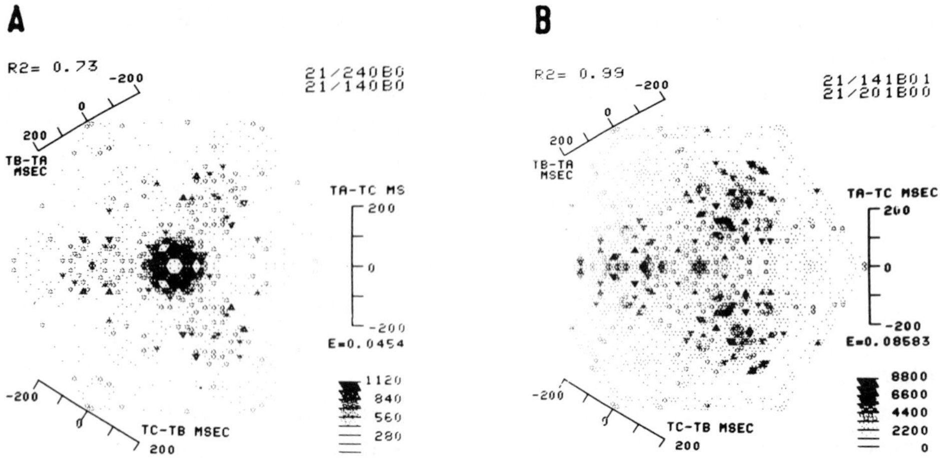

Fig. 5. Modification of single-neuron firing pattern by behavioral state. The hexagons in **A** and **B** show firing patterns of a single neuron in the auditory cortex of a monkey, recorded during each of two behavioral paradigms in an auditory discrimination task. The rate of firing is grouped to eight grey levels. The scale at the lower right marks these levels in percent of the expected rate. **A**: Three-spike auto-correlation, computed from the firing of the neuron during performance of the behavioral paradigm 1, where tone stimuli initiated right shifts of the lever. **B**: similar auto-correlation for the same neuron, computed from the firing during performance of the behavioral paradigm 2, where tone stimuli initiated left shifts of the lever. R_2 = mean firing rate; E = expected number of counts in each triangular bin. (From Vaadia and Abeles 1987).

auditory discrimination-reversal task (from Vaadia and Abeles 1987). In the first behavioral paradigm, presentation of a tone burst stimulus was associated with shifting a lever to the right, while presentation of a noise burst was associated with shifting the lever to the left. In the second paradigm, which was regularly alternated with the first, the contingencies were reversed: left shift after tone burst and right shift after noise burst. Fig. 5A shows the unit activity upon presentation of a tone stimulus during performance of the first behavioral paradigm, while Fig. 5B shows the same neuron's response to the same tone stimulus during the second paradigm. A comparison of these two snowflakes reveals markedly different temporal firing patterns under the two behavioral conditions. In the first condition, the neuron tended to fire in burst of three spikes in response to the tone stimulus (Fig. 5A). This tendency, however, was strongly decreased when the same tone stimulus was associated with the opposite motor response, as expressed by the lack of dark bins around the center in Fig. 5B. Note also that, while the firing patterns of the neuron clearly differ in the two cases, the firing rate is not very different (0.73 spikes/sec as compared to 0.99 spikes/sec).

Conclusion

The above discussion of single-neuron firing codes was by no means intended to be exhaustive. Several other single-neuron neural coding schemes have been pursued, with varying degrees of success. For an early overview of potential single-neuron codes we refer to the classical work of Perkel and Bullock (1968). As a more recent example we mention the work of Richmond and Optican, who proposed a rate code in the visual cortex, which explicitly takes into account the full time course of the firing rate profile (e.g. Richmond and Optican 1987; Optican and Richmond 1987).

Summarizing the findings on single-unit activity in the cortex, both in terms of firing rates and firing patterns, we conclude that:

1. Usually, single-neuron activity consists of a transient response, followed by a long lasting epoch of increased firing rate. The activity may be related to external events, such as sensory stimuli or specific movements, but also to other aspects of behavior, such as intentions to make movements or sensorimotor associations. A single cortical neuron may be active for hundreds of milliseconds to several seconds after the stimulus has disappeared, so that 'something must keep it going'.
2. Higher order neurons show selectivity in a manner which can only be explained by convergence from simple to more complex features. This convergence can be envisaged in at least two different ways, one leading to highly specific grandmother neurons, the other to neurons that can participate in more than one functional group (assembly?). The existence of two independent components of activity as in Fig. 2 suggests that a single neuron may participate in more than one process.
3. If neurons are involved in computation and coding only when their firing rates are elevated, it turns out that most cortical neurons are idle for most of the time. Searching for alternative coding schemes, it could be shown that the temporal firing pattern of single cortical neurons may also serve as a potential neural code.

Cortical activity at the level of multiple-neuron spike trains

In spite of the success in the search for codes in cortical single-neuron activity, there is obviously room for alternative proposals. Clearly, the brain is more than just a collection of single neurons, each living in 'splendid isolation'. They also exert influences onto each other through their anatomical connections. Just as in physics the 'ideal gas' theory of non-interacting particles was considered a first and quite adequate approximation, later approaches emphasized the importance of incorporating the interactions among these particles. Similarly, researchers for a long time have looked for codes which reside in the activity of ensembles of neurons.

One of the first to formulate this approach was Hebb (1949). He suggested that the coherent activity within functional groups of neurons ('cell-assemblies'), mediated by anatomical, presumably plastic connections, forms the basis of the neural code. The groups, he hypothesized, are formed by modifications of synaptic strength that obey what later became known as Hebb's rule: "When an axon of cell A is near enough to excite a cell B and repeatedly or persistently takes part in firing it, some growth process or metabolic change takes place such that A's efficacy, as one of the cells firing B, is increased." (Hebb 1949).

Hebb's hypothesis concerning the functional role of cell assemblies in central processing was adopted widely among theoretically inclined researchers. In fact, it lay the conceptual foundation for most of the current work on 'neural network theories' of brain function (e.g. Braitenberg 1978; Edelman 1981; Abeles 1982a; Palm 1982; Hopfield 1982; Hopfield and Tank 1986; Palm and Aertsen 1986; Rumelhart et al. 1986; Amit 1989). However, there are very little experimental data that challenge the cell assemblies hypothesis. Almost all the above models assume that 'learning' is based on selective modifications of the connectivity among neurons, and that 'computations' are carried out by selective activation of groups of interconnected neurons. According to these hypotheses, the neural code resides in correlated activity within and between neuronal groups. Hence, neither the study of the overall activity in large populations of neurons, nor the recording of single-neuron activity, one at a time, allow for a critical test of the assembly concept. In order to gain an understanding of the processes taking place within and between hypothetical neuronal assemblies, the experimental methodology must involve simultaneous recording of many neurons in parallel, preferably in awake, behaving animals. This enables one to observe simultaneously and separably the activities of many neurons, while they are participating in meaningful processing and computational tasks, and to analyze these activities for possible signs of (dynamic) interactions (Gerstein et al. 1989). Indeed, recent years have shown a growing interest in the simultaneous recording and analysis of spike trains from groups of up to some 10–30 neurons (Abeles 1982a, 1991; Gerstein et al. 1983; Krüger 1983; Eggermont 1990). Associated with this, new computational tools were developed to analyze and interpret the large flow of information coming from such 'multi-neuron' experiments.

Ideally, one should study the activity in a cell assembly by recording the activity of all the neurons in the region in which the cell assembly resides. With the current technology of 'spike sorting' devices, one can hope to record spike activity of a few single neurons (up to six) through one microelectrode (e.g. Abeles and Goldstein 1977) and up to 30 neurons by using multiple electrodes (Krüger 1983; Gerstein et al. 1983). At best, therefore, we can tap only a few members of a hypothetical neuronal network. Nevertheless, it is appropriate to examine how the available physiological data support different concepts and models of neural codes, in quest of an optimal research strategy.

Multiple-neuron firing as a neural code

Several attempts have been made to extend the notion of single-neuron firing rate as a coding mechanism to the activity exhibited by ensembles of neurons. The most notable examples of this approach of *multi-neuron firing rates* as a code can be found in the study of the motor cortex (e.g. Georgopoulos et al. 1988, 1989) and the coding of saccadic eye movements (e.g. van Gisbergen et al. 1987; Lee et al. 1988). Briefly, the firing rates of the various members of the ensemble, usually all neurons in an activated patch of neural tissue, are combined into a 'population vector', which ultimately specifies the direction of the movement to be made. Each single neuron contributes an elementary component to this population vector, the direction of which is determined by the neuron's specificity in terms of the associated movement, and its magnitude by the neuron's firing rate. Related approaches have been proposed for the visual cortex, with the population vector being defined either in the external, visual space (e.g. Vogels 1990) or in an internal, neural activity space (see the contribution of Gerstein and Gochin in this Volume).

Also the *firing patterns* in multi-neuron activity have been invoked in several population coding schemes. An early attempt is found in the concept of 'multi-unit receptive field', introduced by Stevens and Gerstein (1976). A vector-type approach, with the population vector defined in sensory space but based on the instants of multi-unit spike firings rather than their rates, was proposed for the auditory system by Johannesma (1981; see also Gielen et al. 1988; Hesselmans and Johannesma 1989); similar ideas were later applied in the visual system (Bialek et al. 1991). A transition between a rate and a pattern code was proposed for the visual cortex by Krüger (1991; see also Krüger and Becker in this Volume); similarly to Gerstein's proposal, his population vector is defined in neural activity space.

Alternative pattern codes, which do not resort to the notion of a population vector, but instead look at the detailed temporal pattern of multi-unit firing were investigated by Legendy and Salcmann (1985) and Frostig et al. (1985). Pattern codes, based on the notion of 'synfire chains' (Abeles 1982a) were studied by Abeles and Gerstein (1988; see also Abeles 1991). More recently, and inspired by recent findings on oscillatory firing behavior in the cat visual cortex (Gray and Singer 1989; Gray et al. 1989; Eckhorn et al. 1988 and in this Volume), several models have been proposed which invoke the notion of 'dynamic linking' (von der Malsburg 1981, 1986) as a mechanism by which multi-neuron activity reflects information about the visual world. In most of these models, the linking of neurons into functional groups is mediated by the synchronization of oscillatory activity (e.g. Sporns et al. 1989; Sompolinsky et al. 1990, 1991; König and Schillen 1991; Schillen and König 1991; Eckhorn et al. 1990, 1991). An alternative model, which emphasizes synchronization rather than oscillation as the principal information carrying device was proposed by Neven and Aertsen (1992; see also Johannesma et al. 1986; and Erb and Aertsen in this Volume).

Response properties of neighboring cortical neurons

Many of the above mentioned multi-unit coding schemes rely essentially on the idea of 'functional maps'. Briefly, this concept is used to describe findings that the functional properties of neurons are distributed over the cortical surface in a topologically ordered way. In particular, it is also used to indicate that neurons at anatomically neighboring positions have 'neighboring' functional properties. The most notable examples of functional maps in the cortex are the columnar systems proposed for the somatosensory cortex (Mountcastle 1957, 1977) and the visual cortex (Hubel and Wiesel 1968, 1977; see also the contributions of Bonhoeffer and Grinvald, Löwel and Braitenberg in this Volume). In order to investigate to what extent this concept holds as a general organizational principle for cortical representations, we examined in two sets of experiments the relations between the firing behaviors of neighboring neurons in the primary auditory cortex and in the granular frontal 'association' areas (Vaadia et al. 1991). Typical examples of our findings are given in Figures 6 and 7, which show the activity of two sets of adjacent neurons recorded simultaneously in each of these two cortical fields.

Figure 6 shows the multi-neuron activity, recorded by five microelectrodes arranged in a circle, from the primary auditory cortex of an alert Rhesus monkey. Three electrodes recorded more than one isolated neuron each (units 2 and 3; units 4 and 5; and units 7, 8 and 9). Each of the nine raster-display bands depicts a single neuron's activity, recorded over a number of trials of 1.2 seconds each. Individual traces are locked in time to the onset of a stimulus (at time=0), which consisted of 3.4 kHz tone bursts of 300 msec duration at an intensity of 68 dB SPL. This result clearly demonstrates that a number of neurons within the recording area shared certain functional properties and responded to the same stimulus (neurons 1, 4, 5, 6 and 7). However, it is also evident that the response patterns of some of these neighboring neurons differed, and that some of them did not respond at all to the stimulus. For example, while units 1 and 5 responded very strongly to the tone stimuli, the activity of units 2 and 8 was virtually unaffected. Notice also that this strong variability of firing behavior was seen even among neurons that were recorded by the same electrode (for example, units 7, 8 and 9). The distance separating these neurons is probably less than 100 μm (Abeles et al. 1975). The dogma of columnar organization of the auditory cortex implies that all the neurons in the same column share the same best frequency. Although the results shown in Fig. 6 are consistent with this dogma, they evidently do not support the simplistic interpretation that the neurons within a column are all activated in unison.

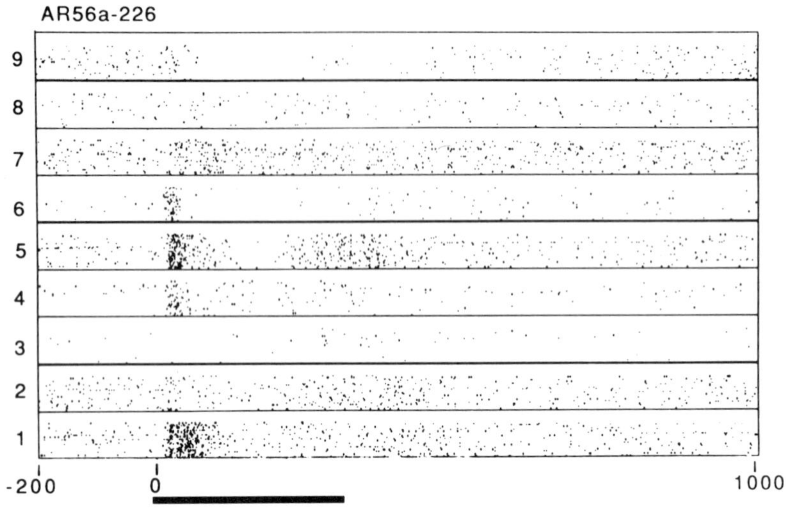

Fig. 6. Raster displays of the responses to tone bursts of 9 neurons in the primary auditory cortex of the Rhesus monkey. The stimulus (a tone burst of 3.4 kHz at 68 dB SPL) is marked by a black bar under the abscissa. The neurons were recorded by 5 microelectrodes. The first electrode recorded unit 1; the second: units 2 and 3; the third: units 4 and 5; the fourth: unit 6; and the fifth: units 7, 8 and 9. Note that neurons 1, 4, 5, 6 and 7 respond to the stimulus, whereas some of the neighboring neurons, e.g. 2 and 8, do not respond at all. This strong variability of firing behavior was seen even among neurons that were recorded by the same electrode (for example, units 7, 8 and 9) (From Vaadia et al. 1991)

The study of neuronal activity in the 'non-specific' association areas poses some difficulties. The functional organization is not very well known and the majority of neurons do not respond at all to sensory stimuli. It is important to study these areas, however, if we wish to examine the mechanisms involved in higher brain functions. To examine the properties of adjacent neurons related to higher functions, one should carefully select and match a recording area with an appropriate, controlled behavioral task. Previous studies in primates have demonstrated that the projections to the prefrontal cortex are segregated in the form of vertical columns (Goldman and Nauta 1977; Goldman-Rakic 1987), and that areas within the frontal cortex are related to higher brain functions (Butters and Pandya 1969; Passingham 1975; Niki and Watanabe 1976, 1979; Evarts et al. 1984; Petrides 1986; Watanabe 1986a,b; Goldman-Rakic 1987; Fuster 1989, and many

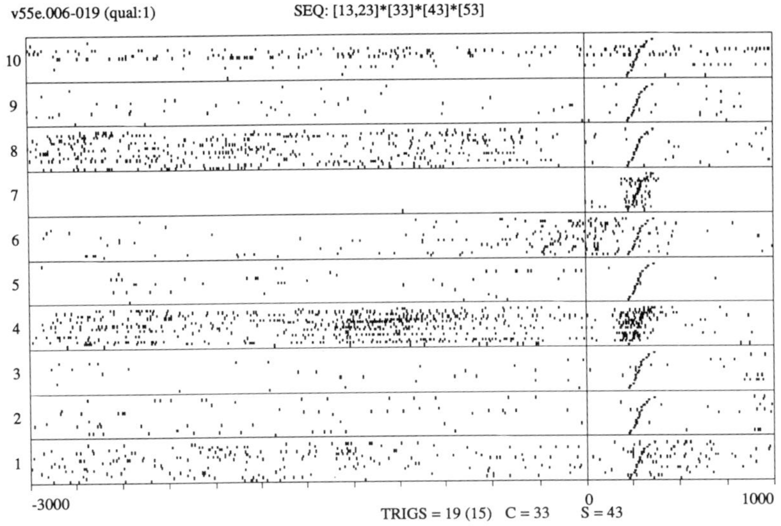

Fig. 7. Raster displays of the activity of 10 neurons in the frontal cortex of a monkey during performance of a localizing task. The rasters show 4 seconds of activity centered around the onset-time of the GO-signal. The trials are sorted (from bottom to top of each strip) according to the reaction time (the time from the onset of the GO-signal to the initiation of arm movement (marked by small crosses). The activity was collected from correct trials where the auditory spatial cues were presented in the left (contralateral) hemifield, at 15° from the midline. The units were recorded by 5 microelectrodes. The first electrode recorded unit 1; the second: units 2 and 3; the third: units 4 and 5; the fourth: units 6 and 7; and the fifth: units 8, 9 and 10. Note the task-related activity of the units 1,4,6,7, while the neighboring units (2,3,5,9) were practically unaffected by behavioral events. (From Vaadia et al. 1989)

others). It was also found that many neurons in the vicinity of the arcuate sulcus responded to both auditory and visual stimuli, when the stimulus served to cue the direction of movements (Vaadia et al. 1986). The combined results of some of the above studies suggest that neuronal activities related to sensory analysis, sensorimotor association, and preparation or execution of movements may be found in the same area. Thus, the frontal cortex seems to be a good place to study neuronal interactions in behaving animals.

In order to study the activity of neighboring neurons in this area, monkeys were trained to perform a spatial task with delay, in which the monkey had to localize auditory and visual stimuli (for details see Vaadia et al. 1991). Figure 7 presents an illustrative example of the neuronal activity in a group of ten neurons in the frontal cortex, that were recorded simultaneously while the monkey was performing the localizing task. The raster-display shows those trials in which the relevant spatial cue was an auditory stimulus, presented at 15° in the contra-lateral hemifield. Each of the 10 strips shows a raster display for the activity of one unit. The vertical line at time 0 marks the onset of the 'GO' signal, which instructed the monkey to make an arm movement towards the location where the auditory stimulus was presented. The units were recorded by 5 microelectrodes (electrode 1: unit 1, electr. 2: units 2 and 3, electr. 3: units 4 and 5, electr. 4: units 6 and 7, and electr. 5: units 8, 9 and 10). Observe that this Figure reveals many similarities with the auditory cortex recording in Figure 6. In particular, it demonstrates that, while the firing rates of some units were clearly affected by the 'GO'-signal during performance of the task, other neurons, even those recorded at the same recording site by the same microelectrode, were not affected at all.

Conclusion

The pattern revealed in Figures 6 and 7 was found to repeat at many other recording sites. Neighboring units could be activated under similar conditions, but could also have different response properties. Moreover, responsive neurons were intermingled with non-responsive neurons. Summarizing, we conclude that:

Neighboring neurons may be functionally related and share common features. However, even when neurons were recorded by the same microelectrode, they were not all activated in unison. These findings suggest that the functional organization of each small volume of cortex allows for the co-existence of functionally distinct neurons, which may participate in several different processes.

Interactions between neighboring cortical neurons

In order to assess the extent to which neurons with similar response properties organize into functional groups, we analyzed the interactions taking place between these neurons. The analysis of interactions among neurons usually consists of cross-correlating spikes from pairs (sometimes triplets) of neurons and inspecting the results for possible signs of 'functional' or 'effective' connectivity (Moore et al. 1966; Perkel et al. 1967, 1975). Recent developments have expanded the scope of these studies. Methods were developed in an effort to reveal global cooperativity in groups of neurons (Gerstein et al. 1985; Gerstein and Aertsen 1985; Aertsen et al. 1986, 1987) and to study in detail the dynamic properties of the correlation between two neurons (Gerstein 1988; Aertsen et al. 1989).

Figure 8 illustrates different types of cross-correlograms obtained from pairs of neurons in the auditory cortex and the frontal cortex of awake monkeys during 'non-performance' periods, i.e. when no stimuli were delivered and the monkey did not perform the task. Fig. 8A shows an example of *uncorrelated* activity: the firing probability of the first cell did not change significantly before or after the firing of the other. About 30% of the neuron pairs recorded from the same microelectrode showed such uncorrelated activity (Vaadia et al. 1991). In some cases a narrow peak confined to one side of the origin could be observed (Fig. 8B). The interpretation that these correlograms reflect a *direct excitatory connection* between the two neurons is supported by the finding that most of these one-sided peaks were found among neurons that were recorded by the same microelectrode, but never among neurons that were more than 600 μm apart. Signs of a *direct inhibitory connection* (a one-sided trough) were found in only very few cases. This is not surprising, however, in view of the low sensitivity of cross-correlation for inhibition under conditions of low firing rates (Aertsen and Gerstein 1985), as typically found in this part of the cortex (Abeles et al. 1990). In the sample of neuron pairs that were recorded by one microelectrode, signs of such 'direct connections' (excitatory and inhibitory) were found in about 20% of the cases, most of them weaker than the example in Fig. 8B (Vaadia et al. 1991).

By far the most common type of interaction found (30% of all pairs; Vaadia et al. 1991) was a more or less symmetrical peak straddling the origin. This type of interaction came in two variants, distinguished by the width of the two-sided peak: *wide* (more than 200 ms; Fig. 8C) and *narrow* (15-100 ms; Figs. 8D,E). Cross-correlograms of this type could emerge when the two neurons shared common excitatory or inhibitory inputs. Two-sided peaks could also emerge when the two neurons excited each other (although this interpretation is highly unlikely for the wider peaks). In most cases the peak gradually

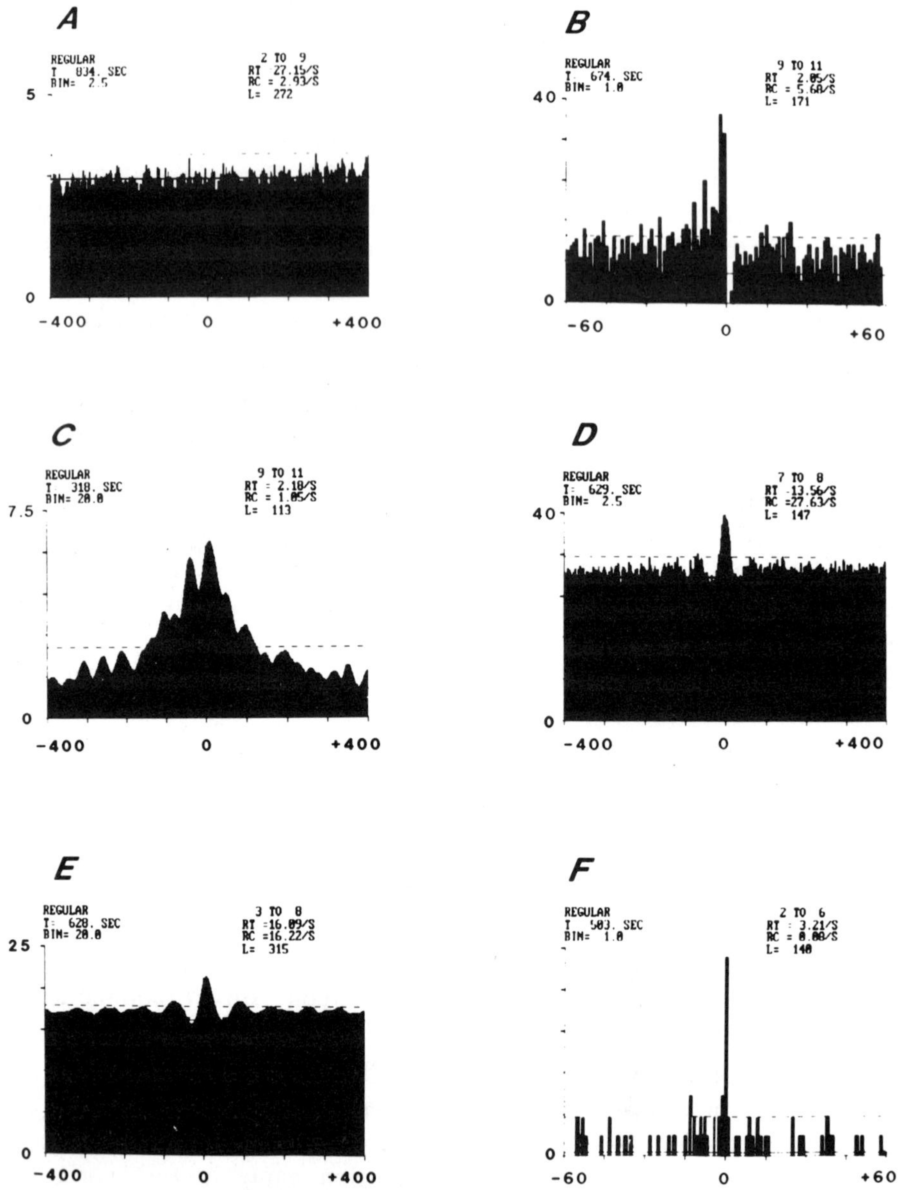

Fig. 8. Cross-correlograms between pairs of neurons in the auditory cortex and the frontal cortex of awake monkeys during 'non-performance' conditions. The abscissa describes the time (ms) around the firing of one neuron, the ordinate describes the firing rate (spikes/s) of the other neuron. The labels on each correlogram give the total data collection time (T), the average firing rate of the two neurons (RT and RC), the bin size (BIN), and the number of data sections (L). For each correlation,

decayed with increasing time interval to the reference spike. In a few cases, there were weak signs of periodicity in the cross-correlograms, as demonstrated in Fig. 8E. The periodicity was in all cases at a frequency of less than 14 Hz. Interestingly, the probability of finding 'narrow' two-sided peaks decreased rapidly with the distance between the cells: according to a preliminary investigation (Lavner 1989) such interaction was found among 30-40% of the pairs recorded by the same microelectrode, as opposed to only 3-8% of the pairs that were 500-600 μm apart. In contrast to this, the probability of finding 'wide' two-sided peaks did not show a clear dependence on pair distance for distances up to 1 mm; within that range the overall frequency of occurrence was 10-20%. Finally, several previous studies reported 'ultra-narrow' peaks of 1 msec or less in cross-correlograms (Toyama et al. 1981; Allum et al. 1982; Murphy et al. 1985; Lurito et al. 1988). An example of such an 'ultra-narrow' peak is shown in Fig. 8F. This correlogram indicates that some spikes of the two units were highly synchronized. This type of cross-correlogram was very infrequent in our studies. A possible explanation may lie in the technological difficulty of detecting two spikes that occur at the same time using a single electrode.

The *width* of the two-sided peak reflects the degree of synchronization of the two neurons and, hence, the time-scale of the processes that affect them. Whether 'narrow' and 'wide' peaks reflect different type of interactions is an still open question. Nevertheless, it is reasonable to hypothesize that the narrow peaks reflect local direct co-activation of relatively small groups of neurons, while the wide peaks reflect a more general co-activation of larger groups of neurons in a relatively wide-spread cortical area. Ultra-narrow peaks were sometimes found at time delays different from zero, which suggests that groups of neurons can fire in precise synchrony and transmit information with high temporal accuracy.

The *area* under the two-sided peak was on the average 0.06 spikes. This area, which equals the correlation coefficient, indicates to what extent the two neurons tend to discharge in synchrony. The low values

---

a band of 99% confidence limits for the equivalent, independent Poisson processes (Abeles 1982b) is shown by broken lines. **A**: Uncorrelated activity. **B**: 'One-sided' narrow peak. (Note the time scale: 60 ms) **C**: 'Two-sided' wide peak. **D**: 'Two-sided' narrow peak. **E**: 'Two-sided' peak with slight signs of periodicity. **F**: 'Ultra-narrow' peak at time 0 (time scale: 60 ms). (From Vaadia et al. 1991)

that we usually measured suggest that most impulse discharges were not correlated. That is, most of the spikes fired by two neurons that shared a common excitatory input originated from EPSPs of other excitatory inputs, which drove each of the neurons independently. This finding confirms the results of previous studies, where triple cross-correlograms (compare the 'snowflakes' in Fig. 5) were used to demonstrate that a single neuron may share common-input with an adjacent neuron from one source, while another input drives the same neuron in unison with another neuron (Abeles 1983; Abeles et al. 1983; Frostig et al. 1983; Vaadia and Abeles 1987).

Conclusion

From these and many similar findings we conclude that:

1. The interactions among adjacent neurons as revealed by cross-correlation analysis are mostly of the 'two-sided', less often of the 'one-sided' type.
2. Usually the observed interactions between neuron pairs are weak, in the sense that many of their spikes are not correlated, even among neurons that have similar functional properties.
3. It is likely that the neurons receive some correlated inputs and other independent inputs. We speculate that the three types of 'two-sided' peak width in cross-correlograms reflect three different mechanisms of neuronal interactions. The 'ultra-narrow' peaks reflect the activity in 'synfire chains', the 'narrow' peaks reflect local co-activation of neurons, and the 'wide' peaks reflect a more general asynchronous mechanism affecting large cortical areas.
4. Oscillating interactions (40-70 Hz) have been reported between cells in the cat visual cortex, that respond with oscillatory firing to adequate visual stimuli. Although oscillatory single-neuron firing in that frequency range was also observed in the somatosensory cortex, not a single case of oscillatory interaction was found there. Oscillations in that frequency range are conspicuously absent in the auditory cortex and the frontal cortex, both in single-neuron firing and in neuronal interactions.

Modifications of neuronal interactions

Modifications in relation to sensory or behavioral events

One of the consequences of Hebb's cell assembly hypothesis would be that neurons organize into functional groups, depending on the momentary computational demand. This would imply that the interactions among neurons should be variable, in particular that they should be modified in relation to behavioral state, or to the presentation of relevant sensory stimuli. Such dependencies on sensory stimulation, arousal levels and behavioral state have indeed been observed (e.g. Dickson and Gerstein 1974; Gassanov et al. 1980; Abeles et al. 1983; Eggermont et al. 1983; Frostig et al. 1983; Eckhorn et al. 1988; Gray and Singer 1989; Aertsen et al. 1987; Krüger and Aiple 1988; Aertsen and Gerstein 1991; Vaadia et al. 1991). We present here two illustrative examples of such modification of interactions by behavioral and stimulus events, one from the auditory cortex, the other from the prefrontal cortex.

Figure 9 shows an example where the spike correlation between two cortical neurons was influenced by a sensory stimulus (from Ahissar et al. 1992). The Figure illustrates the different interactions between two neurons in the auditory cortex of a monkey during presentations of two sound movements in opposite directions. A statistically significant peak can be seen in the first cross-correlogram, computed for the intervals when the stimulus was moving from right to left (Fig. 9A). The position of the peak indicates that the probability of detecting a spike of neuron 9 was increased for about 30 msec after neuron 3 fired a spike. However, when the sound stimulus was moving in the opposite direction (from left to right; Fig. 9B), the interaction between the same two neurons was distinctly different. The correlation in this case was very weak and seems to reflect an opposite interaction, namely, a weak direct inhibitory connection, again from neuron 3 onto neuron 9. Note that the PST histograms of these neurons do not show any such sensitivity; both of them responded with a very similar on-response to the two stimuli (Figs. 9C to 9F). Joint-PST analysis (see next Section) for these two neurons showed that both the peak (Fig. 9A) and trough (Fig. 9B) in the corresponding cross-correlograms originated from spikes fired during the on-response of the two neurons; no significant correlation was observed during the remainder of the response.

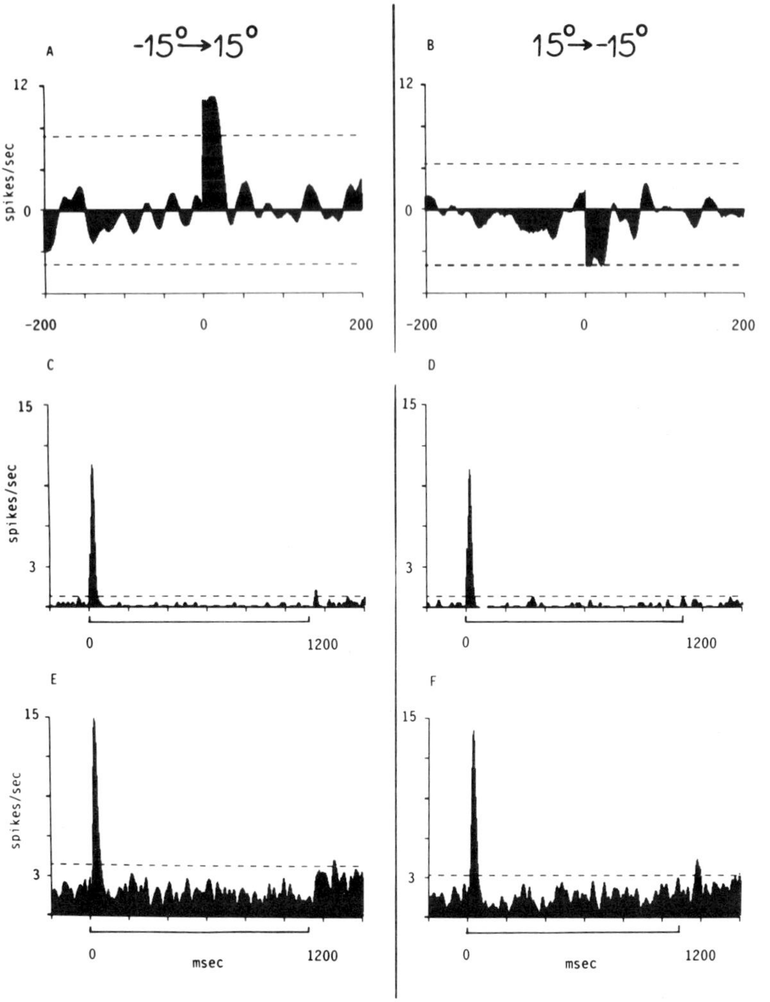

Fig. 9. Modification of interactions in the auditory cortex by sensory stimuli. Example of direction sensitivity, expressed only in the interaction between two neurons, and not in any one of the two single-neuron response profiles. **A-B**: Difference-correlograms of units 3 and 9, computed from data segments recorded during presentation of moving stimuli: A) rightwards (-15° to +15°); B) leftwards (+15° to -15°). **C-F**: PST-histograms showing the responses of units 3 (C,D) and 9 (E,F) to the two stimuli moving in opposite directions (N=291 stimuli for rightward movements; N=295 stimuli for leftward movements). Correlograms and PST-histograms were smoothed, using a gaussian with sigma=15 ms. (From Ahissar et al. 1992)

An example of an interaction that was modified in relation to behavior is presented in Figure 10. It shows the correlation between the spike trains of two prefrontal cortex neurons, collected from two different time sections while the monkey was engaged in the delayed-localization task (cf. Fig. 7). The spike trains in Fig. 10A were recorded during intervals of 1 second, during and immediately following the presentation of a visual stimulus at 30° on the left. The data in Fig. 10B were collected from sections of inter-trial intervals (ITI; 3 seconds each). Comparison of these two correlograms shows that there is a marked difference in the interactions during the two behavioral conditions. An irregular, but very distinct, two-sided peak of the narrow type can be observed when the monkey was presented with the visual stimulus, while the spike trains recorded during the inter-trial intervals show no correlation at all. We note that in the actual trials, these two conditions were separated in time by at most a few seconds.

Dynamical properties of neuronal interactions

It is quite conceivable that these changes of interaction induced by sensory and behavioral events are due to rapid modulations of discharge synchronization among the neurons. Unfortunately, the ordinary cross-correlogram, representing a time-averaged count of near-coincident spikes, does not allow to examine the time course of such possible changes. Recent developments in analysis methodology, however, have overcome this problem. In particular, the *Joint-PSTH* (Aertsen et al. 1989; Palm et al. 1988) was designed to highlight the detailed time structure of firing correlation among two neurons, and its possible time-locking to a third event, such as a stimulus or behavioral event. Moreover, appropriate normalization of the Joint-PSTH enables us to distinguish between contributions due to stimulus- or behavior-induced modulations of the single-neuron firing rates, and those from interneuronal correlation, the latter reflecting the *'effective'* or *'functional connectivity'* among the neurons involved.

Figure 11 shows an example of the results of such Joint-PSTH analysis and the dynamic changes of pair interaction revealed by it. Data were collected from two different time sections of spike trains from two frontal cortex neurons during performance of the same localization task as used in Figure 7. The first section comprises 600 ms immediately following the GO-signal (Fig. 11A), the second one covers an interval of 600 ms, starting 900 ms after the monkey's hand left the target key (after it hit the correct location, and the monkey

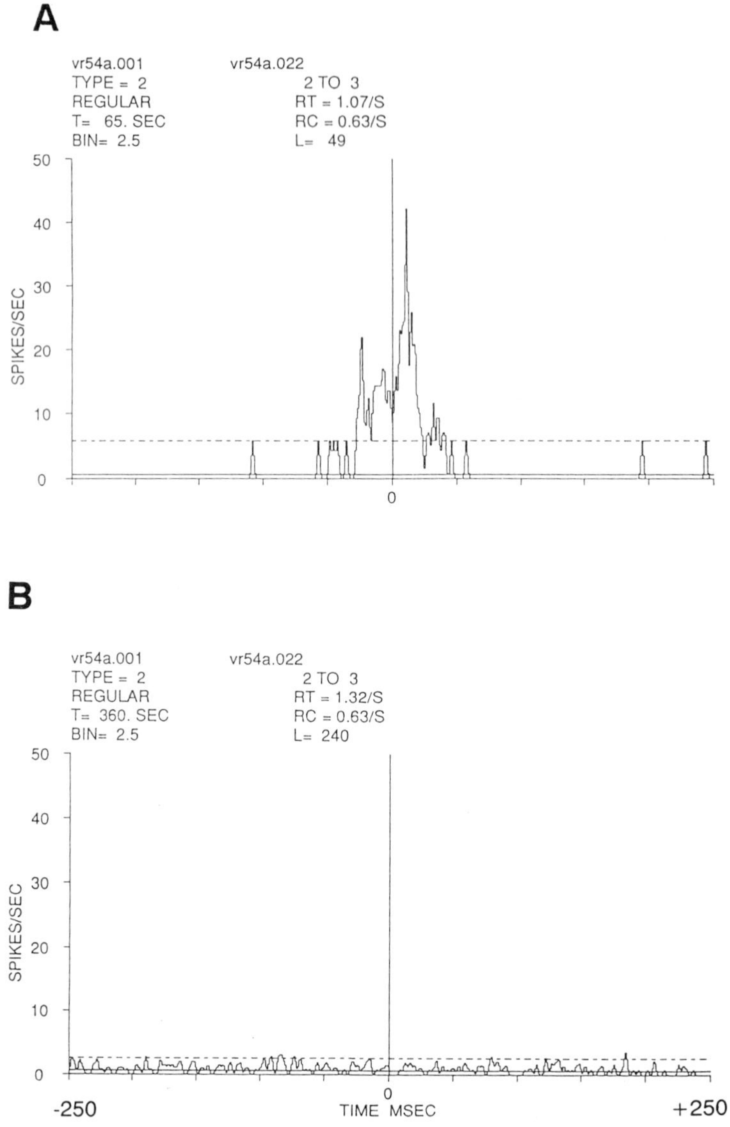

Fig. 10. Modification of interactions in relation to behavioral state. Two cross-correlograms of one pair of neurons recorded in the prefrontal cortex of the monkey during performance of the delayed localization task. The cross-correlogram in **A** was computed from sections of activity, recorded during intervals of 1 second, during and immediately following the presentation of a visual stimulus at 30° on the left. The cross-correlogram in **B** was computed from sections of inter-trial intervals (ITI; 3 seconds each). Observe the marked difference in the interactions during the two behavioral conditions. Note that in the actual trials, these two conditions were separated in time by at most a few seconds.

received its reward) and returned to its resting position (Fig. 11B). Comparison of the normalized Joint-PST histograms in both panels reveals considerable differences in the interaction patterns among the two neurons, both in the time-averaged correlograms and, even more so, in the detailed time course of the correlation, displayed along the diagonal. Following the GO-signal (Fig. 11A), the time-averaged correlation is characterized by a strong, 'bi-phasic' interaction pattern: a narrow peak for negative delays (left of the origin), accompanied by a wider trough for positive delays (right). Interestingly, the positive peak does not reflect an ongoing and stable interaction, but is the net result of two extremely short-lasting instances of discharge synchronization (cf. the diagonal histogram in Fig. 11A), occurring in coincidence with the onset and offset of firing of one of the two neurons (compare the PST-histogram along the y-axis), with no interaction whatsoever outside these two short intervals. Similarly, the negative interaction changes dramatically as time proceeds. The time tourse of modulation, however, is quite different: a sharply increasing and gradually decaying negativity, with the dominant contribution originating from the onset phase of the first neuron, shortly after the first peak of positive interaction, when also the second neuron (PST-histogram along the x-axis) elevates its firing rate. During the second time section, however, separated from the first one by a mere 1.5 s, these same two neurons exhibit a completely different type of correlation (Fig. 11B). In contrast to the earlier result, the overall interaction now is characterized by an asymmetric, damped-oscillation-type correlation, with the main peak straddling the origin. Again, inspection of the diagonal region reveals distinct signs of dynamic modulation of the interaction. Although in this case the increased noise level (presumably due to the considerable reduction in firing rates of both neurons) prohibits an unequivocal parsing into separate components, there are hints of two non-overlapping oscillatory subpatterns (extending roughly from 900-1100 ms and from 1200-1400 ms), possibly associated with concurrent features in the firing rate of one of the neurons (compare the PST-histogram along the x-axis).

This example clearly demonstrates that the neurons' activities may exhibit rapid modulations of discharge synchronization that are related to the behavioral state. These modulations may switch the neurons' firing behaviour from being mutually incoherent into a particular coherent state of joint synchrony, or, alternatively, from one particular pattern of mutual coherence into a different one. Each such pattern

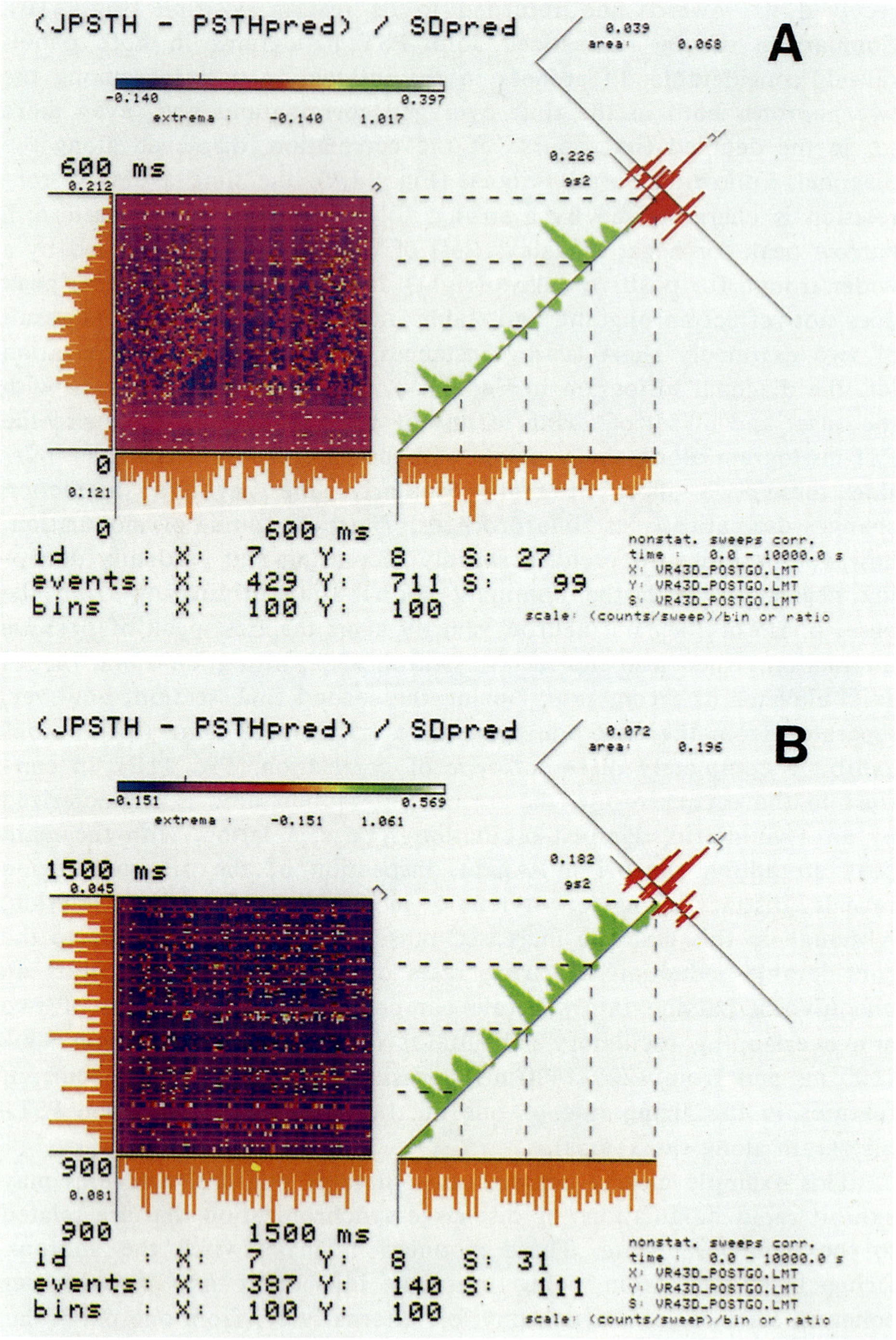
A
(JPSTH - PSTHpred) / SDpred
-0.140 0.397
extrema : -0.140 1.017
0.039
area: 0.068
0.226
gs2
600 ms
0.212
0
0.121
0 600 ms
id : X: 7 Y: 8 S: 27
events: X: 429 Y: 711 S: 99
bins : X: 100 Y: 100
nonstat. sweeps corr.
time : 0.0 - 10000.0 s
X: VR43D_POSTGO.LMT
Y: VR43D_POSTGO.LMT
S: VR43D_POSTGO.LMT
scale: (counts/sweep)/bin or ratio
B
(JPSTH - PSTHpred) / SDpred
-0.151 0.569
extrema : -0.151 1.061
0.072
area: 0.196
0.182
gs2
1500 ms
0.045
900
0.081
900 1500 ms
id : X: 7 Y: 8 S: 31
events: X: 387 Y: 140 S: 111
bins : X: 100 Y: 100
nonstat. sweeps corr.
time : 0.0 - 10000.0 s
X: VR43D_POSTGO.LMT
Y: VR43D_POSTGO.LMT
S: VR43D_POSTGO.LMT
scale: (counts/sweep)/bin or ratio

may last for only a few tens to hundreds of milliseconds. Finally, the observed modulations in synchronized firing may be, but are not necessarily associated with changes in either of the neurons' individual firing rates.

Interactions among larger groups of neurons

So far we only addressed the issue of correlation between two neurons at a time. An important question in view of the hypothesis that neurons dynamically organise into functional groups, is whether correlations also exist between larger groups of neurons, and, if so, whether such group correlations follow a similar pattern as the pair correlations do, particularly regarding their dependence on behavioral state. In order to study the global firing correlations among entire groups of simultaneously recorded neurons, we used the *gravitational clustering* analysis (Gerstein et al. 1985; Gerstein and Aertsen 1985; Aertsen et al. 1986, 1987; Aertsen and Gerstein 1991). This conceptual framework and analysis technique was explicitly designed to deal with population activity, in particular for the detection of co-activation of larger numbers of neurons. We give here only a brief description and refer to the original literature for more details.

Fig. 11. Dynamics of neuronal interaction. Joint-PSTH analysis of two simultaneously recorded neurons from the frontal cortex of a monkey during performance of the 'delayed localization' task. The color-coded, normalized Joint-PSTH matrices in both panels represent the time-dependent correlation of firing among the two neurons, after normalization for stimulus-induced modulations in single-neuron firing rates. The latter are assessed by the PST-histograms shown along the horizontal and vertical axes. The diagonal band of the normalized Joint-PSTH matrix reflects the near-coincident firing correlation as it evolves in the course of time; it is shown once again in the diagonal histogram in the right-hand part of the Figures (lower left to upper right). Finally, the normalized cross-correlogram is obtained by integrating along the diagonal; it is shown in the second histogram in the right-hand part of the Figures (upper left to lower right). Data was collected from two different time sections of spike trains: **A**: Time section of 600 ms immediately following the GO-signal; **B**: Interval of 600 ms, starting 900 ms after the monkey's hand left the target key (after hitting the correct location, and the monkey received its reward) and returned to its resting position. Notice the clear differences in correlation during these two time sections, separated from each other by only about 1.5 s. Further explanation in text.

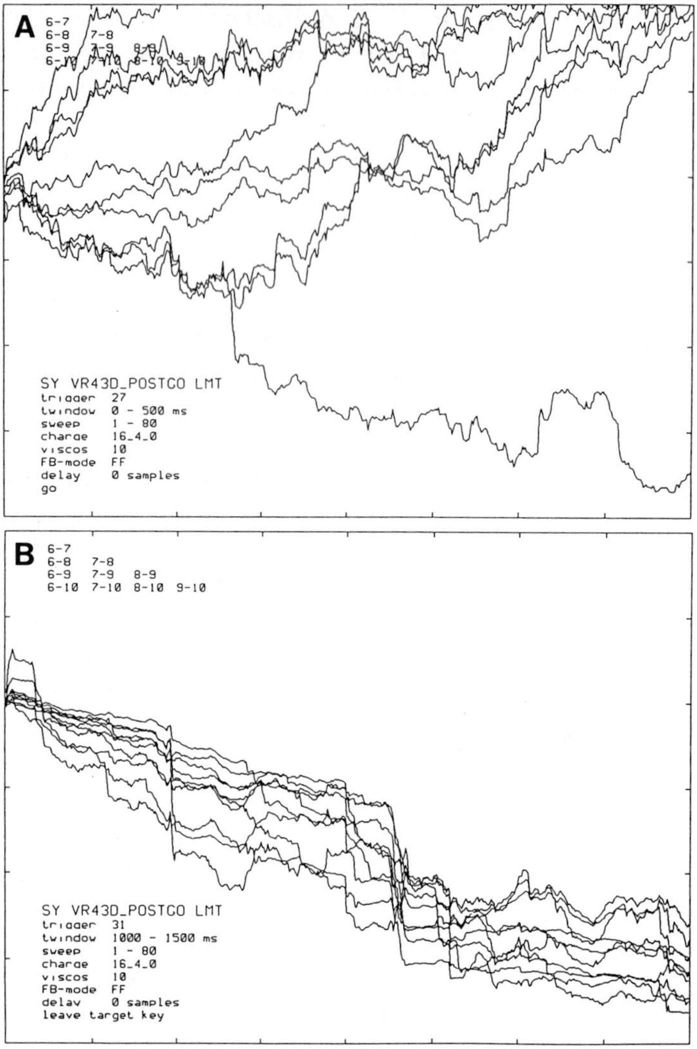

Fig. 12. Modification of interactions among groups of neurons in relation to behavioral state. 'Gravitational Clustering' analysis of correlation among the activities of 5 neurons in the frontal cortex of a monkey during performance of the 'delayed localizing task'. Each set of curves represents the group correlations during a particular sequence of 0.5 second long intervals of spike activity, parsed from a single recording session, the difference being that the first series of intervals (**A**) was time-locked to the GO-signal, while the second series (**B**) was time-locked to the behavioral event of the monkey leaving the target key. Clearly the clustering patterns and, hence, the organization of correlation are distinctly different in these two cases, showing that correlations among groups of neurons in frontal cortex may be altered drastically and in rapid succession, depending on the stimulus context and behavioral state of the animal. Further explanation in text.

Suppose we measure spike trains from N neurons. Each one of these N neurons is represented by a point particle in a fictitious N-space. To each such particle, we associate a time-varying 'charge', determined by the respective neuron's spike train. As a result, the particles will mutually exert forces that cause them to 'move'. The charge functions are defined such that the forces lead to aggregation of those particles which correspond to coherently firing neurons, with each single cluster signifying the member neurons of a particular cell assembly. The time dependence of clustering conveys information on the static ('strength') as well as the dynamic aspects of coherent activity. The resulting configurations can be investigated directly by resorting to high-dimensional cluster analysis techniques, or visually, by appropriate projection of the N-space onto a more convenient 2-space representation. If cell assemblies are dynamic entities, related to stimulus context or behavioral state, the particles associated with the member neurons of such an assembly would aggregate during the stage which calls the assembly to action, and move away from each other to regroup in different clusters, when other assemblies are called upon the stage.

Preliminary results from gravitational analysis of frontal cortex recordings indicate that (a) global correlations among larger groups of neurons in frontal cortex do exist, and that (b) these group correlations may indeed be altered drastically and in rapid succession, depending on the stimulus context and behavioral state of the animal. An example of such group correlation and its behavioral dependence is given in Figure 12. The plots show the pairwise inter-particle distance in the gravitational representation as a function of time, with each single curve representing the firing correlation among a particular pair in the set of simultaneously recorded neurons. The temporal development of clustering is signified by a downward slope of some of the curves: the larger the downward slope, the stronger the positive correlation (and upward for negative correlation). The two panels represent the firing correlations among five well isolated single frontal cortex neurons, recorded simulteously during performance of the localization task. Each of the two panels corresponds to a particular sequence of 0.5 second time intervals of spike activity that were collected from a single recording session. The two panels differ in that the respective time sections were time-locked to different stimulus or behavioral events: similarly to the results in Fig. 11, Fig. 12A describes the correlations during the 0.5 second immediately following the GO-signal, while Fig.

12B covers the interval between 1 and 1.5 second after the monkey's hand left the target key to return to its resting position. Observe how the clustering patterns (and hence, the group correlations) are distinctly different in these two cases. Following the GO-signal (Fig. 12A), only one pair of neurons shows positive correlation (the single descending curve), whereas the remaining particles either remain noisily stationary (i.e. no correlation between the corresponding neurons) or even have a weak tendency to diverge, suggesting a negative correlation. In contrast, during the return movement (Fig. 12B) *all* curves exhibit a strongly similar descent, indicating a collective aggregation into a single cluster. Evidently, during this second interval *all* five neurons temporarily join into a common mode of coherent firing; further analysis (not shown here) reveals that both immediately before and after this particular 0.5 second interval, this collective behavior is very much weaker or altogether absent. It should be born in mind that the selected time sections were separated on the average by only about 1-1.5 second, so that indeed this change of correlation is a very rapid one.

These and similar results (Aertsen and Gerstein 1991; Vaadia et al. 1991) imply that the observed changes in correlation are not simply due to task-related changes in single neuron firing rates, but rather reflect interesting, task-related and highly dynamic changes of interaction among these neurons. We stress that the changes in assembly organization, signified by these changes in firing correlation, could not have been revealed by any single unit analysis of the individual neurons involved.

Conclusion

1. Interactions between neuron pairs as well as between larger groups of neurons can be modified in relation to external events, like sensory stimuli, or to the behavioral state. Such modification may occur on a very short time scale, within a fraction of a second.
2. The activities of pairs of cortical neurons may exhibit rapid modulations of discharge synchronization, that are related to the behavioral state. These modulations may switch the neurons' firing behaviour from being mutually incoherent into a particular coherent state of joint synchrony, or, alternatively, from one particular

pattern of mutual coherence into a different one. Each such pattern may last for only a few tens to hundreds of milliseconds.

3. The modulations in synchronized firing between pairs of cortical neurons may follow a time course which is independent of the firing rate profiles of any of the single neurons involved.

Discussion

Most of the above results could not possibly have been predicted from single neuron measurements. Nevertheless, studies of functional properties of single neurons are still very important. They provide a range of important parameters for each element in the hypothetical 'neuronal network' (maximal rate, response properties, statistical properties of the spike train, etc.). In addition, they provide a description of the functional organization of the cerebral cortex. Thus, single-unit studies can tell us where and when certain processes take place. Moreover, a research strategy that combines the study of the individual properties of single neurons with an analysis of the relations they have with each other allows for a confrontation of different hypotheses, using the same experimental data.

Our observations support the hypothesis that several different neural encoding schemes may be operative in the cortex simultaneously. We postulate that the neural code for higher brain function resides both in the firing activities of single neurons, as well as in the coherent activity of groups of neurons. Our findings further suggest that these 'neuronal groups' are dynamic entities, defined not only by anatomical connections, but also by the everchanging level of correlation among the activities of their member neurons. The salient result of direct observation of the activity in groups of neurons in the working cortex is that the interactions among these neurons may be *context-dependent* and *dynamic* on several different time scales. This suggests that the usual concept of neurons with static interconnections of fixed or only slowly changing efficacy (during learning, for example) is no longer adequate. Instead, we should distinguish between *structural* (or anatomical) connectivity on the one hand, and *functional* (or effective) connectivity on the other. Whereas the former can be described as (quasi) stationary, the latter may be highly dynamic, with time constants of modulation in the range of tens to hundreds of milliseconds. Thus, it appears that dynamic cooperativity is an emergent property of neuronal assembly organization in the brain.

We hypothesize that the cooperativity and the degree of synchronization among cortical neurons can control the synaptic efficacy of the connections between them. This hypothesis predicts that the effectiveness of interactions among neurons may depend on environmental or internal factors that change the degree of synchronization. Considering that a neuron in the cortex makes contacts with thousands of other cells (Braitenberg and Schüz 1991), it becomes evident that when such a neuron is momentarily co-activated with one set of cells, part of its connections will become effective for a corresponding brief period of time. However, when some time later, due to a change in stimulus context or behavioral state, the same cell is co-activated with another set of neurons, a partly or even altogether different subset of its connections will become effective. Thus, there is no need for the synaptic contacts to be particularly strong: the corresponding connections become effective through synchronous activity with other neurons (Abeles 1982a, 1991). Computer simulations (Erb et al. 1986, 1989, 1990) and analytical calculations (Aertsen and Preissl 1991) on artificial neural networks with various types of architectures have demonstrated that considerable and rapid changes in effective connectivity may, in fact, occur without any associated changes in anatomical connectivity. Rather, such changes in effective connectivity may be a reflection of the dynamics of the activity in the entire network, both regarding the rates (Boven and Aertsen 1990) and the internal coherence (Bedenbaugh et al. 1988, 1990) of firing. Thus, the highly dynamic interplay of activity and connectivity in the cortex gives rise to an ongoing process of functional reorganization. Everchanging groups of neurons, each one recruited for brief periods of time, become co-activated and again de-activated, following each other in rapid succession. It is our conjecture that this dynamic reorganization provides the mechanism which underlies our capacity to rapidly change our sensory perceptions, motor behaviour and sensori-motor associations.

Acknowledgements

The results reported in this paper are based on experiments and analyis performed in the Dept. of Physiology at the Hebrew University in Jerusalem. The contributions by Moshe Abeles, Ehud and Merav Ahissar, Hagai Bergman, Benny Karmon, Yizhar Lavner, Eyal Margalit and Israel Nelken are gratefully acknowledged. In the context of a joint research project, additional analysis was carried out at the Max-Planck-Institut für biologische Kybernetik in Tübingen; we thank Stefan Rotter for his contribution. This research received support from the United States-Israel Binational Science Foundation (grant # 88-00250/1), the German Ministry for Science and Technology (BMFT), the German-Israel Foundation for Research and Development (GIF), and the Graduiertenkolleg Neurobiologie Tübingen. In the context of this joint research project, one of the authors (AA) spent the year 1990-91 on sabbatical leave in the Dept. of Physiology at the Hebrew University; this stay was supported by the Lady Davis Foundation and the Minerva Foundation.

References

Abeles M, Assaf J, Gottlieb Y, Hodis H, Vaadia E (1975) Speculation on a neural substrate for immediate memory. Sensory Physiology and Behavior 15:117-126

Abeles M, Goldstein MH (1977) Multiple spike train analysis. Proc. IEEE 65:762-773

Abeles, M. (1982a) Local cortical circuits. An electrophysiological study. Springer, Berlin,

Abeles M (1982b) Quantification, smoothing, and confidence limits for single units' histograms. J Neurosci Meth 5:317-325

Abeles M (1983) The quantification and graphic display of correlations among three spike trains. IEEE Trans Biomed Engin BME-30:236-239

Abeles M, de Ribaupierre F, de Ribaupierre E (1983) Detection of single unit responses which are loosely time-locked to a stimulus. IEEE Trans Syst Man Cyber SMC-13:683-691

Abeles M, Gerstein GL (1988) Detecting spatiotemporal firing patterns among simultaneously recorded single neurons. J Neurophysiol 60:909-924

Abeles M, Vaadia E, Bergman H (1990) Firing patterns of single units in the prefrontal cortex and neural network models. Network 1:13-35

Abeles M (1991) Corticonics. Neural circuits in the cerebral cortex. Cambridge University Press, Cambridge, UK

Aertsen AMHJ, Gerstein GL (1985) Evaluation of neuronal connectivity: sensitivity of cross correlation. Brain Res 340:341-354

Aertsen A, Gerstein G, Johannesma, P (1986) From neuron to assembly: Neuronal organisation and stimulus representation. In: Palm G, Aertsen A (eds) Brain Theory. Springer, Berlin, pp 7-24

Aertsen A, Bonhoeffer T, Krüger J (1987) Coherent activity in neuronal populations: analysis and interpretation. In: Caianiello, ER (ed) Physics of Cognitive Processes. World Scientific Publishing, Singapore, pp 1-34

Aertsen AMHJ, Gerstein GL, Habib MK, Palm G (1989) Dynamics of neuronal firing correlation: modulation of "effective connectivity". J Neurophysiol 61:900-917

Aertsen AMHJ, Gerstein GL (1991) Dynamic aspects of neuronal cooperativity: fast stimulus-locked modulations of 'effective connectivity'. In: Krüger J. (ed) Neuronal Cooperativity. Springer, Berlin, p 52-67

Aertsen A, Preissl H (in press, 1991) Dynamics of activity and connectivity in physiological neuronal networks. In: Schuster H (ed) Nonlinear dynamics and neuronal networks. VCH Verlag, Weinheim

Ahissar E, Vaadia E (1990) Oscillatory activity of single units in a somatosensory cortex of an awake monkey and their possible role in texture analysis. Proc Natl Acad Sci USA 87:8935-8939

Ahissar M, Ahissar E, Bergman H, Vaadia E (1992) Encoding of sound source location and movement: activity of single neurons and interaction between adjacent neurons in the monkey auditory cortex. J Neurophysiol (in press)

Allum JHJ, Hepp-Reymond MC, Gysin R (1982) Cross-correlation analysis of interneuronal connectivity in the motor cortex of the monkey. Brain Res 231:325-334

Amit D (1989) Modeling brain function. Cambridge University Press, Cambridge, UK

Barlow HB (1972) Single units and sensation: A neuron doctrine for percepteral psychology. Perception 1:371-394.

Bedenbaugh PH, Gerstein GL, Boven K-H, Aertsen AMHJ (1988) The meaning of stimulus dependent changes in cross correlation between neuronal spike trains. Soc Neurosci Abstr 14:651

Bedenbaugh PH, Gerstein GL, Aertsen AMHJ (1990) Dynamic convergence in neural assemblies. Soc Neurosci Abstr 16:1224

Bialek W, Rieke F, de Ruyter van Steveninck R, Warland D (1991) Reading a neural code. Science 252:1854-1857

Boven K-H, Aertsen A (1989) Dynamics of activity in neuronal networks give rise to fast modulations of functional connectivity. In: Eckmiller R et al. (eds) Parallel processing in neural systems and computers. Elsevier Science Publishers, pp 53-56

Braitenberg V (1978) Cell assemblies in the cerebral cortex. In: Heim R, Palm G (eds) Theoretical Approaches to Complex Systems. Lecture Notes in Biomathematics, Vol. 21. Springer, Berlin Heidelberg New York, pp 171-188

Braitenberg V, Schüz A (1991) Anatomy of the cortex. Statistics and geometry. Springer, Berlin

Butters N, Pandya D (1969) Retention of delayed alternation : Effect of selective lesions of sulcus principalis. Science 165:1271-1273

Dayhoff JE, Gerstein GL (1983) Favored patterns in spike trains. I. Detection. J Neurophysiol 49:1334-1348

Dayhoff JE, Gerstein GL (1983) Favored patterns in spike trains. II. Application. J Neurophysiol 49:1349-1363

Deeke L, Kornhuber HH, Lang W, Lang M, Shreiber H (1985) Timing function of the frontal cortex in sequential motor cortex in motor and learning tasks. Human Neurobiol 4:143-154

Dickson JW, Gerstein GL (1974) Interactions between neurons in auditory cortex of the cat. J Neurophysiol 37:1239-1261

Donchin E (ed) (1984) Cognitive Psychophysiology. The Carmal Conferences. Vol. 1. Erlbaum Pub., New Jersey

Eckhorn R, Bauer R, Jordan W, Kruse W, Munk M, Reitboeck HJ (1988) Coherent oscillations: a mechanism of feature linking in the visual cortex? Multiple electrode and correlation analysis in the cat. Biol Cybern 60:121-130

Eckhorn R, Reitboeck HJ, Arndt M, Dicke P (1990) Feature linking via a synchronization among distributed assemblies: simulations of results from cat visual cortex. Neural Computation 2:293-307

Eckhorn R (1991) Stimulus-specific synchronisations in visual cortex: linking features into global figures? In: Krüger J (ed) Neural Cooperativity. Springer, Berlin Heidelberg New York, pp 184-219

Edelman GM (1981) Group selection as the basis for higher brain function. The organization of the cerebral cortex. In: Proc of a neuroscience research program colloquium. Schmitt et. al. (eds) The MIT Press, Cambridge, pp 536-563

Eggermont JJ (1990) The correlative brain. Theory and experiment in neural interaction. Springer, Berlin

Eggermont JJ, Epping WJM, Aertsen AMHJ (1983) Stimulus dependent neural correlations in the auditory midbrain of the grassfrog (Rana temporaria L.). Biol Cybern 47:103-117

Erb M, Palm G, Aertsen A, Bonhoeffer T (1986) Functional versus structural connectivity in neuronal nets. In: Strukturbildung und Musteranalyse, Proc. 9th Cybernetics Congress (DGK) Göttingen (FRG), p 23

Erb M, Aertsen A, Palm G (1989) Functional connectivity in neuronal systems: context-dependence of effective network organization does not require synaptic plasticity. In: Elsner N, Singer W (eds) Dynamics and plasticity in neuronal systems. Thieme, Stuttgart, New York, p 445

Erb M, Aertsen A, Palm G (1990) Stability in physiology-oriented neuronal network models. In: Elsner N, Roth G (eds) Brain - Perception - Cognition. Thieme, Stuttgart, New York, p 527

Evarts EV, Shinoda Y, Wise SP (1984) Neurophysiological approach to higher brain function. Wiley Intersciences Press, New York

Frostig R, Gottlieb Y, Vaadia E, Abeles M (1983) The effects of stimuli on the activity and functional connectivity of local neuronal groups in the cat auditory cortex. Brain Res 272:211-221

Frostig R, Frostig Z, Frysinger R, Schechtman V (1985) Multineuron analysis reveals complex patterns of interaction among neurons. Soc Neurosci Abstr 11:1020

Fuster JM (1973) Unit activity in the prefrontal cortex during delayed response performance: neuronal correlates of transient memory. J Neurophysiol 36:61-78

Fuster JM (1989) The prefrontal cortex. Anatomy, physiology, and neuropsychology of the frontal lobe. Raven Press, New York

Gassanov UG, Galashina AG, Bogdanov AV (1980) A study of neuron systems activity in learning. Neural Mechanisms of Goal-Directed Behavior and Learning 341-352

Gerstein GL, Bloom MJ, Espinosa IE, Evanczuk S, Turner MR (1983) Design of a laboratory for multi-neuron studies. IEEE Trans Systems, Man and Cybernetics SMC-13:668-676

Gerstein G, Perkel D, Dayhoff J (1985) Cooperative firing activity in simultaneously recorded populations of neurons: detection and measurement. J Neurosci 5:881-889

Gerstein G, Aertsen A (1985) Representation of cooperative firing activity among simultaneously recorded neurons. J Neurophysiol 54:1513-1527

Gerstein GL (1988) Information flow and state in cortical neural networks: Interpreting multi-neuron experiments. In: von Seelen W, Shaw G, Leinhos UM (eds) Organization of neural networks. VCH Verlag, Weinheim (FRG), pp 53-75

Gerstein GL, Bedenbaugh P, Aertsen AMHJ (1989) Neuronal Assemblies. IEEE Trans on Biomed Engin 36:4-14

Georgopoulos AP, Kettner RE, Schwartz AB (1988) Primate motor cortex and free arm movements to visual targets in three-dimensional space. II. Coding of the direction of movement by a neuronal population. J Neurosci 8:2928-2937

Georgopoulos AP, Lurito JT, Petrides M, Schwartz AB, Massey JT (1989) Mental rotation of the neuronal population vector. Science 243:234-236

Gielen CCAM, Hesselmans GHFM, Johannesma PIM (1988) Sensory interpretation of neural activity patterns. Math Biosci 92:15-35

Goldberg ME, Segraves MA (1987) Visuospatial and motor attention in the monkey. Neuropsychologia 25(1A):107-118

Goldman PS, Nauta WJH (1977) Columnar distribution of cortico-cortical fibers in the frontal association, limbic and motor cortex of the developing Rhesus monkey. Brain Res 122:393-413

Goldman-Rakic PS (1987) Circuitry of primate prefrontal cortex and the regulation of behavior by representational knowledge. In: Mountcastle VB, Plum F (eds) The Nervous System, Vol. V, Handbook of Physiology. Am Physiol Soc, Bethesda, MD, pp 373-417

Gottlieb Y, Vaadia E, Abeles M (1989) Single unit activity in the auditory cortex of a monkey performing a short term memory to tones task. Exp Brain Res 74:139-148

Gray CM, Singer W (1989) Stimulus-specific neuronal oscillations in orientation columns of cat visual cortex. Proc Natl Acad Sci USA 86:1698-1702

Gray CM, König P, Engel AK, Singer W (1989) Oscillatory responses in cat visual cortex exhibit inter-columnar synchronisation which reflects global stimulus properties. Nature 388:334-337

Hebb D (1949) The organization of behavior. A neuropsychological theory. Wiley, New York

Hesselmans GHFM, Johannesma PIM (1989) Spectro-temporal interpretation of activity patterns of auditory neurons. Math Biosci 93:31-51

Hopfield JJ (1982) Neuronal networks and physical systems with emergent collective computational abilities. Proc Natl Acad Sci USA, 79:2554-2556

Hopfield JJ and Tank DW (1986) Computing with neural circuits: A model. Science 233:625-633

Hubel DH, Wiesel TN (1968) Receptive fields and functional architecture of monkey striate cortex. J Physiol 195:215-243

Hubel DH, Wiesel TN (1977) Functional architecture of macaque monkey visual cortex (Ferrier Lecture). Proc Roy Soc London, Vol. B. 198:1-59

Johannesma PIM (1981) Neural representation of sensory stimuli and sensory interpretation of neural activity. In: Szekely Gy, Labos E, Damjanovich S (eds) Neural communication and control. Adv Physiol Sci 30:103-125

Johannesma P, Aertsen A, van den Boogaard H, Eggermont J, Epping W (1986) From synchrony to harmony: Ideas on the function of neural assemblies and on the interpretation of neural synchrony. In: Palm G, Aertsen A (eds) Brain Theory. Springer, Berlin Heidelberg New York, pp 25-47

König P, Schillen TB (1991) Stimulus-dependent assembly formation of oscillatory responses. 1: Synchronisation. Neural Computation 3:155-167

Krüger J (1983) Simultaneous individual recordings from many cerebral neurons: techniques and results. Rev Physiol Biochem Pharmacol 98:177-233

Krüger J, Aiple F (1988) Multimicroelectrode investigation of monkey striate cortex: spike trains correlations in infragranular layers. J Neurophysiol 60(2):798-828

Krüger J (1991) Spike train correlations on slow time scales in monkey visual cortex. In: Krüger J (ed) Neuronal Cooperativity. Springer, Berlin, pp 105-132

Lavner Y (1989) Functional interactions between cells in the prefrontal cortex of behaving monkeys. M.Sc. Thesis (in Hebrew), Hebrew University, Jerusalem

Lee C, Rohrer WH, Sparks DL (1988) Population coding of saccadic eye movements by neurons in the superior colliculus. Nature 332:357-360

Legendy C, Salcmann M (1985) Bursts and recurrences of bursts in the spike trains of spontaneously active striate cortex neurons. J Neurophysiol 53:926-939

Lurito JT, Schwartz AB, Petrides M, Kettner RE, Georgopoulos AP (1988) Crosscorrelations between motor cortical cells simultaneously recorded during reaching task in the monkey. Soc Neurosci Abst 14:142.5

Moore GP, Perkel DH, Segundo JP (1966) Statistical analysis and functional interpretation of neuronal spike data. Ann Rev Physiol 28:493-522

Moore GP, Segundo JP, Perkel DH, Levitan H (1970) Statistical signs of synaptic interactions in neurons. Biophys J 10:876-900

Mountcastle VB (1957) Modality and topographic properties of single neurons of cat's somatic sensory cortex. J Neurophysiol 20:408-434

Mountcastle VB (1977) An organizing principle for cerebral function: the unit module and the distributed system. In: Edelman GM, Mountcastle VB (eds) The Mindful Brain. MIT Press, Cambridge (MA), pp 7-50

Murphy JT, Kwan HC, Wong YC (1985) Cross-correlation studies in primate motor cortex: Synaptic interaction and shared input. Can J Neurol Sci 12:11-23

Neven H, Aertsen A (1992) Rate coherence and event coherence in the visual cortex: a neuronal model of object recognition (submitted)

Niki H, Watanabe M (1976) Pre-frontal unit activity and delayed response: Relation to cue location versus direction of response. Brain Res 105:79-88

Niki H, Watanabe M (1979) Prefrontal and cingulate unit activity during timing behavior in the monkey. Brain Res 171:213-224

Optican LM, Richmond B (1987) Temporal encoding of two-dimensional patterns by single units in primate inferior temporal cortex. III. Information theoretic analysis. J Neurophysiol 57:162-178

Palm G (1982) Neural assemblies. An alternative approach to artificial intelligence. Springer, Berlin

Palm G, Aertsen A (1986) Brain Theory. Springer, Berlin

Palm G, Aertsen AMHJ, Gerstein GL (1988) On the significance of correlations among neuronal spike trains. Biol Cybern 59:1-11

Passingham RE (1975) Delayed matching after selective prefrontal lesions in monkeys (macaca mulata). Brain Res 92:89-102

Perkel DH, Gerstein GL, Moore GP (1967) Neuronal spike trains and stochastic point processes. II. Simultaneous spike trains. Biophys J 7:419-440

Perkel DH, Bullock TH (1968) Neural Coding. Neurosci Res Progr Bull Vol. 6

Perkel DH, Gerstein GL, Smith M, Tatton WG (1975) Nerve-impulse patterns: a quantitative display technique for three neurons. Brain Res 100:271-296

Perrett DI, Rolls ET, Caan W (1982) Visual neurons responsive to faces in monkey temporal cortex. Exp Brain Res 47:329-342

Petrides M (1986) The effect of periarcuate lesions in the monkey on performance of symmetrically and asymmetrically reinforced and auditory go, no-go tasks. J Neurosci 6:2054-2063

Richmond BJ, Optican LM (1987) Temporal encoding of two-dimensional patterns by single units in primate inferior temporal cortex. II. Quantification of response waveform. J Neurophysiol 57:147-161

Rumelhart DE, McClelland JL, and the PDP Research Group (1986) Parallel distributed processing. Explorations in the microstructure of cognition. MIT Press, Cambridge, Mass.

Schillen TB, König P (1991) Stimulus-dependent assembly formation of oscillatory responses. 2: Desynchronisation. Neural Computation 3:167-178

Sompolinsky H, Golomb D, Kleinfeld D (1990) Global processing of visual stimuli in a network of coupled oscillators. Proc Natl Acad Sci USA 87:7200-7204

Sompolinsky H, Golomb D, Kleinfeld D (1991) Cooperative dynamics in visual processing. Physical Rev A 43:6990-7011

Sporns O, Gally JA, Reeke GN Jr, Edelman GM, (1989) Reentrant signaling among simulated neuronal groups leads to coherency in their oscillatory avtivity. Proc Natl Acad Sci USA 86:7265-7269

Stevens JK, Gerstein GL (1976) Interactions between cat lateral geniculate neurons. J Neurophysiol 39:239-256

Toyama K, Kimura M and Tanaka K (1981) Crosscorelation analysis of interneuronal connectivity in cat visual cortex. J Neurophysiol 46:191-201

Vaadia E, Benson DA, Hienz RD, Goldstein MH, Jr. (1986) Unit study of monkey frontal cortex: active localization of auditory and visual stimuli. J Neurophysiol 56:934-952

Vaadia E, Abeles M (1987) Temporal firing patterns of single units, pairs and triplets of units in the auditory cortex. J Isr Med Sci 23:75-83

Vaadia E, Kurata K, Wise SP (1988) Neuronal activity preceding directional and nondirectional cues in the premotor cortex of rhesus monkeys. Somatosensory and Motor Res 6:207-2309

Vaadia E, Bergman H, Abeles M (1989) Neuronal activities related to higher brain functions - theoretical and experimental implications. IEEE Trans on Biomed Engin 36:25-35

Vaadia E, Ahissar E, Bergman H, Lavner Y (1991) Correlated activity of neurons: a neural code for higher brain functions? In: Krüger J (ed) Neuronal Cooperativity. Springer, Berlin, p 249-279

van Gisbergen JAM, van Opstal AJ, Tax AA (1987) Collicular ensemble coding of saccades based on vector summation. Neurosci 21:541-555

Vogels R (1990) Population coding of stimulus orientation by striate cortical cells. Biol Cybern 64:25-31

von der Malsburg C (1981) The correlation theory of brain function. Internal report 81-2. Max-Planck-Institute for Biophysical Chemistry, Göttingen (FRG)

von der Malsburg C (1986) Am I thinking assemblies? In: Palm G, Aertsen A (eds) Brain Theory. Springer, Berlin Heidelberg New York, pp 161-176

Watanabe M (1986a) Prenatal unit activity during delayed conditional go/nogo discrimination in monkey I. Relation to stimulus. Brain Res 382:1-14

Watanabe M (1986b) Prefrontal unit activity during delayed conditional go/nogo discrimination in monkey II. Relation to go and nogo responses. Brain Res 382:15-27

Wise SP, Mauritz KH (1985) Set related neuronal activity in the premotor cortex of rhesus monkeys: effects of changes in motor set. Proc R Soc Lond B 223:331-354

Novel Strategies to Unravel Mechanisms of Cortical Function: From Macro- to Micro-Electrophysiological Recordings

Amos Arieli

The Weizmann Institute of Science, Rehovot, Israel

Background

At what resolution in time does cortical activity make sense? It is clear that different processes occur on different time scales: the micro-seconds to milliseconds scale characterizes direct sensory events, like spatial localization of auditory or visual stimuli (Pulfricht effect). The tens to hundreds of milliseconds scale characterizes attention processes like spotlight of attention, while different states of alertness can last many seconds.

It seems that there is a direct relationship between the time scale and the spatial resolution in cortical activity. The activity involved in a direct sensory process is well defined in small areas; for example an orientation column. On the other hand, an attention process involves huge populations and maybe even the whole cortex.

When we come to investigate the cortex, different electrophysiological phenomena relate to different resolutions in space and time. Two different electrophysiological phenomena have been recorded quite extensively. The first is the recording of action potentials (*spikes*) which reflects the output of single cortical neurons with a time resolution of milliseconds. The second is the recording of the Electroencephalogram (*EEG*), a slow continuous wave which reflects the activity of thousands of neurons and is correlated to the state of the animal (Adrian and Matthews 1934; Elul 1969, 1972; Gevins and Shaffer 1980; Jasper 1981).

Many neurophysiological experiments today are based on spike recordings (Abeles 1982; Krüger 1983). However, comparisons of the quantitative results from psychophysical experiments with studies of single neurons clearly indicate that many aspects of motor function, perception, or other cognitive functions, result from the coordinated action of thousands of neurons yielding a performance greatly exceeding that shown by any individual neuron (Dudai 1989; Georgopoulos et al. 1988; Gray et al. 1989). Thus, while the study of single neurons has revealed their remarkably selective response properties and the functional architecture of some cortical areas, it has become increasingly evident that we should move on to the study of neuronal populations.

Studies of global neuronal activity were popular up to 30 years ago, but their popularity declined as soon as the studies of single neurons became feasible. The study of global neuronal activity was carried out using surface electrodes to record the Electro-Cortico-Gram (*ECoG*), or microelectrodes to record Local-Field-Potentials (*LFP* defined as the local EEG recorded from the tip of the microelectrode). Due to the limited spatial resolution of the recorded waves and due to our lack of understanding of the relation between these waves and the brain cell activity under the electrode, such studies did not advance our knowledge regarding the spatio-temporal organization of activity in neuronal populations.

There is a considerable gap between the knowledge of cortical complexity and the research tools that have been available until now to the investigators. Traditional tools have not allowed detailed examination of the dynamic organization of the cortical neuronal activity in time and space. This gap is one of the reasons for the very limited knowledge about the nature of the processing in the brain.

Research Goal

The aim of this research is to understand the spatio-temporal organization underlying the function of cortical neuronal populations. To accomplish this goal, it is essential to bridge the gap between the recordings of single neurons (microelectrode recordings) and the recordings of large populations of neurons (EEG, LFP or optical recordings).

In the following presentation I will consider two different techniques: multi-microelectrode recordings and real-time optical imaging.

A: The relationships between spike acitivity, LFP and ECoG and the way they reflect the dynamic organization of neuronal populations in the cortex

This work was done together with Prof. M. Abeles and Dr. E. Vaadia (Arieli et al. 1985; 1986).

To approach these questions, experiments were performed in alert muscle relaxed cat. All operations were done under full anaesthesia and the recording began 24 hours later when the cat was fully recovered and alert. Spikes were recorded simultaneously from up to 9 neurons using 6 microelectrodes placed within a 1 mm radius in the cat auditory cortex (using optical methods, I found similar results in the visual cortex). LFPs were recorded from the same microelectrodes, and the ECoG was recorded from above the penetration site. All data were sampled, stored and displayed online by a computer.

A few words regarding our current knowledge about the EEG. The major part of the EEG is the consequence of synaptic input from the thalamus to the cortex, especially to pyramidal neurons. The pyramidal neurons are oriented perpendicular to the surface of the cortex and parallel to each other. This arrangement produces a large electric field that can be recorded from the surface of the brain and from the scalp (Creutzfeldt and Houchin 1974; Elul 1962; Llinas and Nicholson 1974; Scherrer 1976). An EPSP on the apical dendrite near the surface of the brain will produce an inward current into the dendrite and a negative wave on the surface of the cortex, while an EPSP near the soma will produce an outward current in the apical dendrite and a positive wave on the surface. The thalamus projects its activity over large cortical areas, and a high correlation exists between the activity in the thalamus and the EEG in the cortex (Lopes da Silva et al. 1973, 1980; Steriade and Deschenes 1984; Verzeano and Negishi 1960). After cutting the connections to the cortex there is no normal pattern of EEG in the cortex, although the thalamus continues to produce the same patterns of activity (Andersen and Andersson 1979; Creutzfeldt and Houchin 1974; Frost 1974; Steriade and Deschenes 1984). Although the EEG is an effective research tool that reflects the activity in the brain, it is important to emphasize that the extracellular currents expressed in the EEG are a few hundreds times smaller than the intracellular currents, and therefore do not effect the activity of the neurons. In order to understand the relations between LFP and spike activity, the LFP was averaged around the time of the spikes of a single neuron (defined as *Spike Triggered Averaging*). The results showed that:

1. In 88% of the neurons recorded, a significant correlation was found between the occurrence of a spike and the LFP recorded from the same electrode (defined as the *triggering electrode*). In the majority of cases, the average wave is composed of a dip accompanied by a peak (*"typical wave"*).The spike appears near the climax of the dip (Fig. 1). This result indicates that the synaptic activity in the nearest vicinity of the electrode is time-locked to the activity of the neuron (Creutzfeldt and Houchin 1974).

2. The LFPs from different electrodes may have different shapes. However, whenever spikes occur, there is a tendency for a given neuron to have the same shape in the LFPs recorded from different electrodes (Fig. 2). The LFP and the EEG in Fig. 2 were averaged by spikes from unit 1 and 7. The average LFP was triggered by 310 spikes of unit 1 (recorded from channel 1). A significant wave lasting a long time (at least 0.5 sec. before spike and 0.5 after spike) can be observed. A similar wave is seen in all the other traces, except in the ECoG. The average LFP triggered by 312 spikes of unit 7 has a different shape, which is seen in other traces as well.

3. In 64% of the neurons, in addition to the typical wave, an extended positive wave (0.5-1 second) is recorded after the spike occurs. This wave begins and ends in all the neurons where it occurs, at the same time, and it always appears in the average ECoG recorded from the surface of the cortex in an opposite phase. In contrast, the typical wave appears on the surface, if at all, in a weak form and in the same phase (Fig. 2 ECoG).

The question arises: why do we see the average wave in other electrodes? There are two main possibilities:

(a) *Passive transition* - the average wave in the triggering electrode (Fig. 3 E(1)) is produced in the vicinity of the electrode (Fig. 3, radius r1) but is seen at long distances (Fig. 3, radius R1).

(b) *Active transition* - the wave is a consequence of a common input into a large cortical area (the wave is produced both in area r1 and in area r2).

In order to distinguish between these possibilities we have to examine the relations between the average wave in the triggering electrode and the spike activity recorded from other electrodes. If a correlation exists, then the average wave should be produced by a common input to a large area - Active transition. The reason is that the LFP itself cannot influence the activity of neurons. Therefore, spikes which were recorded from distant electrodes (E(2)) and found to be in correlation with the LFP in the triggering electrode (E(1)), result from direct synaptic input to this area (r2). The pattern of this input has a similar shape as the LFP in the triggering electrode (r1). If, on the other hand, the LFP is produced in one area (r1) and is seen at long distances (R1) then the spikes of a neuron in adjacent electrodes (E(2)) would not be influenced by the average wave.

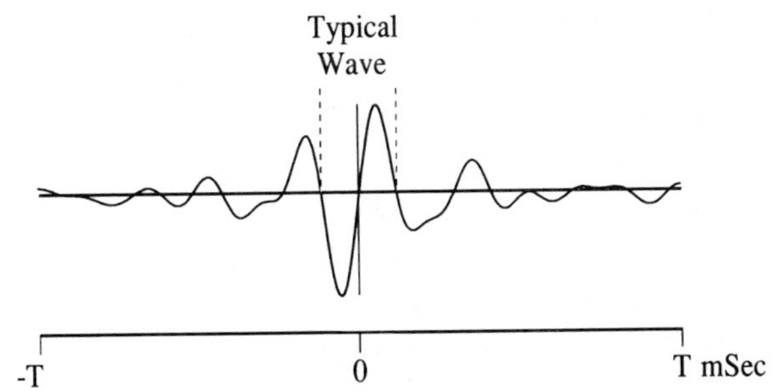

Fig. 1. Schematic description of the "typical wave" in the average LFP triggered by spikes of a single neuron

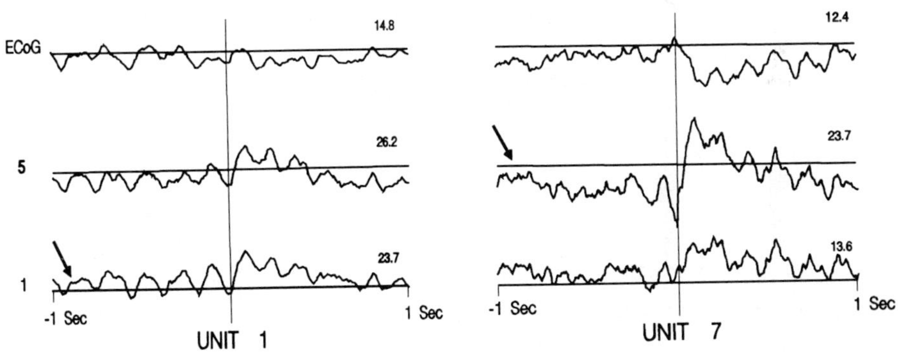

Fig. 2. Two examples, from the same recording, of average LFP and ECoG triggered by spikes of a single neuron: LEFT - average triggered by 310 spikes of unit 1, recorded from Channel 1 (arrow). RIGHT - average triggered by 312 spikes of unit 7, recorded from Channel 5 (arrow). The RMS (IV) is indicated on each trace

Fig. 4 shows the Cross-Renewal-Density (*CRD*) between the time thatspikes occured in neuron 1 or 7, and the time that spikes occurred in all other neurons recorded from other electrodes. If there is no correlation, the spike rate in other neurons would not be influenced by the fact that a spike occurred in neurons 1 or 7 and the result will be a flat CRD. In each trace there is a change in spike rate. The upper trace is the sum of all the other traces (CRD between neuron 1 and neurons 2,3,4,5,6,7 or between neuron 7 and neurons 1,2,3,4,5,6). This CRD suggest that relatively large areas (as big as 2 mm) are working in coordination.

The lower trace in Fig. 5 shows the average LFP in the trigger electrode around spike 1 or 7. The CRD between spikes from unit 1 or 7 and the spikes of neurons from other electrodes is displayed in the upper trace. There is similarity between the two waves: a peak in the CRD lies opposite to a trough in the average LFP. This is in agreement with previous findings that a negative wave in the EEG expresses intracellular depolarization (Creutzfeldt et al. 1966; Frost and Gol 1966; Frost 1974; Jasper 1965). During synchronous EEG (patterns of homogeneous shape observed on extended areas of the cortex typically found in light sleep) the similarity may be extended to long latencies up to 750 msec after a spike occurred. The prolonged decrease in the spike rate is similar to the prolonged positive wave in the average LFP.

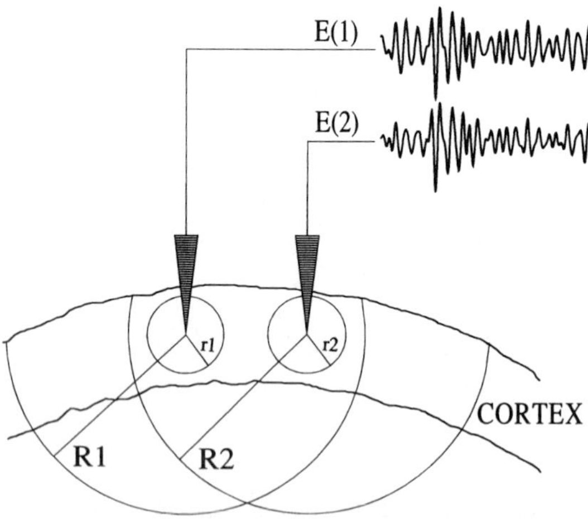

Fig. 3. Schematic description showing active and passive transition of the LFP

These results mean that whenever a spike occurs in a single neuron, there is a tendency in other neurons, recorded in different electrodes, to alter their firing rate. This tendency follows the change in amplitude of the average LFPs triggered by the same neuron. Whenever a spike occurs in a single neuron, there is a tendency in a second neuron to alter its firing rate (the CRD between each pair in Fig. 4). Usually this tendency does not follow changes in the average LFP. However, the tendency of all the neurons to change their spike rate, does follow the average LFP (Fig. 5). (The cross-correlation between spikes of pairs of neurons may have different shapes. However, the shape of the sum of all cross-correlations is very similar to the average LFP triggered around the spikes of the same neuron). This result indicates

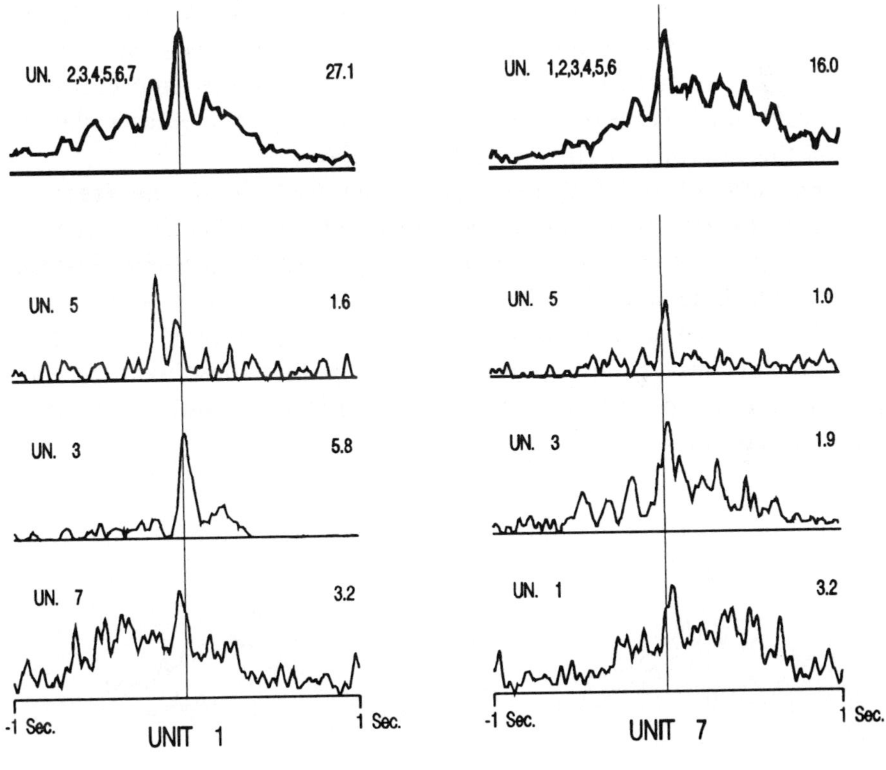

Fig. 4. Two examples of Cross-Renewal-Density between spikes of a single neuron (left - unit 1, right - unit 7 recorded simultaneously) and the spikes of the other neurons. The maximal spike rate (spikes/seconds) is indicated on each trace

that different neurons tend to fire in different, but fixed, temporal relation to the LFP, rather than all neurons altering their firing rates in the same direction at the same time.

In 53% of the neurons a reversed correspondent shape was found between the sum of the different CRDs and the average LFP. In 96% of the neurons a correspondence in shape was found in the prolonged positive wave.

These results imply that the similarity between the average LFP in two electrodes is the consequence of activity in the vicinity of each electrode, and is not due to passive conduction to long distances. There is a combination of depolarizing input - a prolonged depolarizing input to the upper cortical layers (probably through the nonspecific thalamocortical system), in addition to depolarizing input to the vicinity of the cell body (probably through the specific thalamocortical system) (Jasper 1965; Jones 1981; Macchi and Rinvik 1974; Steriade and Deschenes 1984). The prolonged positive wave increases the level of the activity of all neurons in the area, starting a short time before the typical wave until its termination. The typical wave increases the tendency of the neurons to fire in bursts of spikes.

In the state of quiet sleep most of the EEG is in the frequency range of 0-13 Hz. In an alert state most of the EEG is in the frequency range of 14-70 Hz (Noda and Adey 1970; Paisley and Summerlee 1984; Steriade and Deschenes 1984). In both alert and sleeping states, the average spontaneous LFP/EEG (if significant) is composed mainly of slow waves. This points to the fact that these average waves emphasize mainly processes that are also typically found in the cortex being in a state of rest.

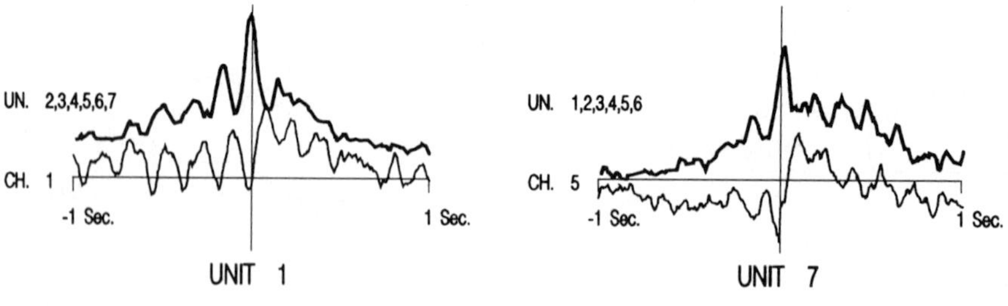

Fig. 5. Two examples of average LFP triggered by spikes of a single neuron (lower trace) and Cross-Renewal-Density between spikes of the same neuron and spikes of the other neurons (upper trace)

In summary, the results indicate that the EEG is generated by very large populations of neurons. Within these populations many weak common inputs exist, each of which drives only some of the neurons in the population. Application of the same analysis to asynchronous EEG further shows that during synchronization there is no increase in the number of the synchronized neurons and in their spike rate. There is, however, an increase in the duration of the coherent activity.

As to other processes that were typically found in an alert cortex, I will only state the conclusions without showing the results:

1. Adjacent areas (1 mm) receive synchronized thalamic input similar in shape and intensity, which changes as a function of distance.
2. The activity of all the neurons is greatly influenced by the intensity of this input, but there is no rhythmical regularity in its intensity and there is no fixed order in the targets that are affected by this input.
3. There is a constant inhibition of neuronal activity that is proportional to the degree of synchronicity of the incoming input.

B: The spatio-temporal organization of neuronal assemblies in the visual cortex revealed by real-time optical imaging

In order to overcome the limitations of classical electrophysiological recordings I used optical imaging techniques in the laboratory of Prof. A. Grinvald. The following presentation is based on the research done together with him (Arieli et al. 1987; Arieli and Grinvald 1988; Grinvald et al. 1989 a,b; Lieke et al. 1989).

Real-time optical imaging is achieved by staining the cortex with a voltage sensitive dye, which binds to the external surface of excitable membranes. The dye acts as a molecular transducer that transforms changes in membrane potential into an optical signal. The resulting changes in the fluorescence of the stained neurons correlate linearly with their electrical activity. Optical imaging of cortical activity provides information about intracellular electrical activity of neuronal populations, including the extensive dendritic and axonal arbors of cortical neurons. Real-time optical imaging offers milli-second time resolution, and spatial resolution of 100 - 200 microns. Thus, optical imaging offers three major advantages: (a) Good spatial resolution.

(b) It provides information about activity in the dendritic arbors, which have important functions in receiving inputs to the neuron. This is unlike single unit or intracellular recording techniques which record from neuronal somata only. (c) Simultaneous recording from 124 sites is feasible.

It is well known that even in primary sensory areas, where sensory input is processed, there is a large amount of on-going (spontaneous) activity - without a sensory stimulus. Little is known about the spatio-temporal organization of this activity, its interactions with stimulus-evoked activity, and its significance to the function of neuronal assemblies.

We have defined a *neuronal assembly* as a group of neurons that cooperate to perform a given neuronal computation. The activity of neurons in an assembly is time-locked (coherent). However, the neurons that comprise an assembly may be spatially intermixed with neurons in other neuronal assemblies that are performing different computational tasks. Therefore, to visualize activity in only one assembly, the spikes of a neuron that is part of that assembly can serve as a source of synchronization for selective visualization. With sufficient averaging, triggered on the spike time of a given reference neuron in an assembly, activity of neurons in other, irrelevant, neuronal assemblies are averaged out.

We have performed a series of experiments in which the spatio-temporal structure of on-going activity and evoked activity were recorded from the same cortex. The visual cortex (area 17,18) of an anesthetized cat was stained with the dye RH-795 (developed and synthesized by R. Hildesheim, at the Weizmann Institute). The cortical activity was monitored continuously for 70 seconds by recording the optical signal from 124 sites simultaneously, the EEG, the LFP and spike activity (from two isolated neurons). Cortical activity was evoked with visual stimuli consisting of a drifting gratings with a fixed orientation.

The spike triggered averaging analysis confirmed the result (see Fig. 1) that single neurons had a tendency to fire at a negative - positive peak of the LFP. In most cases the average optical signal near the electrode site had a positive peak at the same time, indicating that many neurons next to the electrode site were firing coherently. Fig. 6 shows LFP and three optical traces from different cortical loci. The first optical trace (Op. 1), recorded 200 micron away from the electrode site, shows population activity very similar to the LFP: depolarization in the optical recording opposite to a trough in the average LFP. The two other traces show that different components of the LFP originate in different sites on the cortex.

Average optical traces from 124 different loci triggered by spikes of single neurons during on-going activity shows both homogeneity and heterogeneity of the spatio-temporal pattern of on-going optical activity. There is a significant wave over a large area (at least 2 x 2 mm) that coincides with the spontaneous firing of any single neuron recorded.

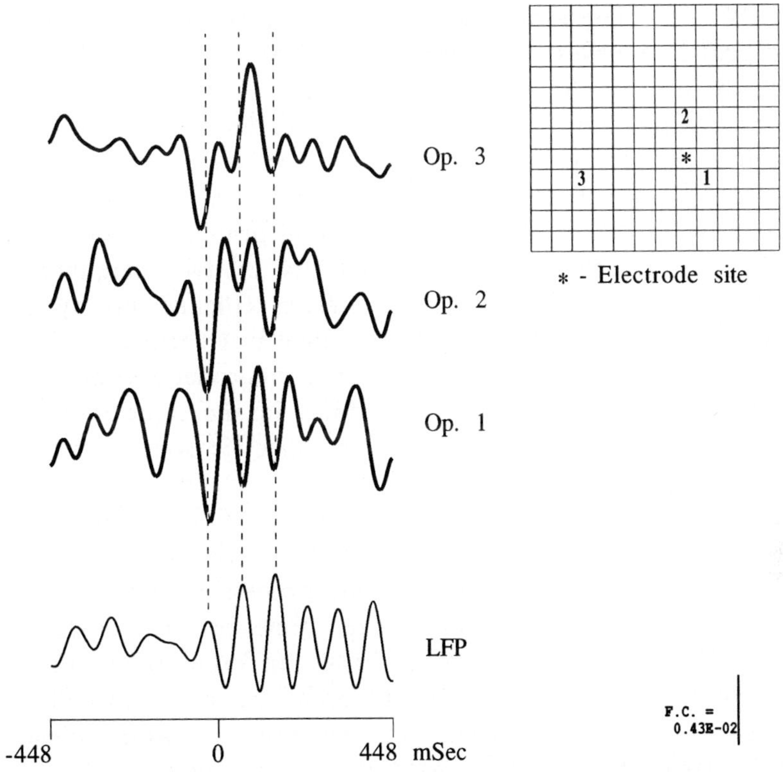

Fig. 6. Spike Triggered Averaging of spontaneous optical and electrical activity triggered by 35 spikes of a single neuron. The scale at the bottom shows the time around the occurrence of the spike. The average LFP shows that the neuron had a tendency to fire at a negative wave followed by a positive wave of the LFP. Three optical traces from different cortical loci are shown at the top. The square in the photodiode matrix marked by "electrode site" is above the penetration site from which the spikes were recorded

Such spatio-temporal maps raise the question: What is the relevance of these waves to cortical activity - or how big is the amplitude of these waves in relation to a different but known phenomena.

Most interestingly, we found that the amplitude of on-going coherent activity recorded optically (per spike used for averaging) was of the same order of magnitude as that produced by activity evoked with an optimal visual stimulus. This result has been a great surprise to investigators who have been studying the cortex primarily with single unit electrodes.

Analysis of segments of the data, grouped together according to the shape of the LFP, indicated that the patterns varied during the recording session (70 sec.). Therefore, these patterns must be dynamic over a short time scale. In order to illustrate the time dependency of the averaged activity spread, the average waves were divided into frames, each one showing the amplitude spread at a given time relative to spike occurrence. Following the different frames we found coherent (time-locked) on-going activity but not synchronous activity - different areas are active at different times, confirming previous results.

We also found that the spontaneous activity of two neighboring neurons, with very similar functional properties (picked up by the same electrode), can be correlated with non-identical cortical regions, suggesting that these neurons belong to different neuronal assemblies.

In conclusion, different neuronal assemblies in the same area can be selectively visualized by the choice of the specific source of synchronization.

The existence of a number of significant modulations in the average waveform is an expression of a process which occurs over a large area several times during the recording. This process includes several events which occur consecutively in a fixed time pattern. Different neuronal assemblies tend to be active at fixed, different times during the process. Neighboring neurons in different neuronal assemblies might participate at different times in the process, while distant neurons may be active at the same time during the process.

During more alert periods, the input which influences the activity of neuronal assemblies does not have a fixed form which repeats itself at different times and in different areas.

Let me conclude my remarks by observing that the results of my research support, in a general way, the approach by R. Elul as expressed in the following quotation: "The thalamus is scanning the cortex. The implication is that the EEG frequency reflects the scanning frequency, and the EEG amplitude reflects the ensemble size. (...) The meaning of reduced amplitude and increased frequency of the EEG ('activation') is, then, a spatial construction of overall (cortex and thalamus) ensemble size in order that a more localized (and smaller) subset may be sequenced more frequently. Increased temporal resolution is obtained by restricting overall nonspecific connectivity. When the environment makes no demands on the organism, its brain can 'idle' its scans now encompassing a spatially expanded or more distributed number of elements but sequencing at slower rate" (Elul 1977).

References

Abeles M (1982) Local cortical circuits - an electrophysiological study. In: Braitenberg V (ed) Studies of Brain Function, Springer-Verlag, Berlin Heidelberg New York

Arieli A, Vaadia E, Abeles M (1985) Local and surface Electrocorticogram demonstrate dynamic organization of cell population in the cortex. European Neuroscience Association, p1

Arieli A, Vaadia E, Abeles M (1986) The behavior of neuronal populations in the cortex. Soc Neurosci Abstr 12:348

Arieli A, Frostig RD, Lieke E, Hildesheim R, Grinvald A (1987) Cortical components of the EEG revealed by real-time optical imaging of neuronal activity in cat cortex. Soc Neurosci Abstr 13:52

Arieli A, Grinvald A (1988) Dynamic patterns of on-going coherent activity in neuronal assemblies revealed by real-time optical imaging in cat cortex. Soc Neurosci Abstr 14:1122

Adrian ED, Matthews BHC (1934) The Berger rhythm: Potential changes from the occipital lobes in man. Brain 57:355-385

Andersen P, Andersson SA (1974) Thalamic origin of cortical rhythmic activity. In: Creutzfeld OD (ed) Handbook of Electroencephalography and Clinical Neurophysiology, Elsevier, 2C:90-114

Creutzfeldt OD, Watanabe S, Lux HD (1966) Relations between EEG phenomena and potentials of single cortical cells: II. Spontaneous and convulsoid activity. Electroenceph Clin Neurophysiol 20:19-37

Creutzfeldt OD, Houchin J (1974) Neuronal basis of EEG waves. In: Creutzfeld OD (ed) Handbook of Electroencephalography and Clinical Neurophysiology, Elsevier, 2C:5-54

Dudai Y (1989) On the complexity of internal representations. In: The Neurobiology of Memory - Concepts, Findings, Trends, Oxford University Press, pp 141-153

Elul R (1962) Dipoles of spontaneous activity in the cerebral cortex. Exp Neurology 6:285-299

Elul R (1969) Gaussian behavior of the Electroencephalogram changes during performance of mental task. Science 18:328-331

Elul R (1972) The genesis of the EEG. Int. Rev. of Neurobiol 15:228-272

Elul R (1977) Oscillating fields and pulse distributions: Relation of neuronal waves to EEG. Neurosci Res Prog Bull 12(1):97-101

Frost JD, Gol A (1966) Computer determination of relationships between EEG activity and single unit discharges in isolated cerebral cortex. Exp Neurology 14:506-519

Frost JD (1974) Physiological bases of normal EEG rhythms. In: Creutzfeld OD (ed) Handbook of Electroencephalography and Clinical Neurophysiology, Elsevier, 6A:150-159

Georgopoulos AP, Kettner RE, Schwartz AB (1988) Primate motor cortex and free arm movements to visual targets in three-dimensional space: (2) Coding of the direction of movement by a neuronal population. J Neurosci 8(8):2928-2937

Gevins AS, Shaffer RE (1980) A critical review of electroencephalographic (EEG) correlates of higher cortical functions. CRC Critical Rev Bioeng 4(2):113-163

Gray CM, König P, Engel AK, Singer W (1989) Oscillatory responses in cat visual cortex exhibit inter-columnar synchronization which reflects global stimulus properties. Nature 338:334-337

Grinvald A, Lieke E, Frostig RD, Arieli A, Ts'o DY, Hildesheim R (1989a) Optical imaging of cortical activity. In: Ottoson D, Rostene WH (eds) Visualization of brain functions, The Wenner Gren Center, Stockholm, pp. 277-289

Grinvald A, Frostig RD, Ts'o DY, Lieke E, Arieli A, Hildesheim R (1989b) Optical Imaging of Neuronal Activity in the Visual Cortex. In: Lam DMK, Gilbert CD (eds) Neural Mechanisms of Visual perception, Gulf Publishing Co, Houston, Texas, pp 117-136

Jasper HH (1965) Intracellular oscillatory rhythms in pyramidal tract neurons in the cat. Electroenceph Clin Neurophysiol 18:541-553

Jasper HH (1981) Problems of relating cellular or modular specificity to cognitive functions: Importance of state-dependent reactions. In: Schmitt FO, Worden FG, Adelman G, Dennis SG (eds) The Organization of the Cerebral cortex, MIT Press, Cambridge, pp 375-393

Jones EG (1981) Functional subdivision and synaptic organization of the mammalia thalamus. In: Porter R (ed) Neurophysiology IV, Intern Rev Physiol 25:174-245

Krüger J (1983) Simultaneous individual recordings from many cerebral neurons: Techniques and results. Rev Physiol Biochem Pharmacol 98:177-229

Lieke A, Frostig RD, Arieli A, Ts'o DY, Hildesheim R, Grinvald A (1989) Optical imaging of cortical activity; Real-time imaging using extrinsic dye-signals and high resolution imaging based on slow intrinsic signals. Annu Rev Physiol 51:543-559

Llinas R, Nicholson C (1974) Analysis of field potentials in the central nervous system. In: Creutzfeld OD (ed) Handbook of Electroencephalography and Clinical Neurophysiology, Elsevier 2B:61-83

Lopes da Silva FH, van Lierop THMT, Schrijer CF Storm van Leeuwen W (1973) Organization of thalamic and cortical Alpha rhythm: Spectra and coherences. Electroenceph Clin Neurophysiol 35:627-639

Lopes da Silva FH, Vos JE, Mooibroek J, van Rotterdam A (1980) Relative contributions of intracortical and thalamo-cortical processes in the generation of Alpha rhythms, revealed by partial coherence analysis. Electroenceph Clin Neurophysiol 50:449-456

Macchi G, Rinvik E (1974) Thalamo-telencephalic circuits: A neuroanatomical survey. In: Creutzfeld OD (ed) Handbook of Electroencephalography and Clinical Neurophysiology, Elsevier, 2A:86-133

Noda H, Adey WR (1970) Firing variability in cat association cortex during sleep and wakefulness. Brain Res 48:513-526

Paisley AC, Summerlee AJ (1984) Relationship between behavioural states and activity of the cerebral cortex. Prog in Neurobiol 22:155-184

Scherrer J (1976) Organization of spontaneous electrical activity in the neocortex. Prog in Brain Res 45:309-325

Steriade M, Deschenes M (1984) The thalamus as a neuronal oscillator. Brain Res Rev 8:1-63

Verzeano M, Negishi K (1960) Neuronal activity in cortical and thalamic networks. J Gen Physiol Suppl 43:177-195

Neuronal Population Coding and the Elephant

George L. Gerstein[1] and Paul M. Gochin[1,2]

[1] Dept. of Physiology, University of Pennsylvania, Richards Bldg. G-4, Philadelphia, PA 19104, USA
[2] Dept. of Psychology, Princeton University, Princeton, NJ, USA

We examine several ways to study representation of external events by a population of neurons. It is useful in the laboratory to consider this as a clustering problem, but it is not clear whether and how the brain accomplishes a similar result. In particular there is a problem in selecting which neurons are to be included in the population analysis.

Introduction

Popular wisdom in neurobiology readily accepts that population codes and computations are essential to the operations of the nervous system. One portion of these concepts that is at least partially accessible to experiment is the relation between stimulus and response at the population level. The desired relationship must be understood in both directions. A population code or representation is the response to the presentation of a stimulus (the direct problem), but equally, this code or representation must be "read" in order to let the organism detect and discriminate the stimulus (the inverse problem).

The basic arguments that suggest the need for population processes are based on (a) the "noisiness" of individual neuron responses to presentations of repeated identical sensory stimuli, and (b) the rather high dimensionality required to describe the various aspects (parameters) of a stimulus.

In the type of single neuron experiments that have been both possible and popular for some thirty years, the usual approach to dealing with the noisy response problem is to make a stimulus time locked average (the PST histogram) over something like thirty to fifty repetitions of the presentation. But of course, behaviorally we can get a reaction from the organism in just a single presentation of the stimulus. Ignoring all the details, this contrast suggests that the nervous system must take an equivalent population average over some number of neurons. This should produce a statistically clean result in one stimulus presentation with the same type of information that we can obtain in the laboratory from the single neuron over many presentations. The assumption that these two forms of average are the same is a restatement of the Ergodic Hypothesis, and of course holds exactly only under conditions of strict stationarity which are rarely if ever obtained in the nervous system.

One of the striking omissions in this type of thinking is the assumption that the ubiquitous variability of response is just noise and that it carries no information. Another assumption is that the "average response" over time or over population exists and is meaningful and available to the operations of the nervous system.

We now examine the dimensionality required for stimulus description in terms of the conventional single neuron experiment. The response is a (noisy) temporal pattern of firing (or of probability for firing) in response to a particular stimulus presentation. As the stimulus parameters are varied, we observe systematic (but noisy) changes in the temporal pattern as well as in the total amount of firing. Can this firing pattern from a single trial be uniquely associated with a particular stimulus (both in the direct and inverse sense)? One approach that uses the entire temporal pattern of the single neuron response is the principal components analysis of Richmond et al. (1987). Here the averaged responses to a limited but orthogonal family of (visual) stimuli are used to calculate a set of principal components. Each response can then be described (or decomposed) into a "spectrum" of contributions from the waveforms of these first few principal components. The effect of this process is to make a multi-dimensional description of the response, which hopefully may be uniquely associated with a similarly multi-dimensional description of the stimulus. The entire complex process is however rather noisy, so that such methods using data from one neuron alone are not likely to match behavioral performance for the inverse problem. A population process must be invoked even if we accept that a biological brain can compute and store something like the principal components of a family of responses.

This paper will examine some of the difficulties in understanding population coding schemes starting from single neuron data, and will also show that population codes can be thought about in several very distinct ways, each of which may be quite incomplete. The elephant in the title refers to the ancient story about the attempts of several blind men to characterize the whole creature, with rather diverse results reminiscent of the neurobiological problem we want to examine. Above all, we will raise some questions about how the nervous system can learn to use population codes for representation and computation.

Computational ideas

It will be convenient at this point to ignore the detailed temporal patterns of a neural response. We can return to them later in a number of ways. For the moment, let us characterize a response from a neuron by its total firing counted over some appropriate time window following the stimulus presentation. In addition we will assume in all the following that response properties are approximately stationary (although with variability across trials), and in particular that there is no plasticity that imposes a systematic evolution of the observed value of the response measure.

Receptive field or parameter space description

One popular description of neural response is to plot the total firing as a function of one or more stimulus parameters. Each stimulus parameter can be treated as an orthogonal coordinate value; this may be an abstraction, or may represent actual spatial or other appropriate variables that are important stimulus parameters. Note that this requires assumptions about which stimulus parameters are chosen to be significant. The usual choices are those descriptors which are "simple" in the laboratory, but of course these may not be the most appropriate for the computations going on in the brain.

The simplest such representation is with a single stimulus parameter. Here we might idealize the receptive field (i.e. the response of each neuron as a function of the stimulus parameter) in the form of a constant multiplying a Gaussian of some variance, and centered at the parameter value where that neuron responds most vigorously. (Obviously more complex shapes of receptive fields do exist.) With a population of such neurons, there is a multiplicity of overlapping receptive fields, i.e. a series of such "hills", each centered at a different value of the stimulus parameter, and possibly with a different width (variance) and height (strength). For each value of the stimulus parameter, these curves define the firing level that results for each neuron. With sufficient neurons, there is a unique "spectrum" of firing in the population for each value of the stimulus parameter, so that the inverse problem is in principle at least quite soluble (see Erickson 1963; Hinton et al. 1986; Vogels 1990 for discussions of accuracy and resolution in the representation).

With two stimulus parameters, the receptive fields could be idealized as possibly non-isotropic hills, each centered at the appropriate (2-dimensional) location on the plane of stimulus parameter values. Again, much more complex receptive field shapes can be observed in experiments. Note that in some cases such a description becomes a map of the receptor sheet, as in considering the x-y location of a stimulus on retina or body surface. However, even in the visual and somatosensory systems which are spatially mapped in an orderly way, other stimulus parameters are at least equally important, and their inclusion in the receptive field definition makes direct map interpretation considerably more difficult. As in the simple one-dimensional case above, each pair value of stimulus parameters calls out firing from the several neurons as defined by the several overlapping Gaussian hills. Again the "spectrum" of firing in the population is unique for the particular stimulus parameter values, so that the inverse problem should be soluble.

Note that in this class of receptive field representation, there is an intrinsic ambiguity for each single neuron in examining the inverse problem. Even in the one-dimensional simple Gaussian receptive field case, a given firing level (the response index) corresponds to two possible values of the stimulus parameter. With higher dimensionality (say N) of receptive field (i.e. more stimulus parameters), we note that the firing level remains a one-dimensional variable, so that at best it can define an N-1 dimensional curve or surface on each of the N-dimensional response hills. It is precisely these ambiguities that are removed for the inverse problem by dealing with the "spectrum" of firing from all available recorded neurons. The useful population for this purpose are only those neurons which show some degree of overlap of receptive fields in the stimulus parameter region of interest. A number of different methods for combining the firing of the observed neurons have been proposed. In those situations where the parameter space describes 2- or 3- dimensional physical space, it has been convenient to use vectorial addition or averaging processes. Such operations in the parameter space yield a single resultant vector that represents the activity "spectrum" of the entire population of observed neurons (Georgopoulos et al. 1988; Van Gisbergen et al. 1987; Lee et al. 1988)

We should now consider the problems caused by the observed firing variability in any one trial or stimulus presentation. The receptive fields we have been discussing above are themselves measured as averages over many trials at each of many values of the stimulus parameters. Therefore there is a measured variance at each point of the receptive field. This means that the inverse problem is in fact much more complex than noted above, since a given observed level of firing of a neuron can at best only be probabilistically assigned to some region of the receptive field. Depending on the direction that the variabilities of the several observed neurons took on this trial, we may get an "inconsistent" spectrum, so that the inverse problem is truly not soluble, or that we get erroneous results.

As a final comment on the receptive field approach to stimulus identification, we should note that it is *only* available to *us* in the laboratory, and that only after a lot of calibration experiments have been done. It seems extremely unlikely that this is a computational process directly available to the nervous system, since it requires storing a response profile over all possible stimulus parameters for each neuron. On the behavioral level however, some familiarity with the range and quality of possible stimuli is usually required for reliable performance, so that the required calibration data might be acquired in the course of experience.

It is appropriate to examine the relation between the receptive field approach to stimulus identification (which involves something like a map in an abstract stimulus parameter space) and the existence of direct sensory maps. Such geometric maps exist in many levels of the visual, somatosensory and auditory systems. In the first two systems they are characterized by a direct (although distorted) spatial mapping of the receptor sheet, so that a stimulus at a given x-y location calls out changed neuron activity in a limited region of a more central sheet in relay nucleus or cortex. Additional stimulus variables are also often represented in such maps, and take the form of stripes within the basic x-y organization. In the auditory system, such systematic x-y organization can represent more complex attributes of the stimulus than location on the receptor sheet, as in the cortical maps of doppler shift or echo delay in the bat. In all such mapped systems we might idealize the result of a spatially punctate (or other limited) stimulus to be a spatial distribution of activity in the population of the neuronal sheet, with neurons at the appropriate map point being the most active.

In this type of mapping, both the direct and inverse problem of stimulus representation within the mapped variables are automatically solved by the limited locus of activity. There would seem no need to invoke complicated population schemes. However, not all neurons in sensory systems are arranged in such orderly maps; for example, in higher levels of the visual system (like infero-temporal cortex) there is no visuotopic order. And even when geometric mapping is present, note that only a very limited number of additional stimulus parameters are mapped (not much more than 2). In general, geometric maps, even when they exist, are not enough for accurate stimulus representation, and it remains necessary to invoke population coding to deal with more complicated stimulus attributes.

Firing space description

There is a different approach to the information representation contained in the firings of a population of observed neurons which is "model free", does not require the calibration implicit in receptive fields, and above all does not require a priori assumptions about significant stimulus variables. Here we create a fictitious N-dimensional space for N observed neurons, and lay off the observed firing level of each of these neurons along its own (for the moment orthogonal) dimension. Thus the population response to each trial or stimulus presentation is represented by a single point in the N-dimensional space, with coordinate values corresponding to the firing levels of each neuron in the whole observed population. With repeated presentations of the same stimulus, the firing variability will create a cloud of points (one for each trial) in the N-space. Repeated presentations of a different stimulus (i.e. different values of the appropriate stimulus parameters) should call out somewhat different firing in the population of neurons, and hence will create a somewhat different cloud of points in the N-space. The extent to which these two clouds do or do not overlap determines the extent to which a single trial can identify the stimulus parameter values. In other words we are now dealing with a standard clustering problem, although there remain a number of difficulties.

For convenience we might calculate the center of gravity of each cluster, and some appropriate variance measure for its size. If the spacing of the centers is larger than the cluster diameters, the stimulus parameters can be uniquely identified by the firing "spectrum" across the population. If the clusters do overlap, the stimuli are only probabilistically distinguishable with this population of neurons.

We may still explore the stimulus parameter space with the N-dimensional firing space representation, although we do not need to decide a priori what the relevant stimulus parameters are. Since each stimulus (with its set of parameter values) corresponds to a particular response cluster, we may use a vector to the cluster center to "describe" the stimulus. A "distance" between (i.e. subtraction of) two such vectors can evaluate what is (or what is not) a significant change in the stimulus. The inner (dot) product of the two vectors can also be used as a measure of stimulus similarity (Di Lorenzo 1989). We may find that the stimulus parameters which are most easily defined in the laboratory for technical reasons are in fact not the most useful and orthogonal for producing distinguishability of the firing clusters in the firing space. Combinations of such "simple" parameters may turn out to be more natural descriptors of the stimulus; the search for appropriate combinations however is generally not trivial, and amounts to an "eigenvector" or principal components analysis in the firing space.

In the simplified form of vector space representation so far considered we have implicitly assumed that the firing variability of each of the neurons is independent. If this is not the case, it may be appropriate to depart from the assumption of orthogonal coordinates (i.e. a cartesian N-space). Under some circumstances we might better describe and separate the point clusters relative to a new, still cartesian, but rotated coordinate system. In such a case the optimal information descriptors in the population are combinations of individual neuron firing rates.

Results

We now illustrate some of the above ideas using data obtained from infero-temporal (IT) cortex of monkeys (Gochin et al. 1991). Separable extracellular recordings of several neurons at a time were obtained by standard methods (multiple tungsten microelectrodes, eye coils to monitor eye position) in a series of sessions with a conscious, attentive monkey. The task required fixation of a target light while various visual patterns were presented at various nearby locations in the visual space. No behavior based on the patterns was required; liquid reward was given for adequate fixation during the trial presentation. The patterns used were of the "Fourier descriptor" type (Zahn and Roskies 1972; Schwartz et al. 1983). These patterns were used only because it has been demonstrated that IT neurons are reactive to them. Further experimental details are given in Gochin et al. (1991).

Known properties of IT cortex neurons are reviewed in Gross et al. (1985). This cortex is generally accepted to be the highest level of the visual form processing system. Individual neurons, which are not retinotopically arranged on the cortex, have extremely large spatial receptive fields which usually include the fovea, but are hard to characterize in terms of any other obvious stimulus parameters or characteristics. The one exception to this seems to be a small population of neurons that appear to be sharply tuned to faces, sometimes even in particular orientations (Gross et al. 1972; Rolls and Baylis 1986). Most IT neurons respond to a variety of complex shapes, frequently with invariance of response to retinal location, stimulus size or contrast. The reponses do show some stimulus selectivity, but this is hard to quantify. These properties have led to the hypothesis that IT function can only be understood in terms of neural assembly processes and ensemble coding (Gross et al. 1985; Rolls 1987).

The receptive field or parameter space description of the ensemble firing of IT neurons is not directly useful because the stimulus parameters that would define an appropriate space can not be specified. Therefore, we now examine the description based on the firing space, as defined above. In the simplest variation of this idea, we will ignore all temporal details of the neuronal firing patterns, and will define the response of each neuron as a simple spike count over some appropriate time window following upon the stimulus presentation in each trial.

We assign an orthogonal cartesian coordinate dimension to each of the simultaneously observed neurons, and for each trial use the several observed spike counts to define a single point in the space. A tutelary example of this process using artificial spike trains is shown in Fig. 1 for two simulated neurons. The points representing individual trials form three clusters according to which of the three stimuli was presented (and which corresponding response spike counts occurred). As in real data, a certain amount of variability was placed into this simulation, so that the clusters show some considerable dispersion.

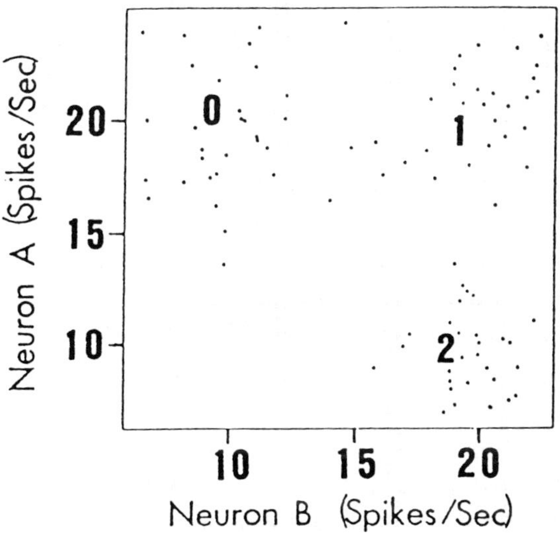

Fig. 1. Linear scatter plot of the joint response of two simulated neurons under three stimulus conditions (*0*, *1* and *2*). Responses were measured as average firing rates over an appropriate time window in each trial. Each point represents a separate trial with the presentation of one of the three stimuli

Note however that neither of these simulated neurons alone can code all three stimuli uniquely: each neuron can distinguish one of the three stimuli, but produces identical activity for the two other stimuli. It is only when the activity of both neurons together in an ensemble code is considered that all three stimuli can be uniquely identified in this firing space description.

In dealing with real IT data, generally more than three neurons were simultaneously recorded. Thus the simple kind of geometry shown in Figure 1 for two neurons is not possible. We need another tool to determine whether there has been clustering of points according to stimulus in the N-dimensional firing space, where N is the number of observed neurons. In this paper we will use non-linear mapping to project the original N-dimensional firing space to a two-dimensional space for visual inspection (Sammon 1969). This algorithm minimizes

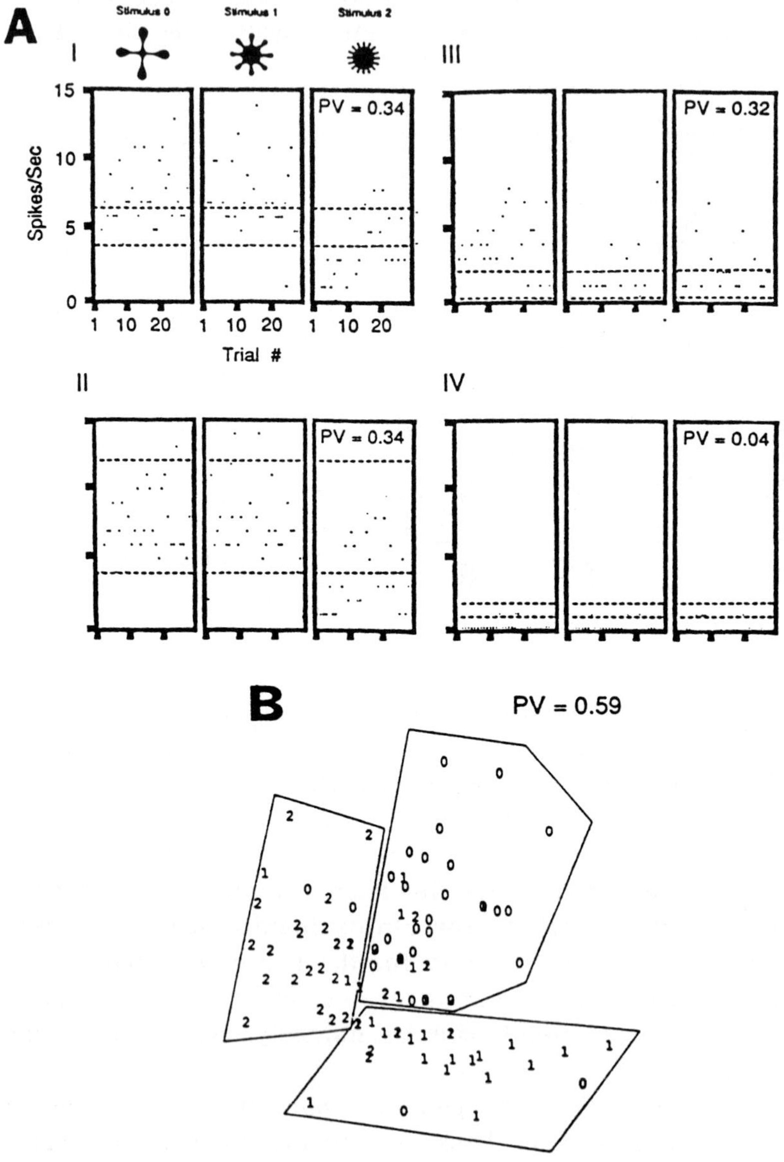

the difference in total interpoint distances between the original and projected spaces in such a way that small interpoint distances are maintained at the expense of large interpoint distances. The distances are computed with a Euclidian metric, and a steepest descent calculation is used to search for the minimum change. The two dimensions with the largest variance in the original N-space are used for the initial (geometric) test projection.

We emphasize that non-linear projection is being used here for illustrative purposes; it is not necessarily the optimal way to detect and quantify clustering in the N-space. However, in spite of its various defects as a method, we will be able to use it as a vehicle to examine some of the inherent problems that the brain faces in using population coding.

We demonstrate the non-linear mapping process in Figure 2 B for four simultaneously recorded IT neurons subjected to three different visual stimuli over 79 trials. Each point in the projection (corresponding to a single trial) has been labelled with its proper stimulus identification (0-2). The apparent (but imperfect) clustering is emphasized by the manually drawn polygons which (more or less) define the region to which a majority of the points of a given stimulus class projects. (Note that since the polygons are defined manually, there is no guarantee that they are in any way optimal for achieving the best segregation of the numbered points; however, the process gives results that seem quite reasonable.) It is now necessary to define a numerical estimate of the quality of stimulus identification and segregation both for the single neuron and for the assembly of neurons analyzed

---

Fig. 2. Analysis of a group of four simultaneously recorded real IT neurons. **A**: Responses at each trial of the individual neurons (*I-IV*) sorted according to which of the three stimuli (0, 1, 2) had been presented. The abscissas identify the successive occurrences of a given stimulus; stimuli were actually presented in a repeating sequence of 0, 1, 2. Reproductions of the three stimuli are shown above the plot for neuron I. The horizontal dashed lines show the locations of the optimal partitions for each neuron. Note that neurons I and II could not distinguish stimulus "0" from stimulus "1", while neuron III could not distinguish stimulus "1" from "2"; neuron IV could not identify any of the stimuli. **B**: Non-linear mapping of the joint response of the four neurons; The numbers represent the stimulus which had been presented in a given trial. The three (manually drawn) polygons delineate the clusters associated with each of the three stimulus conditions

through the N-dimensional firing space and its projection. In both single and assembly situations we can use the following definition of a "partition value":

$$PV = \frac{1}{M}\left[\sum_{i=1}^{s} c_i - \sum_{i=1}^{s}\sum_{\substack{j=1\\ j\neq i}}^{s} \frac{w_{ij}}{(s-1)}\right]$$

where

PV = partition value, which satisfies $0 \leq PV \leq 1$
c_i = number of correctly classified stimulus type i trials
w_{ij} = number of stimulus type i misclassified as type j
s = number of different stimulus types
M = total number of trials over all stimuli.

This metric for the quality of stimulus identification takes account both of errors of incorrect inclusion and of exclusion.

When we apply the metric to the responses of a single neuron, we need to set several (s-1) thresholds on the firing levels in the responses to define the zones that correspond to each of the stimuli. There are no known independent criteria for the correct response of a given neuron to a given stimulus condition. Therefore we exhaustively try all possible boundary assignments and assume that those which produce the highest numerical partition values are the "correct" assignments.

When we apply the metric to the responses of an assembly of neurons as analyzed in the N-dimensional firing space and the non-linear projection method, the stimulus boundaries have already been defined, and application of Equation 1 is straightforward.

The quantification of stimulus identification by the "partition value" for the data shown in Figure 2 gives the rather unsurprising result that PV = 0.59 for the assembly, while the best of the neurons individually achieves only PV = 0.34. Thus, by the particular measure here defined, the neuronal assembly can do a better job of stimulus identification than can any of its constituent neurons. This result is generally true in the IT material reported here, consisting of 13 groups of three to eight simultaneously recorded neurons. However, we note that the group partition values varied over a fairly wide range, so that not all the observed neuronal groups were performing at an equal level in the stimulus identification problem.

As in almost all measurements of both individual and group neuronal response to a precisely repeated stimulus, the material here showed variations from presentation to presentation. It is appropriate to inquire whether this is a confounding factor in the above analysis, and whether there is a significant benefit in observing the simultaneous (rather than sequential) responses of the neurons in a group. In other words, how much do we in the laboratory gain in studying population coding principles by doing technically demanding recordings of simultaneous and separable spike trains. (Of course, for the brain, such parallel information is presumed to always be available, and not technically demanding.) We examined these questions by shuffling the data on stimulus presentation boundaries so that the N-dimensional firing space construction and subsequent non-linear projection and partition value measurement was carried out on different presentations (of each type of stimulus) for each of the observed neurons; this shuffle destroys any detailed timing relations among the observed neurons, and leaves only the stimulus imposed modulations of response. Under this manipulation, partition values for most of our simultaneously recorded neuronal groups were little changed. This suggests that, at least to a first order approximation, we may ignore the simultaneous recording aspect of the data, and study the combined population of all available neuronal data taken using the given family of stimuli.

The somewhat disconcerting result of analyzing all our data as a single lump is shown in the projection of Figure 3A. Clearly, this is a disorganized jumble of numbers which allow no polygons to define stimulus-segregated regions. By contrast, if we reduce the population to the six neuronal groups that had the highest partition values (32 neurons), the projection gives the excellent results of Figure 3B, with PV = 1.0. Thus the population coding performance of a large group of "appropriate" neurons considerably transcends the performance of the several subgroups, which in turn do considerably better than any of the individual neurons. In turn, the inverse problem of population coding (the N firing patterns of a single trial to be uniquely associated with a particular stimulus) can be solved with excellent accuracy *in the laboratory*, provided the "appropriate" group of neurons is observed and analyzed.

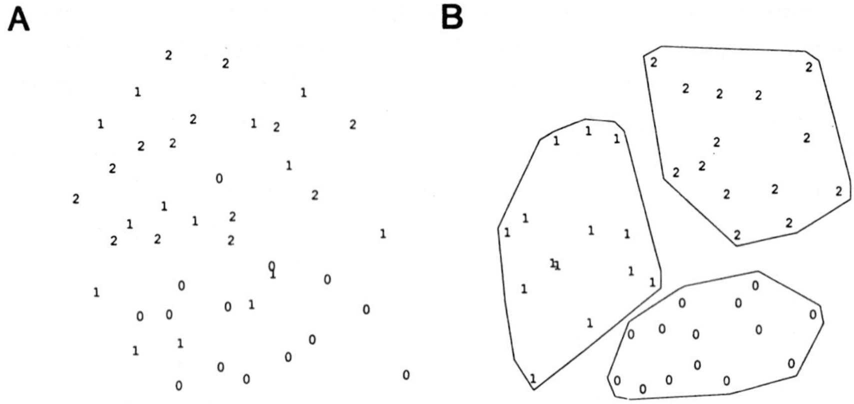

Fig. 3. Analysis of a larger neuronal population formed by combining the (smaller) groups that had been simultaneously recorded. This procedure means that the contributions of any detailed neuronal timing relationships to the population coding process will be ignored. **A**: Non-linear map of the joint responses of all 67 neurons. **B**: Non-linear map of the joint responses of the 32 neurons from the 6 groups with the highest group PVs

Discussion

The result that inclusion of certain neurons into the analyzed population degrades the stimulus identification process in our laboratory analysis requires some explanation. We could at this point call into question the concept of firing space as a descriptor. However, if we accept the firing space, then the degradation, in fact, is an artifact of the particular cluster detection method that we have used. The reasons lie in the preservation of interpoint distances by the projection algorithm. An ideal method would show improved identification as some neurons are added to an initial population (as we have seen above), but would never show degradation for any additional neurons. Practical methods however, would always run into a signal/noise problem as irrelevant neurons are added to the analyzed population.

Consider a two neuron example to clarify this aspect of cluster analysis. Suppose one neuron produces three distinctly different levels of response to the three stimulus types, i.e. its individual performance is already at the PV = 1.0 level. Now suppose that the second neuron in our example population has nothing whatever to do with the stimulus: it fires randomly at various rates, and produces a broad range of counts in the appropriate time windows defined by the stimulus presentations. The firing of this second neuron can be characterized as variable, and not discriminating of the stimulus types. If we construct the two-dimensional firing space for these data with the discriminating neuron graphed along the abscissa and the non-discriminating neuron graphed along the ordinate, we will observe three distinct distributions of points along the abscissa, and much elongated along the ordinate. It is obvious that points lying within a single such cluster may be much farther from each other than they are from points in one of the adjacent parallel, elongated clusters. Hence a distance preserving projection rule like the non-linear projection algorithm is inappropriate and causes an artifactual degradation of the group partition value. A proper clustering analysis method for such data would in effect ignore, or average out the point dispersion along the ordinate, and hence would preserve the excellent stimulus identification that is determined by the clustering along the abscissa. The central point to be taken from all this, however, is that there are some neurons which help in forming a population code, and other neurons which are irrelevant to it. Obviously in the random selection of neurons inherent in normal extracellular experimental methods, typical data will include both types of neurons in a continuum of "relevance" to the problem. (In the example we have described just above, we chose the extreme of a completely "irrelevant" neuron; neurons with sufficiently low PV would pose the same difficulties). Thus the data and several analyses presented above suggest that we may divide our observed neurons into a "useful" and a "noise" or "irrelevant" category.

We have so far only considered the problem of population codes as determined by data analysis in the laboratory. The real problem, however, is to understand how the brain itself could carry out such an N-dimensional clustering process, dealing properly with the selection of those neurons which are to be included and those which are to be ignored or devalued in the calculation.

An extremely useful concept for dealing with ensemble properties of brain networks is the Hebbian Assembly. This is defined (Hebb 1949) as a network of neurons that has formed a significant synaptic connectivity through operation of some form of (possibly modified) Hebb plasticity rules. Such a group of neurons, whose association has formed through use in some specific problem or calculation, may lie spatially interspersed with other neurons which belong to other or to no Hebbian Assemblies. It seems appropriate to examine the possibility that those of our recorded neurons that can be shown to contribute to an improvement in the group stimulus partition value are members of a particular Hebbian Assembly, while those neurons that do not so contribute are members of a different Assembly. If this situation could be verified, it would automatically provide the necessary internal selection mechanism for the "relevant" neurons, since there would be very little connection between the networks of "relevant" and "irrelevant" neurons.

The present existence of such Hebbian Assemblies would leave unknown the mechanisms of their original creation and growth. We are, however, dealing with data obtained during an extremely well practiced and familiar fixation task involving presentation of only a limited family of stimuli. These data were not obtained during the learning phases of the behavioral task where all stimuli and indeed the situation was novel. We additionally should note that the behavioral situation did *not* require discrimination or any other cognitive assessment of the stimuli. Thus we have no independent proof that the nervous system was making a discrimination; we can merely examine whether the proposed coding mechanisms could in principle suffice for the purpose.

Neurons that belong to a particular Hebbian Assembly should by definition exhibit stronger coupling to other members of the same assembly than to arbitrary neurons outside the assembly. The appropriate tools for assessing the strength of interconnections are based on cross-correlation of pairs of spike trains. In its simplest form, the cross-correlation measure will show peaks corresponding to favored timing relations in the two spike trains. The width, shape and temporal offset of such peaks, together with appropriate control calculations can be used to specify an "effective connectivity" between the two observed neurons. This is the simplest possible circuit that would produce the observed cross-correlation; additional interneurons could always be invoked. The components of such a circuit can be parsed into (a) direct connection between the observed neurons, (b) shared input (from unknown sources) to the observed neurons, and (c) stimulus input (i.e. a known source) to the observed neurons. We emphasize that such a circuit is not necessarily the anatomical connectivity, but may be a subset of it. These methods, along with the appropriate controls and various extensions are reviewed in (Gerstein et al. 1983; Krüger 1983; Abeles 1982; Eggermont 1990).

We have used the clustering properties of our observed neuronal population in the firing space, as described above, to define two groups of neurons. The activities in one group can contribute information to a population code. Activities in the other group are irrelevant to the stimulus representation and may introduce noise into the code. If the "relevant" and "irrelevant" neurons are members of separate Hebbian assemblies, we would expect that there will be more and stronger signs of connections within each group than between them. It is of course possible that the "irrelevant" neurons are actually distributed among several different assemblies. In this case we would expect signs of connectivity to appear mainly within the "relevant" group. We will therefore want to examine cross-correlations of spike train pairs selected to be "relevant"-"relevant", "relevant"-"irrelevant", and "irrelevant"-"irrelevant".

Although the data set examined in this paper consists of some 64 neurons, of which 32 neurons were "relevant", the data were actually recorded in various smaller groupings. Thus, for purposes of cross-correlation, we are limited to the pairs within such smaller groupings rather than examining all possible pairs among the full data set. We show separately the counts for direct connection (narrow peaks) and for shared input (broad peaks), but we lump these to calculate the percentage of all cross-correlations in each "relevance" category which show peaks beyond those attributable to stimulus effects. The following Table shows the results.

	"narrow peaks"	"broad peaks"	neuron pairs	total percent
"R"-"R"	11 (18.96%)	11 (18.96%)	58	37.93
"R"-"I"	2 (7.41%)	5 (18.52%)	27	25.93
"I"-"I"	12 (16.67%)	14 (19.44%)	72	36.11

We note first of all from the neuron pairs column that there is some tendency for the "relevant" and the "irrelevant" neurons repectively to cluster spatially, since there are relatively less "mixed" pairs in the simultaneous recordings. (The simultaneous group recordings were obtained with closely spaced electrodes, i.e. from relatively small sample volumes "randomly" placed within IT cortex.)

Examining the total percentages of the last column we have the rather surprising result that the "relevant" neurons have roughly similar overall likelihood of showing connectivity with "irrelevant" neurons as with other "relevant" neurons. There may of course be a sampling problem here, since the overall number of pairs in each category is not all that large. And we note that the percentage of direct connections (narrow peaks) for the "R"-"I" category does seem lower, although with very inadequate statistics. But if we accept the rough equality of percentages in the last column, this means that the "relevant" neurons do *not* clearly form an assembly distinguished in terms of stronger connectivity as measured by the standard cross-correlation tools.

We can now reiterate the central functional problem to which this paper has lead us: How does the brain select the particular neurons whose activity is to be used in a population code? And how is this population code computed and interpreted?

If the brain carries out a computation which is functionally roughly like the clustering operation in the firing space that we have described above, it is clearly advantageous to include relatively few "irrelevant" neurons in the clustering process simply for better signal-noise performance. This is extremely evident in the nonlinear projection method of clustering which we used for illustrative purposes. Obviously more appropriate methods exist (both in the laboratory, and for the brain itself), but they are all subject to the signal-noise problem.

We can attempt to trivialize the non-appearance of Hebbian assemblies among the "relevant" neurons by suggesting that all our data is obtained from a single more or less functionally homogeneous layer in a multi-layer computational process. In such a model, the actual assembly would involve convergence of our observed neurons onto neurons in another layer elsewhere, and that could not be detected unless recordings were also made there simultaneously. This kind of picture, however, seems incompatible with the wide variety of receptive field types and property detectors that are ordinarily found among contiguous cortical neurons; it does seem likely that fairly complex (multi-layer) operations are carried out fully within a given small patch of cortex.

Another possibility is that neurons form dynamic (i.e. temporary) assemblies that are specific to a particular stimulus rather than to the analysis of a particular stimulus-class. This would suggest that we should seek differential patterns of effective connectivity for each individual stimulus condition. Note that such analysis may ignore the "relevant"-"irrelevant" distinction between neurons that we have made above.

The appropriate calculations could not be done for the data reported here for statistical reasons; it was necessary to compute the cross-correlograms for a particular neuronal pair across all stimulus conditions in order to obtain adequate counts. However such analyses have been carried out on recordings from a number of different cortical areas studied in a number of laboratories. The results have been partly reviewed in (Gerstein 1988; Aertsen and Gerstein 1991) and indeed demonstrate the frequent occurrence of stimulus specific effective connectivity, i.e. that organization of observed neurons varies dynamically with stimulus (and context or other ancillary conditions). This situation could be named "grandmother assemblies", where the assembly is called into being by modulation of effective connectivity by the particular stimulus-related activity of both observed and (possibly nearby) unobserved neurons.

Finally, we should remove the restriction on time structure that we imposed early in this paper. We have so far specified response only as the total firing count in an appropriate time window after the stimulus presentation. Clearly this can be generalized without difficulty, so that we consider a sequence of shorter time windows after stimulus (or before behavior). There are the usual statistical problems here, since the shorter these windows are taken in order to improve the time resolution the worse will be the counting statistics. There is a reasonable region of compromise, however; windows of about 100 ms for the IT data presented in this paper clearly show the growth and decay of whatever clustering there is in the response as examined in the firing space description. Even better time resolution has been reported for vectorial operations in the property space description of neuronal firing (Georgopoulos 1989).

Conclusions

At this point these experiments have raised more questions than given answers about population coding. Again we note the logical similarity to the problem of describing the elephant using only local tactile information.

We have seen that neuronal firing across a population, assessed in an appropriate time window, can function as population code in the laboratory. A cluster analysis process can serve as detector and discriminator of what such a code represents. However, adequate performance in this analysis requires that most of the data come from a selected set of neurons (which are by this criterion identified as "relevant" to the process). The inclusion of data from many "irrelevant" neurons always degrades performance by an amount that may depend on the details of the clustering algorithm.

However, the "relevant" neurons do not clearly seem to form a distinguishable assembly. If it existed, such an assembly would be associated with the discrimination process of the particular set of stimuli being presented, and would represent a significant building block of cortical computation.

Cluster analysis is certainly appropriate in the laboratory, but may not at all correspond to the process carried out by the nervous system. We are therefore still left with the problems of (a) determining how the brain actually analyzes population codes, and (b) assuming that there is a signal to noise problem, how the brain selects which neurons to analyze for a given population code discrimination process. It is easy to suggest, but not obviously correct, that experiments which record larger populations, make longer recordings and introduce appropriate discriminative behavioral design represent the desired strategy.

References

Abeles M (1982) Local Cortical Circuits, Studies of Brain Function Vol. 6, Springer, New York

Aertsen AMHJ, Gerstein GL (1991) Dynamic aspects of connectivity: fast stimulus-locked modulations of "effective connectivity". In: J Krüger (ed) Neuronal Cooperativity. Springer, New York

Di Lorenzo PM (1989) Across unit patterns in the neural response to taste: vector space analysis. J Neurophysiol 62:823-833

Eggermont J (1990) The Correlative Brain. Springer, New York

Erickson RP (1963) Sensory neural patterns in gustation. In: Zotterman Y (ed) Olfaction and taste. Pergamon, Oxford pp 205-213

Georgopoulos AP, Kettner RE, Schwartz AB (1988) Primate motor cortex and free arm movements to visual targets in three-dimensional space. II. Coding of the direction of movement by a neuronal population. J Neurosci 8:2928-2937

Georgopoulos AP, Lurito JT, Petrides M, Schwartz AB, Massey JT (1989) Mental rotation of the neuronal population vector. Science 243:234-236

Gerstein GL, Bloom M, Espinosa I, Evanczuk S, Turner M (1983) Design of a laboratory for multineuron studies. IEEE Trans on Systems, Man and Cybernetics SMC-13:668-676

Gerstein GL (1988) Information flow and state in cortical neural networks: Interpreting multi-neuron experiments. In: v.Seelen W, Shaw G, Leinhos R (eds) Organization of Neural Networks. VCH Verlagsgesellschaft, Weinheim, pp 53-86

Gochin PM, Miller ER, Gross CG, Gerstein GL (1991) Functional interaction among neurons in inferior temporal cortex of the awake macaque. Exp Brain Res (in press)

Gross CG, Rocha-Miranda CE, Bender DB (1972) Visual properties of neurons in inferotemporal cortex of the macaque. J Neurophysiol 35:96-111

Gross CG, Desimone R, Albright TD, Schwartz EL (1985) Inferior temporal cortex and pattern recognition. In: Chagas C, Gattass R, Gross CG (eds) Pattern recognition mechanisms. Springer, New York pp 179-201

Hebb DO (1949) The organization of behavior. Wiley, New York

Hinton GE, McClelland JC, Rumelhart DE (1986) Distributed representations. In: Parallel distributed processing. Explorations in the microstructure of cognition. Vol. 1: Foundations. MIT Press, Cambridge, MA. pp 77-109

Krüger J (1983) Simultaneous individual recordings from many cerebral neurons: techniques and results. Rev Physiol Biochem Pharm 98:177-233

Lee C, Rohrer WH, Sparks DL (1988) Population coding of saccadic eye movements by neurons in the superior colliculus. Nature 332:357-360

Richmond BJ, Optican LM (1987) Temporal encoding of two-dimensional patterns by single units in primate inferior temporal cortex. II. Quantification of response waveform. J Neurophysiol 57:147-161

Rolls ET, Baylis GC (1986) Size and contrast have only small effects on the responses to faces of neurons in the cortex of the superior temporal sulcus of the monkey. Exp Brain Res 65:38-48

Rolls ET (1987) Information representation, processing and storage in the brain: Analysis at the single neuron level. In: Changeux JP, Konishi M (eds) The neural and molecular basis of learning. Wiley, New York pp 503-540

Sammon JW (1969) A nonlinear mapping for data structure analysis. IEEE C18:401-409

Schwartz EL, Desimone R, Albright TD, Gross CG (1983) Shape recognition and inferior temporal neurons. Proc Nat Acad Sci 80:5776-5778

Van Gisbergen JAM, Van Opstal AJ, Tax AJ (1987) Collicular ensemble coding of saccades based on vector summation. Neurosci 21:541-555

Vogels R (1990) Population coding of stimulus orientation by striate cortical cells. Biol Cybern 64:25-31

Zahn CT, Roskies RZ (1972) Fourier descriptors for plane closed curves. IEEE C14:271-291

Is Spike Frequency the Critical Factor in Recognising the Visual Stimulus?

J. Krüger and J. D. Becker

Neurologische Universitätsklinik, Hansastrasse 9, 7800 Freiburg, Germany

Our aim was to investigate how visual stimuli could most reliably be recognised on the basis of the spike patterns they evoke in the striate cortex. Recording simultaneously with an array of 30 microelectrodes (Krüger and Bach 1981; Krüger and Aiple 1988) from various cortical layers of five vervet monkeys, we wondered how reliable was spike frequency coding (Adrian 1932), and which was the role of the response time courses.

A well-known instance where frequency coding is assumed is the orientation selectivity of visual cortical cells (Hubel and Wiesel 1968): typically, a burst of spikes is only evoked when a bar stimulus is optimally oriented. The textbook interpretation is that the high frequency of spikes signals the presence of a line whose orientation matches the angular preference of the cell (see e. g. Kuffler et al. 1984). To test this idea, we have examined how moving bars with different orientations could be recognised from the activity of 30 neurones.

The responses to bars moving in 16 different directions were examined. The recognition procedure was straightforward: We characterised each of the 16 stimuli by its average pattern ("template") of responses from the 30 electrodes. Several additional presentations of the same stimuli were then used as tests. With the aid of a correlation measure we compared the single, non-averaged test response patterns with each of the 16 templates. The template found to be most similar to the test pattern defined the recognised stimulus. Our aim was to find out how to obtain the highest score of *correct* recognitions. To this end

- we subdivided the relevant response interval into bins of various widths so that spatio-temporal patterns with different time resolutions could be tested,
- we normalised the spike frequencies in various ways, and
- we subtracted the resting discharge rates.

Starting from the idea of frequency coding, we firstly used only a single bin encompassing the entire relevant response interval. Counting the spikes in this interval confidently reproduced the information contained in the usual orientation tuning plots, but to our surprise, even in recordings where a large fraction of the cells had pronounced orientation and direction selectivities, only 10 to 20 % of the stimuli could correctly be recognised, with the chance level being at 6.25 %. Different normalisations or the removal of non-oriented neurones did not appreciably improve the situation. As a control, we examined the variances of the response patterns: indeed, two presentations of the same stimulus yielded patterns that on the average differed nearly as much from each other as those evoked by two different stimuli.

The score of correct recognitions rose considerably in all monkeys and layers, when the responses to each stimulus at each electrode were characterised by the counts in *several* smaller time-bins. Each response pattern was then represented by a total number of bin counts equalling 30 times the number of bins.

The more detailed circumstances of optimal recognition were as follows: irrespective of the total duration of the response interval, there was a broad maximum of the number of correctly recognised stimuli when the bin widths ranged between 20 and 100 ms. Larger as well as smaller values resulted in a deterioration of the recognition. The distributions of the percentages of correct identification are exemplified in Fig. 1 for layer VI. The four curves indicate that the effect of different normalisations is a minor one (see legend). However, it is remarkable that the rate of correct recognitions barely exceeds the chance level when the time structure is not taken into account (rightmost data points)

A maximum of correctly recognized stimuli was regularly found in a range of time resolutions around 50 ms in all layers and also for other stimuli such as large coloured fields turned on and off.

To emphasize the point we want to make, in a next step we conserved the temporal information but deliberately deteriorated the frequency information: all bin counts >1 were replaced by 1. Essentially the performances were reduced to a half but they clearly remained above the single-bin cases.

The reason for the outcome of our experiments is the following: it is well known that cortical neurones show a considerable response variability unrelated to stimulation. To explain the reliability of

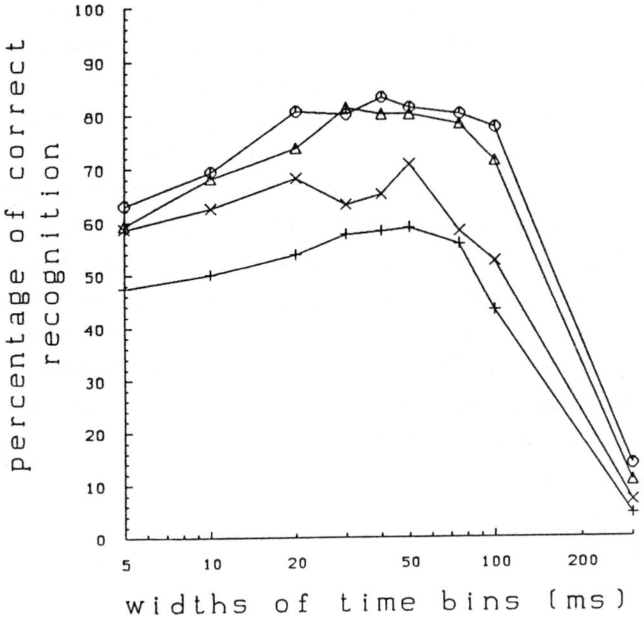

Fig. 1. Percentages of correct recognition for different time resolutions (abscissa) and different normalizations (symbols). The rightmost data points correspond to the case of "spike frequency coding", i. e. one time bin encompasses the entire relevant response interval. Results are shown for four different normalizations, ranging from the most to the least successful ones. The spike train of each neurone was treated independently. Templates and tests were treated identically. Symbols: *o*: non-normalized data; *triangles*: normalization by the square root of the average spike rate; *x*: normalization by the maximal average bin count; +: normalization by the average spike rate. For each of these four cases the subtraction of the ongoing spike rates had very little effect

frequency coding, it is thought that in the nervous system relevant information is carried by signals averaged over several similarly reacting cells (Burns 1968).

However, we reject the implicit association of neuronal variability with noise because most of what appears to be variability is more likely to be significant information from non-retinal sources (Doty 1980; Livingstone and Hubel 1981) which in addition we have found to be highly organised in space (Bach and Krüger 1986).

Extending the ideas of others (Barlow 1972; Eckhorn and Pöpel 1974, 1975; Shaw et al. 1986; Optican and Richmond 1987) we conclude from the present experiments that the neuronal signal contents is segregated into *meaning*, carried by temporal structures of spike trains, and *importance*, carried by spike frequencies. Not only is the information capacity more optimally used but also the segregation offers the opportunity for central instances to modulate the importance of selected components of the meaning without altering the meaning itself. This is possible, as we have seen, because the limited requirements of temporal accuracy allow for considerable differences in spike density.

It is clear that the high frequency portions are the critical structures of spatio-temporal spike patterns since they are most resistant to suppression by extraretinal sources. Therefore we believe, as others have before us, that the essential information about a tilted line is represented by the high frequency responses of optimally stimulated oriented neurones. The new aspect is that one should not *count* these spikes in order to determine the tilt angle.

Acknowlegdements

This work was supported by the Volkswagen Foundation (Schwerpunkt "Synergetik").

References

Adrian ED (1932) The Mechanism of Nervous Action. University of Pennsylvania Press, Philadelphia

Bach M, Krüger J (1986) Correlated neuronal variability in the monkey's visual cortex revealed by a multi-microelectrode. Exp Brain Res 61:451-45

Barlow HB (1972) Single units and sensation: A neuron doctrine for perceptual psychology? Perception 1:371-394

Burns BD (1968) The Uncertain Nervous System. E Arnold Ltd., London

Doty RW (1980) Non geniculate afferents to striate cortex in macaques. Exp Brain Res 41:A10-11

Eckhorn R, Pöpel B (1974) Rigorous and extended application of information theory to the afferent visual system of the cat. I. Basic concepts. Kybernetik 16:191-200

Eckhorn R, Pöpel B (1975) Rigorous and extended application of information theory to the afferent visual system of the cat. II. Experimental results. Biol Cybern 17:7-17

Hubel DH, Wiesel TN (1968) Receptive fields and functional architecture of monkey striate cortex. J Physiol London 195:215-243

Krüger J, Aiple F (1988) Multi-microelectrode investigation of monkey striate cortex: spike train correlations in the infragranular layers. J Neurophysiol 60:798-828

Krüger J, Bach M (1981) Simultaneous recording with 30 microelectrodes in monkey visual cortex. Exp Brain Res 41:191-194

Kuffler SW, Nicholls JG, Martin AR (1984) From Neuron to Brain, 2nd edn. Sinauer Inc., Sunderland Massachusetts pp 68-69

Livingstone MS, Hubel DH (1981) Effects of sleep and arousal on the processing of visual information in the cat. Nature 291:554-561

Optican LM, Richmond B (1987) Temporal encoding of two-dimensional patterns by single units in primate inferior temporal cortex. III. Information theoretic analysis. J Neurophysiol 57:162-178

Shaw GL, Silverman DJ, Pearson JC (1986) Trion model of cortical organization: toward a theory of information processing and memory. In: Palm G, Aertsen A. (eds) Brain Theory. Springer, Berlin pp 177-191

Independence

Horace B. Barlow

Physiological Laboratory, Cambridge CB2 3EG, UK

In my paper in this volume I argue that a representation that is to be efficient at detecting associations should use elements that are normally active independently of each other. Only then is it practical to detect efficiently associations with objects or events represented by *conjunctions* of elements, because it is only when they are independent that the prior probability of such a conjunction can be easily computed. For this reason I can't refrain from drawing attention to the fact that those who have solved the difficult technical task of recording simultaneously from two units and measuring their dependence, often find that the cross-correlograms are virtually flat. This is in a sense disappointing, but it seems to me an astonishing and important fact that is very difficult to explain *without* postulating a mechanism that deliberately encourages independence.

In V1 there are about 100 times as many neurons as input channels. Even if there were no interconnections between neurons this would imply that every neuron shared a large fraction of its input with other neurons, and one would expect correlations on that score. In fact a very large fraction of the excitatory input to a pyramidal cell comes from other pyramidal cells in the vicinity, so how does it come about that this positive interconnection between neurons does not show up in the cross-correlograms? The anti-Hebbian interconnections we postulate seem to provide an explanation that should be explored further by the following types of experiment.

There are two rather definite predictions from the hypothesis proposed. First, the mechanism that promotes independence would be affected by exposure to the strongly redundant patterns that produce pattern specific adaptation. For instance exposure to a grating for a period of a few minutes should increase the mutual inhibition (or decrease the mutual excitation) between two units tuned close to the orientation and spatial frequency of the adapting grating, and this should show up clearly in the cross-correlogram between two such units. Exposure to constant movement in one direction should produce the same effects on directionally selective units.

Experiments testing short term adaptation effects of this sort should be rather easy to perform. It would be more difficult to test the effects of deprivation in the sensitive period, but here again the predictions are clear. It is hypothesised that the derangements of function caused by deprivation results from the inappropriate reinforcement of Hebbian synapses that occurs in the absence of sensory inputs containing their normal statistical structure. It is the decorrelating mechanism, combined with the Hebbian connections, that normally causes units to become selectively sensitive to different regions of the pattern space. Hence one would expect unusual correlations between the firings of units in the cortex of such deprived animals.

Single Cells versus Neuronal Assemblies

Horace B. Barlow

Physiological Laboratory, Cambridge CB2 3EG, UK

Introduction

I wrote a paper almost 20 years ago (Barlow 1972) that was intended to promote the approach to brain function at the level of single neurons, and to act as an antidote to the view that, since there are so many cells in the brain, it is useless to consider what a single one of them does. Though it was aimed at those who advocated the "mass action" approach, in which one records evoked potentials in the hope that the averaged activity of many cells will be meaningful, quite a lot of what I said still seems to me correct and relevant, though what I then regarded as the unenlightened opposition now tends to put its faith in "neuronal assemblies" and "synfire groups" instead of "mass action". Perhaps its therefore worth raising some of the points again.

One can argue that a single cell provides too small a unit for describing brain function since anything of importance depends upon hundreds or thousands of cells acting together. That already seemed implausible in 1972, when it was known with reasonable confidence that single retinal ganglion cells could signal weak lights as well as a whole cat could detect them (Barlow et al. 1971), and I think the view has become totally untenable in the light of the results on cortical neurons obtained by Tolhurst et al. (1983), Parker and Hawken (1985), Barlow et al. (1987), and particularly from the recent results of Newsome et al. (1989) on cells in MT.

Briefly, Newsome et al. recorded from single neurons and tested the behavioural discriminations of awake behaving monkeys while performing the task of discriminating the direction of coherent motion of a small proportion of dots masked by many incoherently moving dots. They found that many cells in MT could detect as low a proportion

(<5%) of coherently moving dots as could the monkey. Now to perform such a task well one must collect together information about motion over just the right area of the visual field, and avoid contamination by information about motions in other directions and from other parts of the visual field. This is precisely what is done by the projective zones of neurons in V1 and V2, together with the cell's own dendritic connections.

Analysis at the single unit level thus gives a satisfactory account of how a difficult task of this sort is done, and it seems absurd to suggest that some mysterious neuronal assembly is doing the same task, and that such an assembly is required to enable the monkey to do it. For such assemblies we have nothing equivalent to receptive field or trigger feature to explain how they gather together the relevant information, and nothing as well defined as a projective zone to tell us the destination of information about their activity. But the concept of a neuronal assembly does bring up interesting possibilities.

Possible importance of joint activity

If you say that a cell is a member of a "neuronal assembly", or a "synfire group", the important new possibility is introduced that the significance of its firing is not fixed, but changes according to the other cells that are concurrently active, just as the significance of one bit in an ASCII code depends upon the other bits active. That is a very important possibility, but it does not seem to me incompatible with a description of a unit's receptive field or trigger feature. It would mean that these could not be as simple as linear weighting functions, and that they might not correspond to simple environmental objects or events, but whatever the complexity of the combinatorial rules governing the unit's activity in the neuronal assembly, a description in environmental terms would still be possible, just as it is possible (though laborious) to describe the significance of a bit in an ASCII code by a list of the alpha-numeric characters that activate it. Furthermore it is such a description that most directly indicates the utility of the bit in the code, and similarly it is such descriptions (i.e. accounts of receptive fields or trigger features) that would most directly indicate the utility of a neural unit to the animal's brain.

Precision of timing

For the reasons given above the idea of assemblies and groups does not seem to me to have been helpful in understanding how the brain deals with spatial patterns or performs other difficult computational tasks, but for the temporal domain the emphasis on precision of timing must be very important. Much of the quantitative work on cortical neurons, including that quoted above, counts impulses over rather long periods (1/2 to 2 secs) and uses that count as the measure of the cell's activity. But there are psychophysical tasks that require precision of timing at least two orders of magnitude better - down to less than a millisecond. This is very clearly indicated by experiments in which the misalignment of moving verniers is detected. A misalignment can be detected with a precision of about 6 seconds of arc, even when the vernier is moving over the retina at about 2 degrees per second (Westheimer and McKee 1975). At that speed this spatial offset is equivalent to a temporal offset of less than a millisecond, and it can be shown directly that such a temporal offset in a moving vernier produces an identical perceptual effect to the equivalent spatial offset (Burr 1979). This judgement is unlikely to be based on discriminating an interval between two impulses in one single neuron, so here is a clear case where the activities of two (or more) neurons must be taken into account.

Sparse coding

The results quoted above from retina, VI, and MT do not prove that pontifical cells or grandmother cells exist, but I think they do prove that single cells are reliable and can perform important tasks. I coined the term "cardinal cell" to encapsulate the idea that "the sensory system is organised to achieve as complete a representation of the sensory stimulus as possible with the minimum number of active neurons". In the neural network literature this type of representation is called "sparse coding" (probably a better term than "cardinal cells", with fewer misleading connotations), and the results on the rarity of activation of cortical cells in ordinary use reported by Vaadia in this meeting certainly seem to support the idea that the cerebral cortex is organised to achieve such a representation.

I think it is true as a matter of historical fact that descriptions of receptive fields and trigger features have been much more informative about the organisation of higher brain functions than have descriptions in terms of assemblies and groups. I take that as an indication that, as you proceed to higher levels, neurons do in fact come to have more and more fixed correspondencies with external objects and events, and that these correspondencies depend less and less on the other neurons that are concurrently active. The results of Perrett et al. (1984; see also Barlow et al. 1990) certainly seem to confirm this. Critics who are upset by this apparent support for grandmother neurones or pontifical cells have usually failed to appreciate the following point.

Images of grandmothers and high priests would be very poor primitives with which to represent the real world, except perhaps for those individuals who live in a retirement home for popes and old ladies. But the concept of cardinal cells or sparse coding includes the idea that the representation must be as *complete* as possible, as well as having few active units at any one time. This means that specifying the selectivities of these higher level units is a very difficult problem, and one that we do not know how to do, but that does not falsify the principle of representation that their specification is thought to achieve.

Sub-cellular levels

Should one perhaps analyse the brain at a finer, more detailed level than that of single unit activities? In 1972 it was already apparent that single synapses or synaptic complexes were capable of complex feature detection (see for example Dowling 1970; Koch et al. 1986). This means that analysis at the subcellular level is necessary to understand biophysical mechanisms, even in the case of such a simple example of pattern recognition as directional selectivity. But it still remains true that what is transmitted to other destinations in the brain is the activity of the whole cell, not the activities of separate synaptic complexes on that cell; hence analysis at the single cell level still gives one the information that is required in order to understand how the brain as a whole works, even though analysis at sub-cellular levels may be required to elucidate the mechanisms by which it does it.

References

Barlow HB (1972) Perception 1:371-394

Barlow HB, Kaushal, Hawken, Parker (1987) J Opt Soc Amer A 4:2366-2371

Barlow HB, Levick, Yoon (1971) Vision Res 11: suppl. 3:87-101

Burr (1979) Vision Res 19:835-837

Dowling (1970) Invest Ophthalmol 9:655-680

Barlow HB, Blakemore C, Weston-Smith EM (1990) (eds) Images and Understanding. Cambridge University Press, Cambridge, pp 94-107

Koch Ch, Poggio T, Torre (1986) TINS 9(5):204-211

Newsome, Britten, Movshon (1989) Nature 341:52-54

Parker and Hawken (1985) J Opt Soc Amer A 2:1101-1114

Perrett et al. (1984) Human Neurobiology 3:197-208

Tolhurst et al. (1983) Vision Res 23:775-785

Westheimer G, McKee (1975) J Opt Soc Amer 65:847

which works, even though working at sub-cellular levels may be required to elucidate the mechanism by which it does it.

References

Neurons as Computational Elements

Horace B. Barlow

Physiological Laboratory, Cambridge CB2 3EG, UK

Introduction

In order to show why the concept of receptive fields has given so much insight into brain function it may help to take a more comprehensive view of the computational task that single neurons perform.

Neurons have *dendrites* that receive input information, and it is the details of these connections, together with the properties of the other neurons that supply the input, that form the cell's *receptive field* or *trigger feature*. But it is other properties of neurons as computational elements that give special significance to receptive fields and trigger features, so I'll start by describing these other properties.

Projective zones

A neuron does not broadcast indiscriminately to all other parts of the brain whenever its dendrites are effectively tickled, but signals selectively to a particular zone, and perhaps to particular cells within that zone. Because it requires tedious anatomical study to find the details of these projective zones, less is known about them than about the receptive fields and trigger features of single neurons, but I believe this capacity to address the result of the dendritic computation to a particular subset of the other neurons in the brain is extraordinarily important.

Distinguishing signal from noise lies at the heart of the tasks where computer programs stumble and make foolish mistakes, while our brains perform with effortless ease. This is true of object recognition, and must also be true of learning and association formation, and countless other tasks requiring skill and judgement such as playing tennis. Now if you consider what limits the performance of *any* difficult detection, discrimination, or learning task you will see that it is likely to be the collection of the appropriate information. This is because the efficient solution of any signal/noise discrimination requires that the detector be matched to the signal to be detected, so that *all* the relevant information is available, and *only* that information, uncontaminated by noise from other sources. Though I am not suggesting they do it perfectly, neurons have the right kind of structure and organisation to perform this task, and their selective addressing capabilities expressed by their *projective zones* are a key factor enabling them to do it (for more on this topic see Barlow 1981, 1986; Communication; The Darwin Lectures H. W. Mellor and P. Johnson-Laird (Ed.), Cambridge University Press, 1990).

Modifiability

The second important feature of a neuron as a computational element is *modifiability by experience*: neurons do not perform fixed tasks, but ones that can be changed according to circumstances. This is not the place to attempt to summarise such changes, but the fact that they take place is important in considering the utility of receptive fields.

Receptive field or trigger feature

Sherrington described the region and type of cutaneous stimulation that would excite the scratch reflex in a spinal dog as its "receptive field", and this is probably the earliest use of the term. As everyone knows Hartline (1940) used it to describe the limited area of retina that excites a specific ganglion cell, and many others have used it in that sense since then. Some people have assumed that inhibitory influences should not be taken into account in defining the receptive field, especially if such inhibition does not produce any detectable effect on the discharge of the neuron in the absence of concommitant excitation. Others have assumed that the term implies a simple weighting function expressing how a neuron linearly combines influences from different points. Neither of these restrictions is implied by Sherrington's usage, and I cannot see any point in limiting use of the term in these ways, though the distinctions about inhibitory influences and linearity are of course very important. Perhaps the term "trigger feature" that Levick, Hill and I introduced (1964) should be used in this more general sense, for it captures the following merit of descriptions at the level of receptive fields.

To discover how the brain performs the difficult tasks it does perform it is important to know what the cells are telling each other. If one had an exact account of the properties of the neurons that act as inputs to a given unit, and of the effectiveness of the synapses from each of them, then one could in principle calculate how that unit would respond to any environmental stimulus. But that would be a clumsy and laborious way to understand what messages it was passing on to the neurons that it, in its turn, communicates with. The concept of the receptive field or trigger feature short-circuits all of that calculation and gives you the required information directly, because it describes what excites a neuron using terms from the environment, rather than attempting an exact neurophysiological description. Thus it tells you directly the fuctional consequence of its pattern of dendritic connections, and that seems to me a valuable simplification.

Changes in receptive fields can be used to describe the plasticity of neurons, so the concept is also valuable in giving an account of a neuron's modifiability (see for instance Barlow et al. 1957; Hubel and Wiesel 1970; Rauschecker and Singer 1981).

When projective zones and modifiability are included in our view of the computational role of neurons the importance of receptive fields becomes quite clear: they summarise what information a particular cell gathers together and this is the crucial factor in determining what tasks the brain can perform efficiently. They will continue to be important in showing us how the brain organises its operations.

References

Barlow HB (1981) Critical limiting factors in the design of the eye and visual cortex. Proc Roy Soc B 212:1-34

Barlow HB (1986) Why have multiple cortical areas? Vision Res 26:81-90

Barlow HB, FitzHugh, Kuffler S (1957) J Physiol 137:338-354

Hartline (1940) Amer J Physiol 130:690-699

Hubel DH, Wiesel TN (1970) The period of susceptibility to the physiological effects of unilateral eye closure in kittens. J Physiol 206:419-436

Levick, Hill, Barlow HB (1964) J Physiol 173:377-407

Rauschecker JP, Singer W (1981) The effects of early visual experience on the cat's visual cortex and their possible explanation by Hebb synapses. J Physiol 310:215-239

Some Quantitative Remarks about the Retina, the Primary Visual Cortex, and Visual Perception in Humans

Christian Wehrhahn

Max-Planck-Institut für biologische Kybernetik, Spemannstrasse 38, 7400 Tübingen, Germany

Introduction

Psychophysics was founded in the middle of the 19th century as a scientific discipline with the goal to relate the mental processes to the physical world. In vision, on the basis of psychophysical experiments, many predictions were made about the physiological mechanisms underlying perception. Physiologists started to study vision independently without the necessity to find a psychophysical interpretation for their results and a lot of physiological as well as anatomical work on the retina and the visual parts of the central nervous system was carried out without direct reference to perception. At the same time an analogous development took place in psychophysics: perception became a subject to be studied in its own right. In this paper I would like to link visual perception and physiology as closely as possible.

Insofar as vision contributes to perception, changes in the electrical activity of the brain can be attributed to the signals transmitted by retinal ganglion cells to the brain. The optics of the eye, the geometrical arrangement of the photoreceptors, the electrical properties of the signals generated by light in the retinal network and many other details need to be considered before a simple understanding of the role of neural function in perception may be achieved. This understanding will still be at a level very far from higher cognitive processes or even consciousness. Those who want to go beyond should refer to Crick and Koch (1990).

Perception and hardware

Patterns of light are imaged by our optical apparatus in the retina on a mosaic of around $1.25 \cdot 10^8$ rods and $6.4 \cdot 10^6$ cones (Osterberg 1935). The three cone classes found in the primate retina preferentially respond to red, green or blue light respectively. Quantal absorption transduces light flux into electric current across the photoreceptor membrane. For the light adapted eye the relation between changes in light flux and changes in current across the membrane is linear within two orders of magnitude (Baylor et al. 1974).

Cones (as well as rods, but we will not consider them here) are connected synaptically to the bipolar cells: they show two properties essential for our present purpose:

1) Bipolar cells specifically respond to a light increment (ON bipolars) or to a light decrement (OFF bipolars).
2) In a primate cone light signals may be discriminated in a range of about 50 steps of intensity at each level of adaptation. Surprisingly, in bipolar cells only up to 15 intensity steps may be reliably discriminated. The cone signals are represented in the bipolar cells band pass filtered in time and space. Generally speaking, the information content of the biploar signal is reduced compared to the cone signal.

Bipolar cells in monkeys make contact with about 1 million retinal ganglion cells per eye connecting the retina to the brain. In an ON-centre ganglion cell an increase in light intensity in the center of its receptive field will elicit a spike discharge. Correspondingly in an OFF-centre ganglion cell a decrease in light intensity will cause the cell to respond. Remarkably (and possibly as a consequence of property 2) described above for the bipolar cells) at any given luminance level a ganglion cell will fire a spike at an almost fixed time delay after being stimulated with a (sufficiently large) light increment or decrement respectively.

The response of a retinal ganglion cell to an increment or decrement in light is either tonic (in seven out of eight cells) or phasic (in the remaining cells) (Silveira and Perry 1991). In the fovea each cone is linked to one ON-center and one OFF-center tonic ganglion cell. Tonic cells always respond specifically to light of a certain range of wavelengths. In contrast, phasic cells appear to be "color blind". The dichotomy between phasic and tonic retinal ganglion cells has intrigued many visual neuroscientists during the last decade (Valberg and Lee 1991; Zeki and Shipp 1988).

The majority of ganglion cells projects to the LGN, the first relay station in the central nervous system. In the LGN the ganglion cell signals are relayed to cells connected mostly to the primary visual area (V1) of the cortex. In the monkey for each relay cell leading from the LGN to the cortex there is one and only one retinal ganglion cell from which this relay cell receives its input (Lee et al. 1983; de Monasterio and Schein 1987).

Cortical processing and perception of motion

The highly deterministic connectivity which makes the retina and the LGN a good subject for biophysical analysis is blurred in the visual cortex. Each LGN cell in the optic radiation has synaptic contacts to 10^3 or 10^4 cortical cells in V1. On the basis of anatomical and physiological evidence mainly uncovered by the Harvard group (reviewed by Hubel 1988) a subdivision of V1 into local structures or hypercolumns was conceived (Braitenberg and Braitenberg 1979; but see von Seelen 1970) and later found (Horton and Hubel 1980). Hubel and Wiesel have used the term hypercolumn to refer to the whole set of columns for analyzing lines of all orientations (and other visual operations) from a particular region in space via both eyes. Each hypercolumn is an elementary computational unit that represents the machinery necessary for analyzing a given area of the visual field. Cytochrome oxidase stains of human V1 show circular or oval patches with a density of 1 patch/0.7 mm^2 (Horton and Hedley-Whyte 1984). The surface of area V1 of one cortical hemisphere in a human was determined to be 26.13 cm^2 (Blinkov and Glezer 1968). We can calculate from this that area V1 in the two hemispheres of a human has around 7500 cytochrome oxidase patches. The distance between adjacent patches seems to be rather constant independent of whether they receive input from the area centralis or more peripheral parts of the retina. Because of the varying cortical magnification factor, this means that there are many more hypercolumns corresponding to the foveal region than to the peripheral parts of the retina. In the foveal region of V1 the distance between adjacent hypercolumns corresponds to 6 min of arc, or 12 cone spacings, thus (foveally) one hypercolumn gets inputs from a region in the retina corresponding to about 150 cones. However, the number of ganglion cells per hypercolumn appears to be the same everywhere in the visual field. Visual resolution measured with psychophysical methods in the fovea and elsewhere in the field of view yields results closely matching the sampling density of the ganglion cells (Thibos et al. 1987). Even if it looks as if the hypercolumns form a kind of perceptual grid, the higher resolution of the retina is maintained in perception.

Each hypercolumn contains cells with nonoriented receptive fields in its center and orientation selective cells in its periphery (Livingstone and Hubel 1984). Size and scatter in the receptive fields of cells recorded in layers 2,3,5 and 6 of the primary visual cortex suggest the beginning of an organization according to functional criteria while at the same time the retinotopic precision still present in the LGN and layers 4B and 4C becomes looser (Hubel 1988).

Physiological recordings from layer 4B of the primate V1 reveal a high percentage of elements which respond selectively to the direction of movement. In primates this is the first stage in the visual pathway where this type of neurons are found. Psychophysically local motion can be mimicked by using two thin adjacent lines which are either flashed or switched on in successsion (apparent motion). There are indications that for sufficiently small angular separations of the two lines the perception generated by this stimulus is very similar to that of a line which moves over a corresponding distance (McKee 1981). The advantage of the apparent motion stimulus is that the two input signals required to perceive motion are clearly defined with respect to their position in space. By changing the time interval between the two onsets (or flashes) the temporal threshold for the correct identification of the imposed direction of motion can be determined. When this temporal threshold is measured as a function of the angular distance between the lines in the case of two adjacent *dark* lines on a bright background, a clear minimum at an angle of 3 min. of arc is found (Rapf and Wehrhahn 1991). However, when the two lines are brighter than the background upon which they are displayed, the threshold as a function of distance has a much wider minimum, corresponding to a separation of 3 to 6 min. of arc. This is very similar to the results of earlier experiments with flashed lines on a dark background (Westheimer and McKee 1977b; Westheimer 1983).

The different functions for dark and bright lines indicate that ON- and OFF-center ganglion cells either have different access to the same motion detecting circuitry, or two different circuitries exist, one receiving its input from the ON-, and the other from the OFF-pathway. In experiments with flashed lines the angular distance of the lines in which the minimum threshold is observed increase with retinal eccentricity proportional to the cortical magnification factor (Wässle et al 1989). The temporal threshold at the respective minima is surprisingly constant. This means that the maximal velocity which can be discriminated reasonably well increases with eccentricity, while the velocity in V1 in terms of the successive activation of the adjacent parts of the cortical tissue is constant. One could speculate that the time delay between the two signals leading to the perception of apparent motion is generated by a neuronal mechanism involving conduction velocity between hypercolumns similarly as Exner (1875) speculated for the retina. Thus the grid defined anatomically by the distance between adjacent cytochrome oxidase patches in V1 might have a perceptual counter-part in the spatial distance for which local motion can be perceived particularly well.

What could be the neuronal circuitry underlying this? The fact that we "sense" motion in a very basic way and use it as the elementary information for numerous complex visual tasks, seems to imply something like a hard wired "module" similar to the "elementary movement detectors" (EMD) hypothesized in the fly (Buchner 1976). If these EMD's exist in mammals, is their development programmed already in the genome or do we learn to see motion early in our life? Single unit recordings from the visual cortex of kittens seem to imply the first possibility. If this is so it should be possible to identify the cellular substrate of this stereotyped circuitry in layer 4B of V1.

Hyperacuity

There are of course many other tasks attributed to our visual system which have been analyzed by psychophysicists. One of these is hyperacuity or vernier acuity which is perhaps the result of an interpolation mechanism evolved to "smooth" visual perception. For many geometrical constellations which involve patterns extending over more than 5 to

6 min of arc hyperacuity achieves an "apparent" resolution about one order of magnitude above that defined by the cone spacing. One example is the "three dot vernier", a pattern consisting of three vertically aligned equidistant dots. Good subjects can discriminate whether the middle dot is displaced to the left or to the right with respect to the two outer dots with an accuracy of 3 sec of arc, provided the distance between the two outer dots is in the region of 5 to 6 min of arc (Westheimer and Hauske 1975). The patterns for which hyperacuity is achieved may consist of either straight or curved lines and/or dots (Westheimer 1979; Westheimer and McKee 1977a). The correlation of the spatial extension necessary for hyperacuity with the width of a cortical hypercolumn is striking.

One more point deserves attention in the context of hyperacuity. The number of patterns in which we are able to perceive the relative localization with hyperacuity is so large that a prewired template for each of them could hardly be imagined. This implies that as a prerequisite of hyperacuity learning on a very fast time scale (around 10 sec) must occur. Until recently neuronal plasticity in the cortex was experimentally shown to exist only on a time scale of weeks or months. Recent experiments indicate the existence of a much faster process that could also be important in hyperacuity. Physiological recordings in the striate cortex of cats unequivocally show that the filter characteristics of striate cortical cells are not necessarily fixed, but can dynamically change according to context (Gilbert and Wiesel 1990). Thus, no hardwired modules are involved in the neural processes underlying hyperacuity.

The tendency to be organized according to functions ultimately connected with perception which was just described for V1 is perhaps even more pronounced in the second visual area (V2). This area is built of stripes of different width whose inputs are provided by different pathways originating from different types of cells in the hypercolumns of V1. The preservation of the retinotopy becomes less and less important for increasingly higher cortical areas.

Time, synchrony, and dynamical linking

What could be the functional basis of the vast processing capabilities present in these areas of the central nervous system? We consider the fact that an average cortical neuron receives input from 10^3 to 10^4 synapses and in turn is presynaptic to as many other cortical neurones. It is not likely that this structure which is more similar to a haystack than anything else follows deterministic rules of connectivity specified for example in the genome (Schüz, this volume). It is also clear that the state of excitation of a cortical cell depends on the level of depolarization present at the site of spike initiation regardless of the position of the many dendritic spines giving rise to the different components of excitation. The important parameter for the instantaneous level of excitation is the time at which the different components appear at the presynaptic sites, because only if they arrive at the same instant at the spike initiating site the cooperative action of all inputs elicits an action potential in the cell. This statement is, however, only true under the assumption that synaptic action only has an instantaneous effect on the level of depolarization and hence the initiation of a spike. The time course of an EPSP or IPSP is in general in the range of several milliseconds. There are, however, receptors for certain neurotransmitters whose time course is rather slow, for example the muscarinic receptor (Vogt et al. 1991). We can interpret this finding as a neuronal mechanism storing the signal amplitude for a short time and hence as something like short term plasticity or learning in the CNS. Physiological experiments in the visual cortex of cats have shown that receptive field properties of orientation selective units can change after a few stimuli (Gilbert and Wiesel 1990).

In a recent experiment psychophysical thresholds were determined for a hyperacuity task consisting of two vertically aligned dots when the two dots were exposed in a synchrony to each other. Under these conditions the high precision observed for a synchronous presentations of the two dots suffers. Neither onset nor offset asynchrony can be tolerated (Wehrhahn and Westheimer 1992). The data suggest that Vernier acuity may be subserved by dynamical linking (von der Malsburg 1985) of cortical excitation generated by the synchronous arrival of signals within a range of cortical locations whose spatial separation is critical for optimal hyperacuity performance.

Thus time or, more specifically, synchronous excitation at many synapses of a cortical cell is very likely to be the most important feature in the input signals to this cell (Abeles 1991). However, a single action potential fired by one cell is probably of minor importance. Many cells, say 10^2 to 10^4, need to be fired to have a significant effect in higher cortical areas and finally in perception and motor responses. Dynamical linking of many cells into a network which in effect might be functional for only a short period, decoupling of these links and reassembling them into other configurations and functional contexts may be an explanation of the difficulties encountered in interpreting cortical structure in functional terms.

Acknowledgments

I thank V. Braitenberg, D. Rapf, T. Wachtler and G. Westheimer for comments on the manuscript.

References

Abeles M (1991) Corticonics. Neural circuits of the cerebral cortex. Cambridge University Press, Cambridge

Baylor DA, Hodgkin AL, Lamb TD (1974) Reconstruction of the electrical responses of turtle cones to flashes and steps of light. J Physiol 242:759-791

Blinkov SM, Glezer II (1968) Das Zentralnervensystem in Zahlen und Tabellen. VEB Gustav Fischer Verlag, Jena

Braitenberg V, Braitenberg C (1979) Geometry of orientation columns in the visual cortex. Biol Cybern 33:179-186

Buchner E (1976) Elementary movement detectors in an insect visual system. Biol Cybern 24:85-101

Crick F, Koch C (1990) Towards a neurobiological theory of consciousness. The Neurosciences 2:263-275

Exner S (1875) Experimentelle Untersuchungen der einfachsten psychischen Prozesse. Pflugers Arch 11:403-432

Gilbert CD, Wiesel TN (1990) The influence of contextual stimuli on the orientation selectivity of cells in primary visual cortex of the cat. Vision Res 30:1689-1701

Horton JC (1984) Cytochrome oxidase patches: A new cytoarchitectonic feature of monkey visual cortex. Phil Trans R Soc Lond B 304:199-253

Horton JC, Hedley-Whyte ET (1984) Mapping of cytochrome oxidase patches and ocular dominance columns in human visual cortex. Phil Trans R Soc Lond B 304:255-272

Horton JC, Hubel DH (1981) Regular patchy distribution of cytochrome oxidase staining in primary visual cortex of macaque monkey. Nature 292: 762-764

Hubel DH (1988) Eye, brain, and vision. Scientific American Library, New York

Lee BB, Virsu V, Creutzfeldt OD (1983) Linear signal transmission from prepotentials to cells in the Macaque Lateral Geniculate Nucleus. Exp Brain Res 52:50-56

Lee BB, Pokorny J, Smith VC, Martin PR, Valberg A (1990) Luminance and chromatic modulation sensitivity of macaque retinal ganglion cells and human observers. J opt Soc Am A7 (12):2223-2236

McKee SM (1981) A local mechanism for differential velocity detection. Vision Res 21:491-500

Osterberg G (1935) Topography of the layer of rods and cones in the human retina. Acta Ophthalmol Suppl 6:1-103

Rapf D, Wehrhahn C (1991) Two distinct substrates for motion perception in man. In: Elsner N, Penzlin H (eds) Synapse - Transmission - Modulation. Thieme, Stuttgart p 565

Schein SJ, de Monasterio FM (1987) Mapping of retinal and geniculate neurons onto striate cortex of macaque. J Neurosci 7:996-1009

Silveira LCL, Perry VH (1991) The topography of magnocellular projecting ganglion cells in the primate retina. Neuroscience 40:217-237

Valberg A, Lee BB (1991) From pigments to perception: Advances in understanding visual processes. Plenum Press, New York.

Vogt BA, Gabriel M, Vogt LJ, Poremba A, Jensen EL, Kubota Y, Kang E (1991) Muscarinic receptor binding increases in anterior thalamus and cingulate cortex during discriminative avoidance learning. J Neurosci 11:1508-1514

von der Malsburg C (1985) Nervous structures with dynamical links. Ber Bunsenges Phys Chem 89:703-710

von Seelen W (1970) Zur Informationsverarbeitung im visuellen System der Wirbeltiere, II. Kybernetik 7:89-106

Wässle H, Grünert U, Röhrenbeck J, Boycott BB (1990) Cortical magnification factor and the ganglion cell density of the primate retina. Nature 341:643-646

Wehrhahn C, Westheimer G (1992) Temporal asynchrony interferes with Vernier acuity (submitted)

Westheimer G (1979) The spatial sense of the eye. Invest Ophthalmol Vis Sci 18:893-912

Westheimer G (1983) Temporal order detection for foveal and peripheral visual stimuli. Vision Res 23:759-763

Westheimer G (1986) The eye as an optical instrument. In: Boff KR, Kaufman L, Thomas JP (eds) Handbook of perception and human performance vol. I: Sensory Processes and Perception. J. Wiley and Sons, New York

Westheimer G, McKee S (1977a) Integration regions for visual hyperacuity. Vision Res 17:89-93

Westheimer G, McKee S (1977b) Perception of temporal order in adjacent visual stimuli. Vision Res 17:887-892

Wiesel TN, Hubel DH (1966) Spatial and chromatic interactions in the lateral geniculate body of the Rhesus monkey. J Neurophysiol 29:1115-1156

Zeki SM, Shipp S (1988) The functional logic of cortical connections. Nature 335:311-317

Cells in the Visual Cortex are not just Local Receptive-Field Filters

Ulla Mitzdorf and B.-H. Li

Institut für Medizinische Psychologie, Goethestr. 31, 8000 München 2, Germany

Introduction

The famous early publications about the receptive fields (RFs) of sensory neurons (Kuffler 1953; Mountcastle 1957; Hubel and Wiesel 1962) have guided sensory neurophysiology for many years. They have stimulated the detailed investigation of this single-cell property, i.e., the search for the optimal sensory stimulus to activate a nerve cell. In many studies, the early findings by Hubel and Wiesel (1962) about the retinotopic organization of the RFs in the primary visual cortex and their highly specific selection of external information (most commonly a properly oriented light bar that moves across the RF) have been confirmed in several species. This led to the commonly accepted concept that the cells in the primary visual cortex act as local RF filters (Barlow, this volume). Visual stimuli that do not match well with the cells' RF structures are blocked by the filters (or at preceding levels in the thalamus or retina). They are not represented in the primary visual cortex or beyond. Diffuse luminance changes belong to this category of "virtually ineffective" stimuli (Hubel and Wiesel 1962).

A completely different view about the effectiveness of visual stimuli arises if evoked potentials are investigated. In this domain of mass action, the most effective stimuli are diffuse (or sparsely structured) luminance changes. Moreover, mass-action responses are not only evoked at retinotopically corresponding sites in the visual cortex. In early studies of evoked potentials in the cat and monkey (Doty 1958; Cowey 1964; Vaughan and Gross 1969) and in a recent current source-density analysis of evoked potentials (Mitzdorf 1987), significant mass activities were revealed at retinotopically noncorresponding sites in the primary visual cortex.

These discrepancies between the domains of single-cell properties and mass-action phenomena can be resolved by viewing single-cell responses from the mass-action standpoint. From this perspective, not the individual cells' response properties, but the simultaneously evoked responses of a representative group of cortical cells indicate the relevance of a stimulus. Thus, the relevant questions here are: First, is a diffuse-light stimulus still inferior to a RF-type moving bar if the respective average responses are considered and the moving-bar stimulus is the same for all cells, as is the case in mass-action recordings and in real life? Second, do visual stimuli presented at sites far distant from the RF elicit significant responses in single cells, as is suggested by mass-action data?

Results from the primary visual cortex of the rabbit

To get answers to both questions, experiments were performed on rabbits. In these animals, conventionally anaesthetized with N_2O and pentobarbital, the action potentials (APs) of individual neurons were recorded. For each cell, the RF was first identified; then the responses to a set of stimuli were obtained quantitatively by collecting peristimulus-time histograms. The applied stimuli were moving bars and edges with different orientations and velocities, high-luminance stroboscopic flashes generated with a gas discharge tube, and mild, abrupt luminance changes (between the two levels 0.5 and 2 cd/m^2) presented on a display. This display was positioned with the RF in its center (RF-centered on/off) and also displaced far beyond the RF (eccentric on/off). The RF-centered on and off stimuli extended well beyond the sizes of the RFs (average stimulus diameter 25°, average RF size 7°). The eccentric on and off stimuli never included the RF site. They were, on the average, 60° eccentric to the RF site and 30° in diameter. Examples for the responses to all these stimuli are shown in Figs. 1 and 2. From these sets of histograms, the response strengths, i.e., the number of extra APs above the spontaneous-activity level contained in a single response, were extracted (see Figs. 1 and 2).

To minimize the number of animals used, only a small sample of response histograms was collected (ranging from 49 cells' RF responses to 17 cells' eccentric on/off responses). This small sample size was

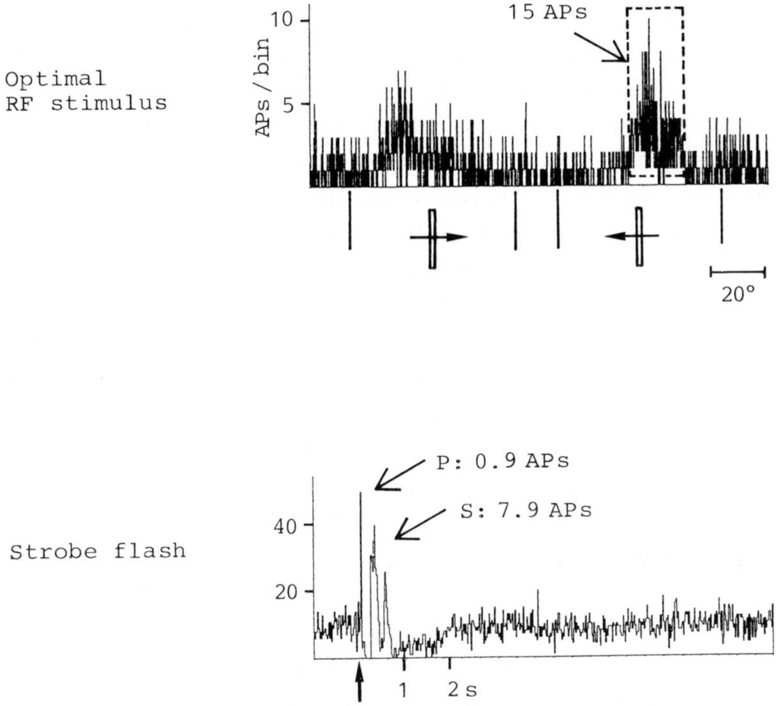

Fig. 1. Upper: a typical response to the optimal RF stimulus; the optimal stimulus for this cell (simple type-2) was a vertical bright bar, moved at 15°/s from temporal to nasal across the RF; bin width 10 ms, 20 responses; lower: a typical response to a strobe flash; a primary response (*P*) is followed by long-lasting inhibition containing however two secondary response components (*S*); bin width 20 ms, 50 responses.

supported by incorporating statistical data from previous studies of large samples in the averaging procedures (Murphy and Berman 1979; Murphy 1985; Swadlow and Weyand 1987; Swadlow 1988). Thereby, also the uncertainties in the final results could be estimated; they range from 10-30%.

At first, the average value of the individual cells' specific RF responses was obtained. This average optimal response has a strength of 11.3 APs per stimulus presentation. These optimal responses cannot be evoked simultaneously in all cells of a group, even if the RF sites coincide, because the respective optimal stimuli differ. Therefore, this value is of purely theoretical interest; it can never be reached in the real situations of information processing.

To obtain the corresponding real average response strength of a cell group, the effect of one RF-type stimulus on all cells of the group must be determined. According to the tuning properties of the individual cells' RFs and their scattered RF sites, the best common RF-type stimulus is a long bright bar moved at an intermediate velocity. Obviously, for many of the individual cells, the orientation, the direction of movement, and the velocity of this common moving bar are not optimal. For the endstopped cells, in addition, it is too long; for those cells which prefer dark bars or edges, its contrast is nonoptimal. All these inadequacies of the common stimulus were taken into account by explicitly considering the orientation tuning properties, direction biases, velocity tuning curves, and contrast preferences of a representative cell sample. The most severe restriction is the constant orientation; it yields a reduction of 55% of the average optimal RF-response. All other specifications of the common stimulus together yield another reduction of 47%. Thus, an average strength of 2.7 APs results for the average response of any cell in the primary visual cortex as this one specific bar stimulus moves across its RF site.

A strobe flash typically caused a primary and one or several secondary responses, as well as long-lasting inhibition (see Fig. 1). The average mass-action response to this stimulus was obtained by taking the adequately weighted average of the individual cells' responses. (Averaging was performed in two steps, first within each cell class, then across cell classes according to the respective percentages from the previous studies). The resulting average response strength per cell is 3.8 APs. It is composed of 0.8 APs in the primary response and 3.0 APs in the secondary responses. Only 14% of the tested cells did not show obvious responses to this stimulus.

The responses to the RF-centered decent luminance increases and decreases were qualitatively similar to the strobe responses. They were usually weaker, slightly delayed in onset, and broader (see Fig. 2; the primary and secondary components were not considered separately in these responses). A slight fraction (about 20%) of the tested cells did not show significant responses. The respective mass-action responses, i.e., the properly weighted average response strengths, are 2.1 APs for the on stimulus and 1.9 APs for the off stimulus.

The majority of the cells also showed obvious responses to the retinotopically noncorresponding eccentric on/off stimuli (88% and 65%, respectively). The responses were well recognizable in histograms of 50 to 200 accumulated single responses. They were usually qualitati-

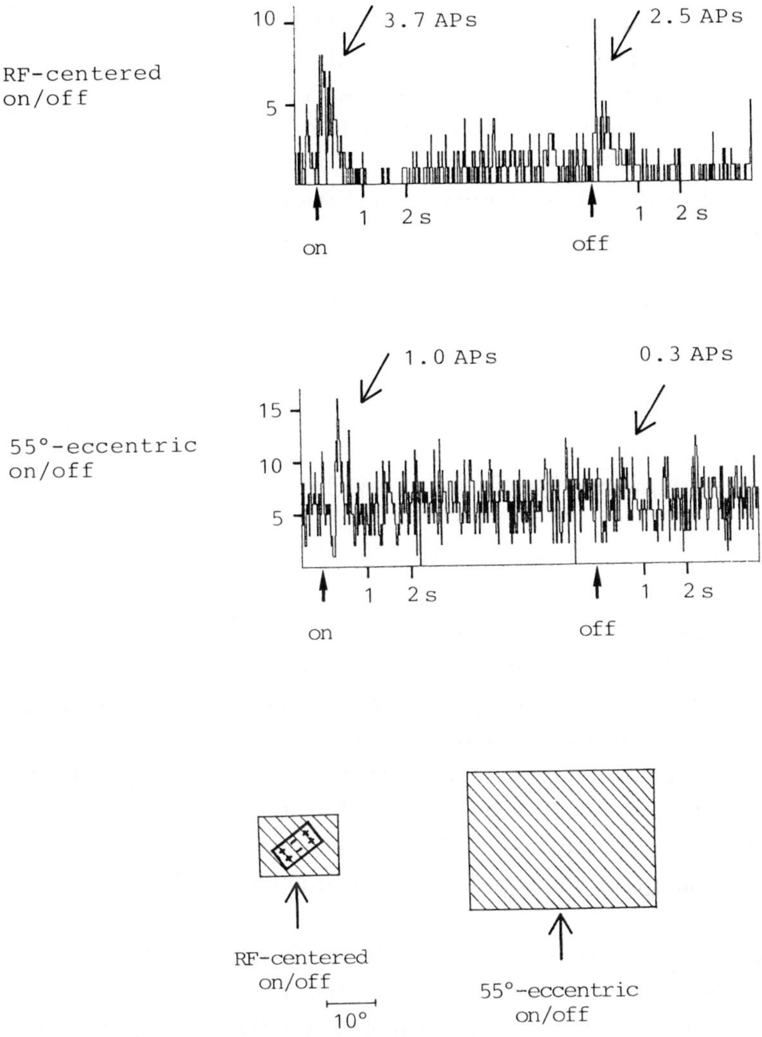

Fig. 2. Typical responses to RF-centered on/off (upper; bin width 20 ms, 20 responses) and eccentric on/off (lower; bin width 20 ms, 50 responses); the RF of this simple type-2 cell and the stimulus areas are indicated below.

vely quite similar to the corresponding responses to the RF-centered stimuli (see Fig. 2). The average mass-action values are 0.6 APs for the eccentric-on response and 0.5 APs for the eccentric-off response. As mentioned above, these responses were evoked by presenting the stimuli at one eccentric site. If they had been presented simultaneously at several eccentric sites, or as an anulus all around, it is very likely that the corresponding average response in the cell group would be several times as large. With such stimulus configurations, the eccentric responses might even exceed the responses to the RF-centered on/off stimuli. Straylight as the cause of these eccentric responses could be ruled out because the eccentrically evoked responses differed qualitatively from those evoked by the RF-centered on/off stimuli in several cells. Moreover, eccentrically presented grating-reversal stimuli were found to cause significant responses also. In these stimuli, the average luminance was kept constant.

Results from the primary visual cortex of the cat

Although the primary visual cortex of the rabbit has, in principle, properties quite similar to the cat primary visual cortex (Murphy and Berman 1975), it differs in several details that might be relevant. The RFs are larger, the orientation sensitivity of the cells is more broadly tuned, and about 30% of the cells are not orientation selective at all. To judge whether these differences are essential for the above-stated mass-action results, the wealth of published data from the primary visual cortex of the cat was reviewed for corresponding data. Data thus obtained allowed to derive analogous mass-action values for all except the eccentric stimuli.

With values for the responses to the cell-specific optimal RF stimuli published by Rose and Blakemore (1974) and Leventhal and Hirsch (1978), the respective average of the optimal responses - 26.0 APs per cell - could be obtained. The strength of the mass-action response to one common moving bar was derived by taking the statistical data about orientation tuning and direction selectivity of the feline neurons into account (Leventhal and Hirsch 1978; Murphy and Burman 1979). The influences of the cells' contrast sensitivity, velocity tuning, and endstopping properties were assumed to be the same as in the rabbit. This assumption leads to an overestimation of the strength of responses in the cat because its cells are more selective. The final result for the average response strength in the primary visual cortex of the cat to a moving-bar stimulus is 1.4 APs. Compared with the individual cells' optimal responses, this mass-action response in the cat is much smaller than in the rabbit (5% versus 24%). This dissimilarity is due to the sharper orientation tuning of the feline neurons.

The average responses to strobe flashes and to mild luminance changes could be derived from early investigations (Baumgartner 1955; Jung and Baumgartner 1955; Creutzfeldt et al. 1968). A strobe flash causes about 3.0 APs per cell, half in the primary and half in the secondary responses. RF-centered on and off stimuli cause 3.6 and 6.1 APs, respectively.

These estimates demonstrate that strong and mild RF-centered contourless luminance changes cause average responses in the cat which equal those in the rabbit (see Table 1). Since the average response to a common moving-bar stimulus in a group of cells is only about half as strong in the cat, the average response to such a diffuse-light stimulus is not only of similar magnitude but even about twice as large in the cat cortex. Although no experimental data are available for the cat for single-cell responses to eccentric stimuli, it is strongly suggested by analogy to the results from the responses to the RF-centered diffuse-light stimuli that the eccentric stimuli would also cause comparably strong activities in the cells in the cat cortex. As mentioned in the introduction, such strong mass activities were found in the primary and secondary visual cortex of the cat (Mitzdorf 1987) and also in the monkey (Cowey 1964).

Stimulus	rabbit	cat
Optimal RF stimuli	11.3	26.0
One moving bar	2.7	1.4
Strobe flash	3.8	3.0
RF-centered on/off	2.1/1.9	3.6/6.1
Eccentric on/off	0.6/0.5	-/-

Table 1. Average strengths of the responses to various types of visual stimuli in the primary visual cortex of the rabbit and the cat (APs per cell per stimulus)

Conclusions and implications of the results

The average response-strength values summarized in Table 1 agree well with the usual findings in both the single-cell domain and the mass-action domain, and a comparison of these results across the domains resolves the discrepancies between the views obtained in either one. The RF-type stimulus is, indeed, the most effective stimulus for the single cell. Influences by a strobe flash or a mild wide-angle luminance change are smaller by factors of 3-9 and can, therefore, be neglected in a first approximation. Such stimuli, when presented at a retinotopically noncorresponding site, are even less effective. If these single-cell activities are inspected from the mass-action point of view, however, then even to a first approximation, the RF-type stimulus loses its predominance. A strobe flash and a mild wide-angle luminance change therefore become as relevant as a moving-bar stimulus or even more effective. Also, the responses to the retinotopically noncorresponding stimuli are of the same order of magnitude now.

The amplitudes of the various mass-action responses, i.e., the average peak firing rates, are even more in favor of the diffuse-light stimuli, because the responses to these abrupt stimuli are more transient than the responses to the moving-bar stimuli. The peak amplitude of the primary response to the strobe flash, for example, is four times as large as the peak amplitude of the mass response to the moving-bar stimulus in both animals.

Thus, the discrepancies between single-cell properties and mass-action responses of the primary visual cortex could be settled. The solution to the problem implied two severe restrictions to the concept of single cells acting as local RF filters, however. First, this concept is only valid to a first approximation. Second, it is restricted to the single-cell domain, i.e., to the response properties of the individual neurons.

Relevance of mass-action responses?

The unfamiliar mass-action aspect of brain activity presented in this chapter collides with the generally accepted single-cell centered concept of cortical information processing. The essence of this processing is thought to be the local feature extraction and the communication between individual cells for further feature specification. This extraction and specification of features undoubtedly is a profound mechanism and has been demonstrated most convincingly for the visual system (e.g. De Yoe and Van Essen 1988). The concept derived from these facts is a severe abstraction from reality, however. It ignores that features or attributes of the external stimuli are not decoded in a perfectly exclusive manner. This is what the above- described mass-action data should definitely bring to our minds. Beyond that, there are indications that mass-action aspects of central processing are of direct functional relevance. It is the domain of mass activities where close correlations with perceptual and behavioral phenomena have been found. To give just a few examples: Perception thresholds correlate precisely with the thresholds of steady-state potentials (Campbell and Maffei 1970) and with a secondary component of transient evoked potentials (Libet et al. 1967). Conditioned significance of stimuli as well as the quality of task performance are related with the coherence or covariance of mass activities across different sites in the central nervous system (John 1972; Gevins et al. 1987). The depth of anaesthesia is inversely related to the mid-latency components of the auditory evoked potentials (Madler and Pöppel 1987). The absence of a sensory stimulus evokes a mass activity if this absence represents a relevant signal (Sutton et al. 1967). Finally, trivial experience is directly related to the present mass-action results: We consciously perceive a strobe flash or a mild wide-angle luminance change as rather strong stimuli, whereas the movement of a small bar or edge may often escape our notice. Although knowledge about coding and decoding mechanisms that act directly and specifically on the macroscopic level is still very sparse, at least the coarsely projecting aminergic modulator systems can be stated as concrete substrates for such macroscopic brain mechanisms, at present.

Acknowledgements

I thank Dr. B. Herzberger for English corrections and Dr. U. Engler for secretarial help. This work was supported by the Deutsche Forschungsgemeinschaft, grants Po 121-13 and SFB 220/D3.

References

Baumgartner G (1955) Reaktionen einzelner Neurone im optischen Cortex der Katze nach Lichtblitzen. Pflügers Arch 261:457-469

Campbell FW, Maffei L (1970) Electrophysiological evidence for the existence of orientation and size detectors in the human visual system. J Physiol (Lond) 207:635-652

Cowey A (1964) Projection of the retina on the striate and peristriate cortex in squirrel monkey, saimiri sciureus. J Neurophysiol 27:366-393

Creutzfeldt O, Rosita A, Ito M, Probst W (1969) Visual evoked responses of single cells and of the EEG in primary visual area of the cat. J Neurophysiol 32:127-139

DeYoe EA, Van Essen DC (1988) Concurrent processing streams in monkey visual cortex. TINS 11:219-226

Doty RW (1958) Potentials evoked in cat cerebral cortex by diffuse and puctiform photic stimuli. J Neurophysiol 21:437-464

Gevins AS, Morgan NH, Bressler SL, Cutillo BA, White RM, Illes J, Greer DS, Doyle JC, Zeitler GM (1987) Human neuroelectric patterns predict performance accuracy. Science 235:580-585

Hubel DH, Wiesel TN (1962) Receptive fields, binocular interaction and functional architecture in the cat's visual cortex. J Physiol (Lond) 160:106-154

John ER (1972) Switchboard versus statistical theories of learning and memory. Science 177:850-864

Jung R, Baumgartner G (1955) Hemmungsmechnismen und bremsende Stabilisierung an einzelnen Neuronen des optischen Cortex. Pflügers Arch 261:434-456

Kuffler SW (1953) Discharge patterns and functional organization of mammalian retina. J Neurophysiol 16:37-68

Leventhal AG, Hirsch HVB (1978) Receptive-field properties of neurons in different laminae of visual cortex of the cat. J Neurophysiol 41:948-962

Libet B, Alberts WW, Wright Jr EW, Feinstein B (1967) Responses of human somatosensory cortex to stimuli below threshold for conscious sensation. Science 158:1597-1600

Madler C, Pöppel E (1987) Auditory evoked potentials indicate the loss of neuronal oscillations during general anaesthesia. Naturwiss 74:42-43

Mitzdorf U (1987) Properties of the evoked potential generators: current source-density analysis of visually evoked potentials in the cat cortex. Intern J Neurosci 33:33-59

Mountcastle VB (1957) Modality and topographic properties of single neurons of cat's somatic sensory cortex. J Neurophysiol 20:408-434

Murphy EH (1985) Effects of pattern deprivation on visual cortical cells in the rabbit: a reevaluation. J Neurophysiol 53:1535-1550

Murphy EH, Berman N (1979) The rabbit and the cat: a comparison of some features of response properties of single cells in the primary visual cortex. J Comp Neurol 188:401-428

Rose D, Blakemore C (1974) An analysis of orientation selectivity in the cat's visual cortex. Exp Brain Res 20:1-17

Sutton S, Tueting P, Zubin J, John ER (1967) Information delivery and the sensory-evoked potential. Science 155:1436-1439

Swadlow HA (1988) Efferent neurons and suspected interneurons in binocular visual cortex of the awake rabbit: receptive fields and binocular properties. J Neurophysiol 59:1162-1187

Swadlow HA, Weyand TG (1987) Corticogeniculate neurons, corticotectal neurons, and suspected interneurons in visual cortex of awake rabbits: receptive-field properties, axonal properties, and effects of EEG arousal. J Neurophysiol 57:977-1001

Vaughan HG, Gross CG (1969) Cortical responses to light in unanaesthetized monkeys and their alteration by visual system lesions. Exp Brain Res 8:19-36

Dynamics of Activity in Biology-Oriented Neural Network Models: Stability at Low Firing Rates

Michael Erb[1] and Ad Aertsen[2]

Max-Planck-Institut für biologische Kybernetik, Spemannstrasse 38, 7400 Tübingen, Germany

We investigated the dynamics of activity in feedback neural network models at low firing rates. The networks were designed to capture the typical features of real cortical networks. Stability analysis of the linearized model and simulations of different degrees of complexity show that stability is only obtained for very fast and sufficiently strong inhibition; otherwise the network activity develops into synchronous oscillations with frequency and amplitude dynamics governed predominantly by the inhibition parameters, but largely independent of (1) the network architecture (uniform, random or structured), (2) the spiking or analog nature of the neural activity, and, albeit to a lesser extent, (3) the linear or nonlinear nature of the neural threshold function. Provided the network connectivity is sufficiently rich and structured, the spike activity exhibits features which resemble those observed in physiological recordings from various cortical areas: cell assembly behaviour with different, simultaneous correlation dynamics (event coherence and rate coherence).

Introduction

In recent years, many different kinds of neural network models have been developed. Addressing a variety of different levels of biological reality, these models occupy a correspondingly wide spectrum of

---

[1] present address: Fak. für Physik, Abt. Biophysik, Philipps-Universität, Renthof 7, 3550 Marburg, Germany

[2] present address: Institut für Neuroinformatik, Ruhr-Universität, P.O. Box 102 184, 4630 Bochum, Germany

mathematical formalizations. They range from sets of coupled differential equations, describing the time course of membrane potentials of interconnected individual neurons, to spin-glass models from statistical physics, dealing with the interactions in populations of binary elements. In the context of a more comprehensive investigation aimed at connecting these different levels of modeling (Erb 1991), we investigated the activity dynamics in physiology-oriented networks of model neurons, both of the spiking and of the analog type. In the present report we focus on the issue of stability of the neuronal activity in a highly interconnected model network, in particular on its dependence on various neuron and network parameters. The model was explicitly designed to capture the typical features of real cortical networks, both in terms of anatomy and physiology. An important constraint in this respect is that of 'sparse' firing, i.e. the activity in the network is required to be of low firing rate, such as typically observed in the neocortex (e.g. Abeles et al. 1990). As will be demonstrated, obtaining stability in such a feedback system of sparsely firing neurons is by no means a trivial problem. In fact, stable solutions could only be obtained for a very confined 'island' in parameter space. Outside this restricted range, the system develops instabilities, certain features of which are reminiscent of phenomena observed in recordings of neural activity in the real cortex.

The network model: formulation and simulation

In order to investigate stability neural networks with feedback, we studied the behaviour of a network of 100 spiking model neurons with fixed synaptic connections (Erb et al. 1990). Figure 1a shows the scheme of the network, the corresponding Equations are given in Figure 1b. In this model the neurons are connected only by excitatory synapses, inspired by neuroanatomical findings that about 90% of the cortical synapses is of this type (Braitenberg and Schüz 1991; Schüz, this Volume). The synapses are modeled as lowpass filters with delayed response, transforming the incoming spike activity into EPSP's. These are summated linearly over the dendritic tree to yield the instantaneous value of the membrane potential at the cell body. The probability of spike generation is modeled by a sigmoid function of this membrane potential; this probability, in turn, is modulated by a refractory mechanism, driven by the recent spike history of the neuron. The final output, a sequence of spikes, is obtained by using the firing probability as the instantaneous rate of a stochastic event generator.

In addition to this basic network of spiking neurons, the 'pyramidal cells', the model comprises an inhibitory mechanism for stabilization. This inhibition consists of two parallel, linear branches: a fast one, with a time constant in the range of that for the excitatory synapses (5 ms), and a slow one with a considerably larger time constant (200 ms). The fast branch is intended to mimic the inhibitory action of the 'stellate cells', the slow branch serves to regulate the overall activity in the network towards a preset value (threshold control; Braitenberg 1978; Palm 1982).

In the present study the overall activity in the net was set to an average firing rate in the order of 20 spikes per second per neuron. Unless otherwise indicated, all numerical calculations as well as the network simulations shown here were performed with the following standard (sub)set of parameter values:

τ_0=4 ms	τ_1=5 ms	τ_2=200 ms	
Δ_0=1 ms		Δ_2=1 ms	
k_0=1		k_2=3	
α=40	μ_0=0	μ_1=0.2	c=0.3

The values of the remaining parameters, in particular D_1 and k_1, were subject to variation, and are given separately in the appropriate Figure captions. The standard values were chosen primarily for reasons of physiological plausiblity. Moreover, in combination with appropriately chosen values for the remaining parameters, the standard set leads to a stable solution under sparse firing conditions, both for spiking and for analog neurons (cf. Figs. 2c-5c; Erb 1991).

One of the striking findings from simulations of this model is that stability at low firing rates appears to be reached only within an extremely confined region of the parameter space. Outside this stable 'island' the network activity either dies, explodes or develops into strong, coherent oscillations. This is illustrated in Figure 2, which shows the lowpass filtered sum activity of the network in response to a stepwise presentation of a random input pattern for three different sets of model parameters. In each of these cases, the connectivity of the network was described by the same random connectivity matrix, with

Figure 1a. Scheme of the Model Network

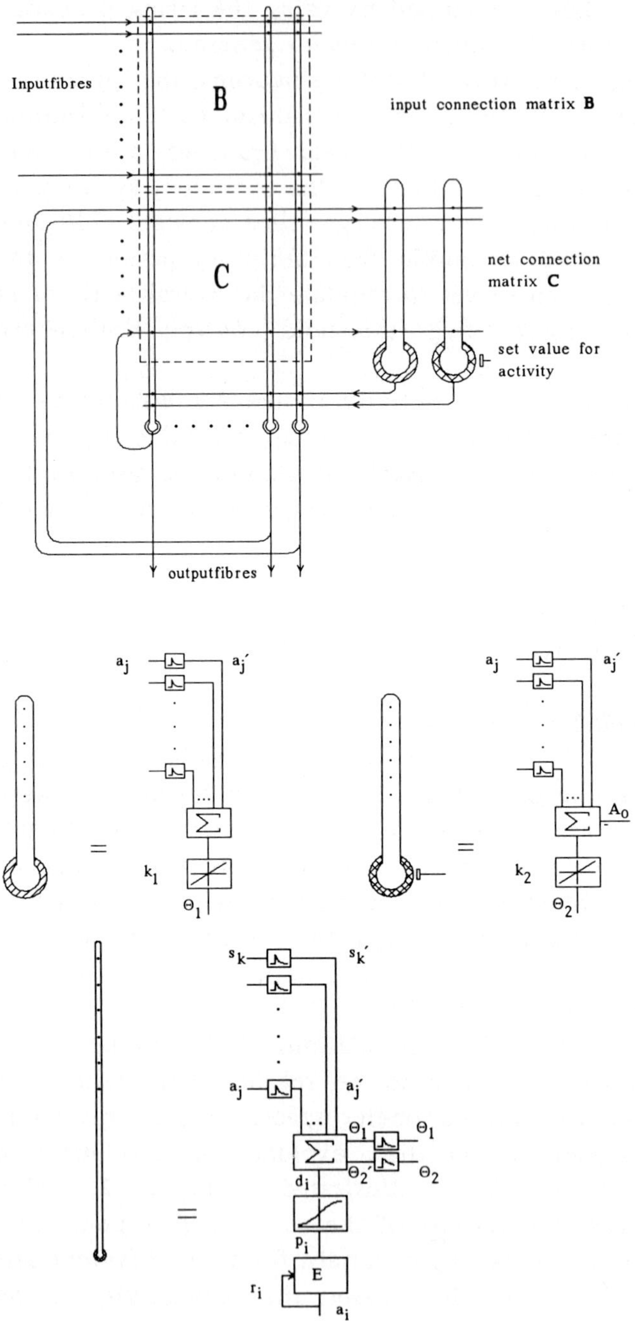

Figure 1b. Equations of the Model

Lowpass filters:

$$\dot{s}_k(t) = -\frac{1}{\tau_{in}} s_k'(t) + \frac{1}{\tau_{in}} s_k(t - \Delta_{in})$$

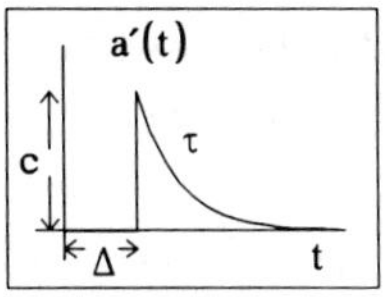

$$\dot{a}_j'(t) = -\frac{1}{\tau_0} a_j'(t) + \frac{1}{\tau_0} a_j(t - \Delta_0)$$

$$\dot{\Theta}_1'(t) = -\frac{1}{\tau_1} \Theta_1'(t) + \frac{1}{\tau_1} \Theta_1(t - \Delta_1)$$

$$\dot{\Theta}_2'(t) = -\frac{1}{\tau_2} \Theta_2'(t) + \frac{1}{\tau_2} \Theta_2(t - \Delta_2)$$

Potentials:

$$\Theta_1(t) = k_1 \cdot \sum_{j=1}^{n} a_j'(t)$$

$$\Theta_2(t) = k_2 \cdot \left(\sum_{j=1}^{n} a_j'(t) - A_0\right)$$

$$d_i(t) = \sum_{j=1}^{n} c_{ij} \cdot a_j'(t) + \sum_{k=1}^{m} b_{ik} \cdot s_k'(t) - \Theta_1'(t) - \Theta_2'(t)$$

Nonlinear characteristic function:

$$p_i(t) = f(d_i(t)) = \lambda_0 + \frac{\lambda_1 - \lambda_0}{1 + e^{-\alpha \cdot d_i(t)}}$$

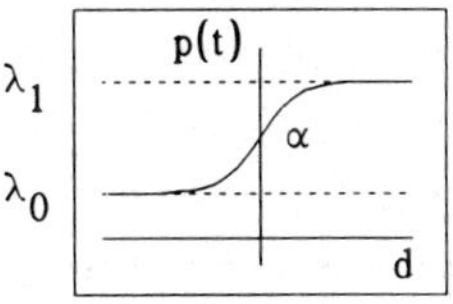

Event generator:

after spike at t_0

$$r_i(t) = \begin{cases} 0 & \text{for } t - t_0 < \Delta_r \\ 1 - e^{-\frac{t - t_0}{\tau_r}} & \text{for } t - t_0 \geq \Delta_r \end{cases}$$

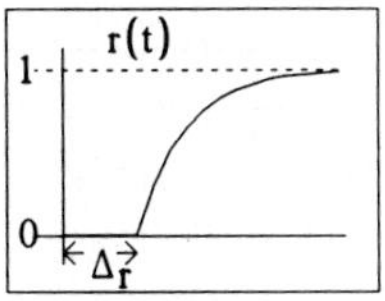

$$a_i(t) = \begin{cases} 1 & \text{with probability } P(1) = p_i(t) \cdot r_i(t) \\ 0 & \text{with probability } P(0) = 1 - P(1) \end{cases}$$

Fig. 1. Scheme (**a**) and Equations (**b**) of the model neural network

constant mean value (0.3) throughout the matrix and uniformly distributed stochastic fluctuations (range ± 0.1). Clearly the network is stable only in the last example (Fig. 2c), whereas the other two (Figs. 2a,b) exhibit various forms of instabilities, differing both in the rate at which the instability develops and decays and in the oscillation frequency.

Stability of linear networks with analog neurons and uniform connectivity matrix

For a quantitative investigation of the stability issue we introduced a number of simplifications. First, instead of actually generating discrete spikes by means of a stochastic event generator, we interpreted the firing probability of each neuron directly as its output activity. Thus, we obtain a deterministic network of so-called ‘analog’ neurons, i.e. neurons with continuously varying ‘firing rates’. Secondly, in order to allow for a formal stability analysis, we studied a linear approximation of the model. Under these conditions it is possible to explicitly formulate the transfer function of the network; this transfer function obviously depends on the various neuron and network parameters. Finally, in order to obtain a more amenable expression for the transfer function, we drastically reduced the complexity of the network connectivity. In the simplified case of a uniform connectivity matrix, i.e. the limiting case (for fluctuations down to zero) of the random connectivity in Fig. 2, the transfer function is given by

$$G_g(s) = \frac{\frac{f'}{\tau_0 s+1} e^{-\Delta_0 s}}{1 - \frac{f'}{\tau_0 s+1} e^{-\Delta_0 s} \left(c - \frac{k_1}{\tau_1 s+1} e^{-\Delta_1 s} - \frac{k_2}{\tau_2 s+1} e^{-\Delta_2 s} \right)}$$

where f' is the slope of the nonlinear characteristic function f at the fixpoint.

Analysis of the pole positions of this transfer function yields a measure for the asymptotic stability of the system. In particular, the pole with the largest real part determines the amplitude dynamics of the network activity: it decides whether the effects of a disturbance will continue to grow or will eventually die out. Clearly, a positive real part signifies an increasing and, hence, unstable solution, whereas a negative real part corresponds to a decreasing, stable solution. Moreover, the imaginary part of this pole specifies the fine grain time course of the network response, in particular its oscillation frequency. Figure 3 shows three examples of such transfer functions, each one for a different set of model parameters. The logarithm of the absolute value of the transfer function, the 'gain' in dB, is coded according to a

Figure 2. Simulation of the Spiking Model

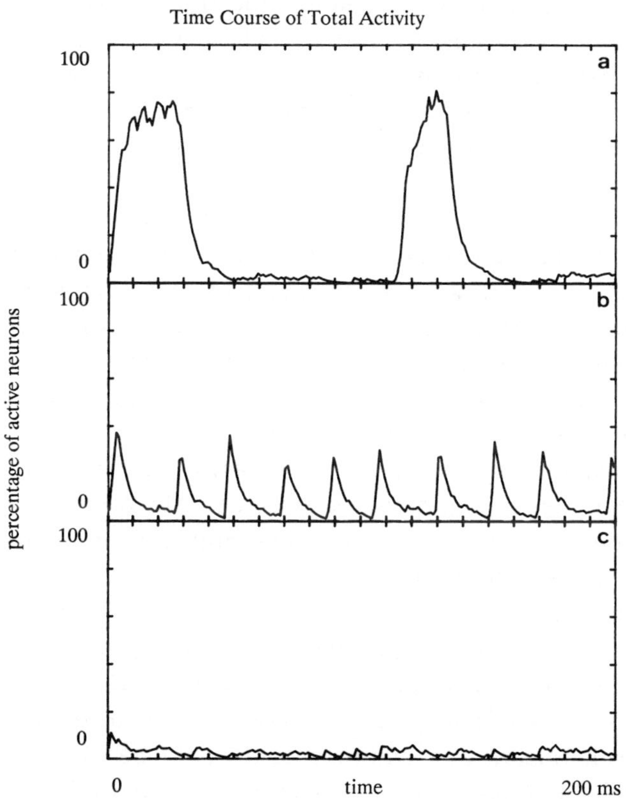

Fig. 2. Lowpass filtered sum activity of the spiking network in response to an input step at t=0 of a random input pattern for three different sets of model parameters (**a**: $\Delta_1=0.1$ ms, $k_1=0.1$, $k_2=3$; **b**: $\Delta_1=1$ ms, $k_1=10$, $k_2=30$; **c**: $\Delta_1=0.1$ ms, $k_1=10$, $k_2=3$). Observe that the network is stable at low rate only in **c**, whereas both in **a** and **b** the network exhibits distinct instabilities, differing both in the time course with which the instability develops and decays and in the frequency of oscillation

grey scale; black spots mark the positions of the poles. For the pole with the largest real part, i.e. the one which lies most to the right, we calculated in each case the growth exponent from the real part, and the oscillation frequency f and period T from the imaginary part. The results are given in Figure 3.

In order to test the predictive value of this stability analysis, we also calculated the step responses of the linearized model for the same three sets of parameter values. The results are shown in Figure 4. Observe that in each case the behavior of the network activity in response to a step input - stable vs. unstable, temporal development of instability, oscillation frequency - agrees very well with the predictions from the pole analysis. In the first two examples, the transfer function has a pole with a positive real part (rightmost black spots in Figs. 3a,b). Accordingly, in both cases the network shows a clearly unstable step response, characterized by a vigorous oscillation (Figs. 4a,b). Observe also that, in accordance with the results of the stability analysis, the first step response (Fig. 4a) exhibits a slower amplitude rise and a higher frequency of oscillation than the second one (Fig. 4b). This reflects the fact that the corresponding pole in the first example (rightmost black spot in Fig. 3a) has a smaller positive real part and a larger imaginary part than its counterpart in the second case (Fig. 3b). In contrast to this, all pole positions in the third example have a negative real part (Fig. 3c). This results in a stable step response with rapidly decreasing amplitude of oscillation (Fig. 4c).

Using this approach of pole analysis, we investigated the influence of the various model parameters on network stability. Unfortunately, the dimensionality of the parameter space is quite high (cf. Fig. 1b), causing an exhaustive exploration to be out of the question. On the other hand, however, the number of truly free parameters, as well as their relevant ranges can be restricted considerably, by using anatomical and physiological plausibility as a constraint. Guided by this criterion, we made a number of exploratory tests in selected subdomains of the parameter space. As it turned out, stability could only be obtained for a very limited range of parameter values. The most crucial of these appeared to be the delay D_1 and the gain k_1 of the fast inhibitory pathway. These were investigated systematically at high resolution, while keeping the others fixed at physiologically plausible and potentially stable values (the standard set defined above). We found that under these circumstances, stability at low firing rate could only be achieved within a very confined 'stability island' (cf. Figs. 3c and 4c as

Figure 3. Logarithmic Plot (dB) of the Absolute Value of the Transfer Function for three Different Parametersets

1: Δ_1 = 0.1 ms k_1 = 40 2: Δ_1 = 0.3 ms k_1 = 10

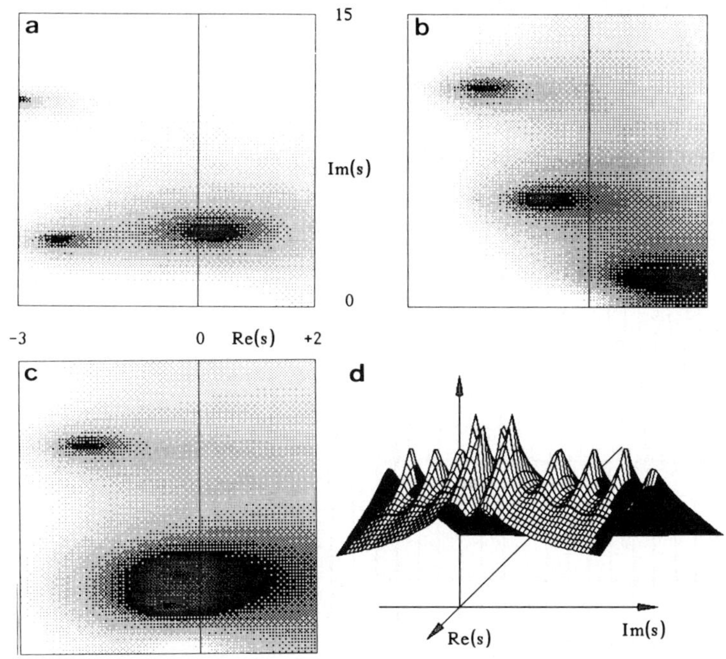

3: Δ_1 = 0.1 ms k_1 = 10 3D-plot for Δ_1 = 0.1 ms k_1 = 10

Results:	$Re(s_p)$	$Im(s_p)$	frequency	period time
1:	0.23	3.54	563 Hz	1.77 ms
2:	0.55	2.53	403 Hz	2.48 ms
3:	-0.36	4.14	659 Hz	1.52 ms

Fig. 3. Transfer function of the linearized network for three different sets of model parameters (**a:** Δ_1=0.1 ms, k_1=40; **b:** Δ_1=0.3 ms, k_1=10; **c:** Δ_1=0.1 ms, k_1=10). The logarithm of the absolute value of the transfer function ('gain' in dB) over a restricted portion of the complex plane is coded according to a grey scale: the larger the value, the darker the grey. Hence, black spots mark the positions of the poles. The growth exponent, the oscillation frequency f and period T, calculated from the real and the imaginary parts of the pole positions are indicated in the Figures. The 3-D plot (**d**) shows the gain for the same parameter combination as in c over an extended range of the complex plane and rotated over 90 degrees. This plot serves to illustrate the multitude and pairwise arrangement of the poles, with the increasing imaginary parts reflecting the various time delays

opposed to 3a,b and 4a,b): the inhibition must be of sufficient but not too great strength and, most critically, should be faster than the excitatory influences (e.g. a 0.1 ms delay for inhibition as compared to 1 ms for excitation). Also, the slope at the operating point of the sigmoid nonlinearity must lie within a certain range; other parameters appear to play a less significant role.

Figure 4. Simulation of the Linear Model

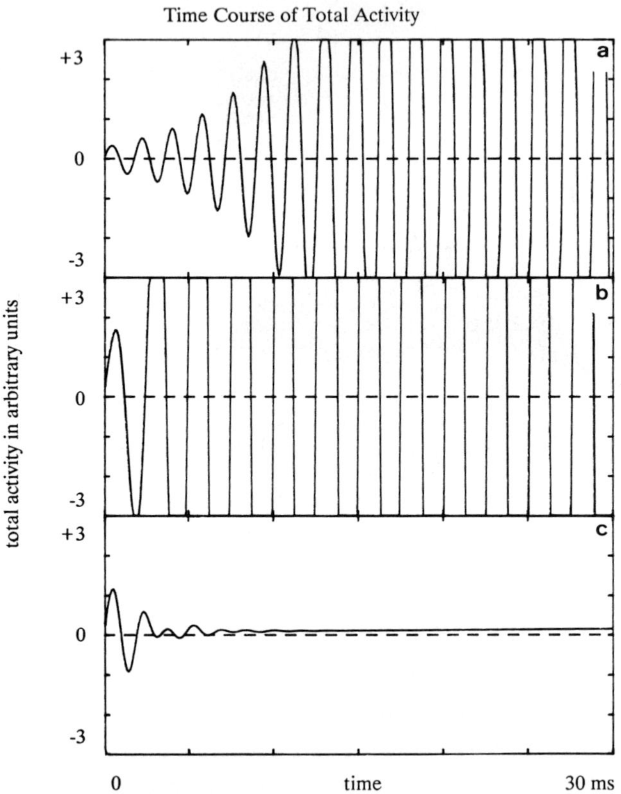

Fig. 4. Lowpass filtered sum activity of linearized network in response to a uniform step input for the same three sets of parameter values as used in Fig. 3. Periods and corresponding oscillation frequencies, directly measured from these step responses are **a**: T=1.81 ms, f=553 Hz; **b**: T=2.64 ms, f=378 Hz; **c**: T=1.67 ms, f=600 Hz. Notice the good correspondence of these values with the corresponding ones in Fig. 3

Stability of nonlinear networks

Clearly, a linear stability analysis can only be expected to reflect the local network behaviour, i.e. the activity dynamics in the vicinity of the fixpoint. For a study of the global dynamics of the network activity, it is necessary to take into account the influence of higher order terms, which come into play because of the sigmoid threshold function of the pyramidal cells (cf. Fig. 1).

After incorporating the non-linear characteristic function into the model network, we again calculated the time course of the network activity in response to an input step. The results are shown in Figure 5 for the same three sets of parameter values used in Figures 3 and 4. Surprisingly, also the behaviour of the nonlinear solutions complies, at least qualitatively, with the predictions from the linear stability analysis. Again, only the third example (Fig. 5c) shows the decay that is indicative of a stable system, whereas the other two (Figs. 5a,b) once more exhibit an unstable, progressively growing oscillation. Observe also, however, that the introduction of the nonlinearity gave rise to a kind of temporal scaling of the step responses: both the rise times of the envelopes and the oscillation frequencies, while approximately retaining their relative magnitude, have clearly grown as compared to their linear counterparts (notice the different time scales in Figs. 4 and 5). In addition, one observes how the amplitude of the oscillations, in contrast to the linear case, is bounded by the saturating nature of the nonlinearity. Moreover, the oscillations exhibit a typical nonlinear distortion, the shape of which is determined by the position of the fixpoint; in our case it is situated in the expansive part of the nonlinearity, due to the imposed constraint of low firing rate (see Erb 1991 for a more elaborate discussion of the nonlinear effects).

Stability of networks with non-uniform connectivity: the emergence of cell assemblies

Thus, an analysis of the pole positions of the transfer function for the simplified model network enables us to make testable predictions regarding the stability of the network, both in the linear and the nonlinear case. The question arises to what extent these predictions remain valid for networks with a more interesting connectivity, in which not all connections are of the same strength. In order to answer this question, we will continue to alleviate, step by step, the simplifying assumptions we made when reducing the full model (Fig. 1) to the linearized transfer function (Equ. 1).

Figure 5. Simulation of the Nonlinear Model

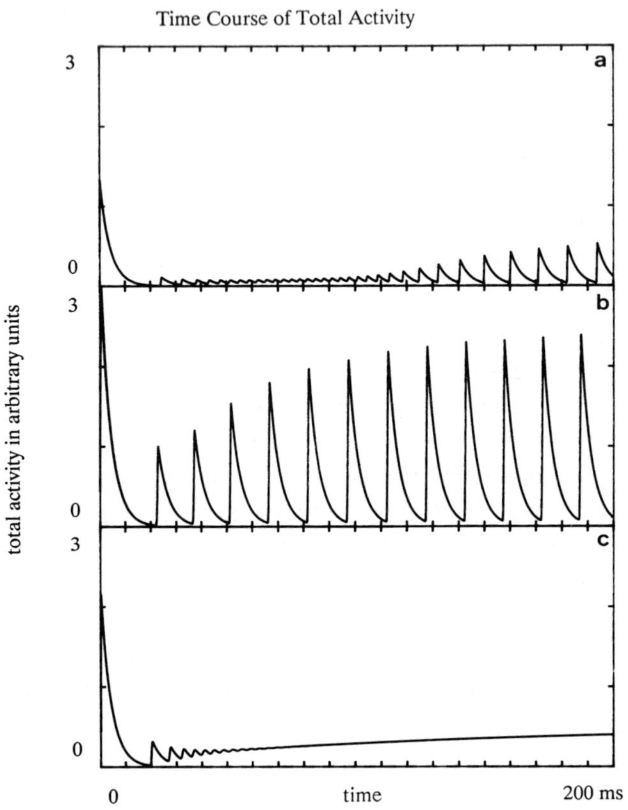

Fig. 5. Lowpass filtered sum activity of the nonlinear network in response to a uniform step input for the same three sets of parameter values as used in Figs. 3 and 4. Observe the qualitative correspondence in the behaviour of the linear and nonlinear solutions: stable vs. unstable, relation between oscillation frequencies and time constants of build-up and decay of oscillation. Notice also the new features introduced by the sigmoid nonlinearity: temporal scaling (compare the different time scales in Figs. 4 and 5), bounded amplitude and distorted waveform of the oscillations.

Deterministic networks of analog neurons

We addressed the issue of nonuniformity of connections by two different approaches. First, we returned to the original, *random* connectivity matrix with constant mean value and uniformly distributed stochastic fluctuations around it (cf. Fig. 2), and gradually increased the fluctuation range. Analysis of the step responses (not shown here) demonstrated that, for a nonlinear network with mean connectivity of 0.3 and fluctuations in the range of %0.1 (i.e. for a dynamic range in the connectivity of a factor of 2), the time course of the summated activity could hardly be distinguished from that in the uniformly connected network (Erb 1991). Moreover, the activity of the individual neurons followed very closely the time course of the summated activity for the entire net. Clearly, the averaging over the many different synaptic connections taking place in each neuron separately gives rise to very similar membrane potential trajectories. Thus, the variability among the activity profiles of different neurons is strongly reduced. As a consequence, under these conditions the individual dynamics and, hence, the mean of the dynamics closely follow the dynamics of the mean. This tendency towards homogeneity in large, highly interconnected networks only breaks down when the dynamic range of the connectivity strengths becomes larger and larger and/or when the connectivity matrix exhibits a clear structure.

In a second approach we investigated the activity dynamics for a *structured* network connectivity. To this end we used a connectivity matrix resulting from a study of associative memory and the performance of different types of learning rules (Erb 1985, 1991; Palm 1986, 1987). In particular, we used a fixed connectivity matrix in which were embedded the memory traces of a set of 10 randomly generated input patterns. The activity in response to a uniform input step for a nonlinear network with this structured connectivity matrix is depicted in Figure 6, again for the same three sets of parameter values as used in the foregoing. Each of the three Figures 6a-c shows the time course of the summated network activity (righthand panel), together with the individual neuron activities (superimposed traces in lefthand panel). Observe that, with the exception of Fig. 6c, the time course of the summated network activity is hardly discernible from the activity in the uniformly connected network (Fig. 5), which once more emphasizes the strong homogenizing effect of averaging.

More interestingly, however, the time courses of the single neuron activities now exhibit two different kinds of nonuniformities. In the first and second example (Figs. 6a,b), the network activity develops into a synchronous oscillation in which *all* neurons are partaking, each one, however, with a somewhat different amplitude as manifested by the broadening of the band of superimposed traces in the lefthand panels. We note that this coherent oscillation is imposed by the global inhibition, which itself is oscillating in counterphase. Interestingly, in

Figure 6. Simulation of the Nonlinear Model with a Learned Matrix

Time Course of Single Neuron Activity and Total Activity

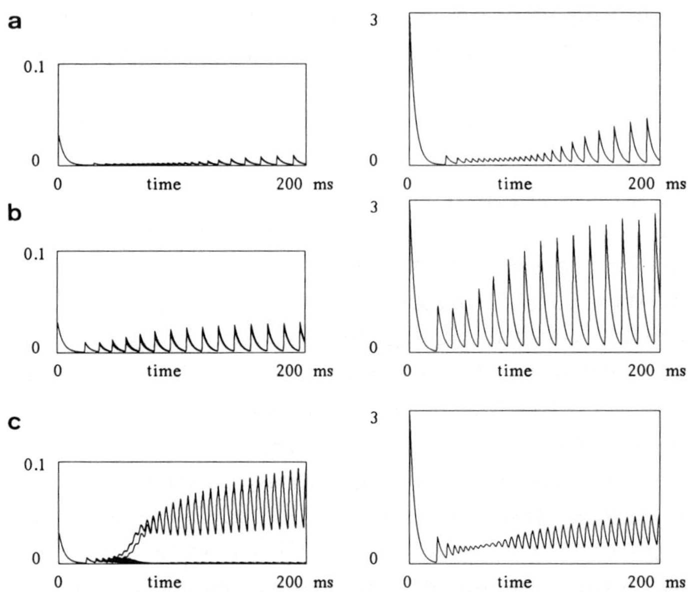

Fig. 6. Dynamic behaviour of the activity in the nonlinear network with analog neurons and structured connectivity matrix. Response to a uniform step input for the same three sets of parameter values as used in Figs. 3 to 5. Time course of the lowpass filtered sum activity (righthand panels) and individual neuron activities (superimposed traces in lefthand panels). Observe the striking similarity of the summated activity with that in the uniformly connected network (Fig. 5). Notice also, however, the different kinds of nonuniformities in the time courses of the single neuron activities. In particular, Fig. **6c** reveals the emergence of a cell assembly: the dynamic instability temporarily dissociates a sub-group, defined through it interconnections, from the network it is embedded in

the third example (Fig. 6c) after a transient, global oscillation in which all neurons participate (0-60 ms), the nonlinearity splits the net into two subgroups: a small group of neurons which increase their firing rates and develop a coherent oscillation, whereas the majority of neurons does not feel addressed by the stimulus and rapidly settles at a very low firing rate. Since the mean activity level in the 'ignited' subgroup (Fig. 6c) is higher than the overall level calculated for the entire network with uniform connectivity (Fig. 5c), the active subgroup develops an unstable oscillation, even at parameter values for which the uniform net was stable. Evidently this last case is the more interesting one from the point of view of information processing. The selective instability provides a mechanism which temporarily dissociates a particular subgroup, defined through it interconnections, from the network it is embedded in. This behaviour closely corresponds to Hebb's notion of a 'cell assembly' (Hebb 1949), and, hence, provides a functional mechanism for signalling the occurrence of some interesting constellation in the 'outside' world.

Stochastic networks of spiking neurons

In a final step, in order to return from the simplified description to the full model, we reinstated the stochastic description with spiking neurons. Using the same structured connectivity matrix as in the deterministic case (Fig. 6), we again measured the step responses. The results for the same three sets of parameter values are shown in Figure 7: the lowpass filtered spike trains for the entire network (righthand panels in Figs. 7a-c) and for the individual neurons (superimposed traces in lefthand panels in Figs. 7a-c and raster displays in Figs. 7d-f). Notice that the activity dynamics in these stochastic, spiking networks resemble those in the deterministic network very strongly. The time course of the *summated* activity, particularly in the first two examples, is quite comparable to that in Figure 6. In addition, we observe similar departures from homogeneity among the *individual* neuron activities as in the deterministic case. Either practically all neurons participate in a coherent global oscillation, albeit with varying amplitudes and differing degrees of synchrony (Figs. 7a,b,d,e) or, alternatively, after a transient oscillation (0-100 ms), the net splits up into separate subgroups: a small group of neurons increase their firing rates, while the majority rapidly settles at a very low rate (Figs. 7c,f).

Figure 7. Simulation of the Spiking Model with a Learned Matrix

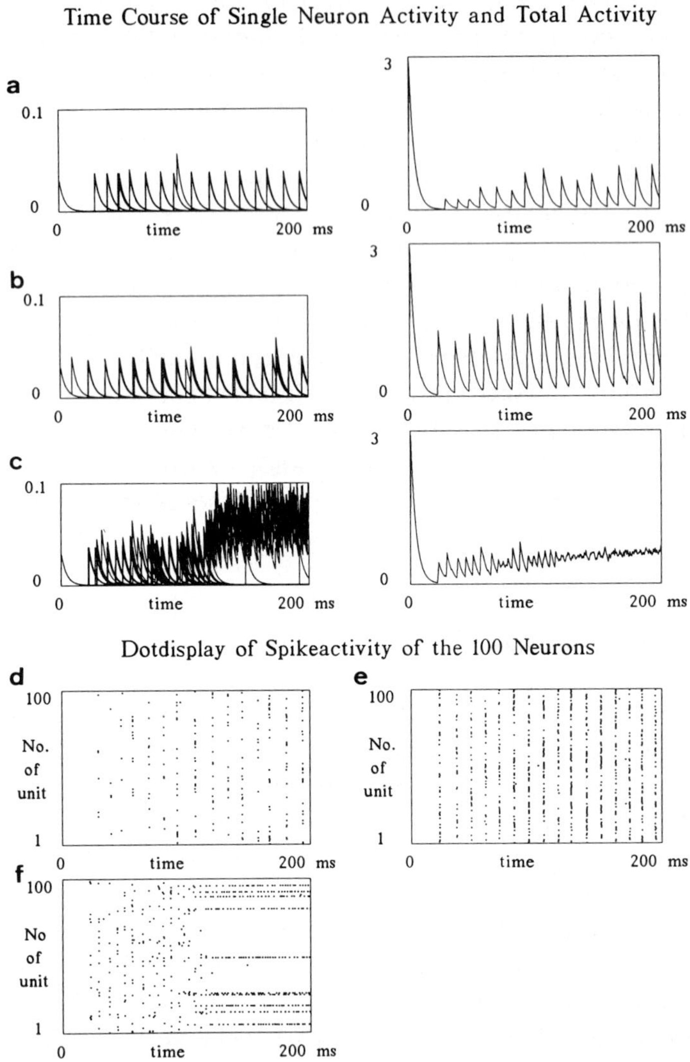

Fig. 7. Dynamic behaviour of the activity in the nonlinear network with stochastic, spiking neurons and structured connectivity matrix. Response to a uniform step input for the same three sets of parameter values as used in Figs. 3 to 6. Time course of the lowpass filtered sum activity (**a-c**: righthand panels) and individual neuron activities (**a-c**: superimposed traces in lefthand panels; **d-f**: raster displays). Observe that the activity dynamics in these stochastic, spiking networks resemble those in the deterministic networks very strongly, both for the sum activity and the single neuron activities. In contrast to the analog network, however, the assembly activity (**c**, **f**) reveals a difference in coherence between spike events and firing rates, demonstrating that this class of networks may exhibit different

Thus, also for stochastically spiking neurons, widespread stimulation of a structured feedback network, after a short epoch of global oscillation, may induce a selective activation and, hence, a temporary dissociation of a particular subgroup from the network.

A more detailed inspection of the activity patterns developed by the analog and the spiking networks reveals a new feature, which is only exhibited by the spiking network. Interestingly, and in contrast to the analog network, the results in Figs. 7c (left) and 7f show that the spike trains of neurons in the activated cell assembly rapidly loose their coherence upon reaching their increased activity level. This fast modulation of spike correlation is not reflected in the firing rates of the neurons involved. These gradually build up and stay at a relatively high level, independently of the reorganization taking place in the precise timing of the individual events. As a consequence, the sum activity of the assembly, after a short epoch of synchronous oscillation following 'ignition', quickly decays to a noisy constant high level. This suggests that the spiking network may be inherently more stable than the analog network with otherwise unchanged parameters, and that when, for some reason, a subgroup instability does develop, it lasts for a rather short time. Indeed, results from additional simulations (not shown here) indicate that in spiking networks with sparse firing, the stability problem is less severe than it appears in the stability analysis of the linearized model with 'analog' neurons.

In addition, this difference in coherence between spike events and firing rates demonstrates that this class of networks may exhibit different correlation dynamics simultaneously, each of them characterized by its own time constant. The correlation among the activities of different neurons may show rapid synchronization of spike trains (*event coherence*) and, simultaneously yet more or less independently, slower co-variations of firing rates (*rate coherence*). Such different correlation dynamics have also been observed in physiological recordings from various cortex preparations (e.g. Krüger and Mayer 1990; Aertsen and Gerstein 1991; Vaadia et al. 1991; Aertsen et al. 1992). A more extensive discussion of their functional significance will be given elsewhere (Neven and Aertsen, in preparation).

---

correlation dynamics simultaneously, each of them characterized by its own time constant: rapid synchronization of spike trains (event coherence) and, simultaneously yet more or less independently, slower co-variations of firing rates (rate coherence)

Discussion

On the basis of a stability analysis of the linearized network model, we found stability at low firing rates only for a very restricted range of parameter values. The most crucial parameters appear to be the delay and the gain of the fast inhibitory pathway. In particular, one needs shorter delays in this pathway than in the excitatory connections (e.g. 0.1 ms delay for inhibition vs. 1 ms for excitation). Such delays are incorporated implicitly in most neural network models, since updating of the membrane potential takes place only one simulation time step after the generation of spikes. Also the slope at the operating point of the sigmoid nonlinearity must be in an adequate range. This can be achieved from outside the network by adjusting either the mean input strength or the set value for the slow inhibition. Other parameters appear to play a less significant role.

The dynamic behaviour of networks consisting of neurons with a nonlinear threshold function was qualitatively comparable to that of the linearized model, indicating that the nonlinearity does not play a crucial role as far as stability is concerned. The same holds for the influence of the connectivity matrix, as long as its dynamic range remains withing certain bounds. Even when the variation among the connection strengths becomes large, the sum activity of the network still basically follows the general pattern described for the simplified model network. Summarizing, we observe very similar dynamics of the summated network activity in all cases studied: a stable solution for a very confined 'island' in parameter space, characterized primarily by very fast and sufficiently strong inhibition, and in the majority of cases a synchronous oscillation with frequency and amplitude dynamics governed predominantly by the inhibition parameters, but largely independent of (1) the network architecture (uniform, random or structured), (2) the spiking or analog nature of the neural activity, and, albeit to a lesser extent, (3) the linear or nonlinear nature of the neural threshold function. Finally, simulations of networks with stochastic, spiking neurons suggest that in such networks the problem of stability at low firing rates may be less severe than in networks of deterministic, 'analog' neurons.

Our finding that stability in sparsely firing feedback networks requires a considerably shorter delay of inhibition than of excitation is in agreement with observations by Abeles (1991), as well as with results of a number of theoretical studies (e.g. Marcus and Westervelt 1989; Amit and Treves 1989; Rubin and Sompolinsky 1989; Golomb et al. 1990). Moreover, it fits well with the notion that inhibition acts locally, i.e. directly on the cell body or on proximal dendrites, whereas excitation is projected onto the dendritic trees, and is more prominent in (long-range) cortico-cortical connections, thus involving longer delays (Braitenberg and Schüz 1991; Schüz, this Volume). Our study further demonstrates that, provided the network connectivity is sufficiently rich and structured, subgroups of neurons may be briefly dissociated from the net by the temporal coherence of the activity patterns that develop upon stimulation. This behaviour is precisely what was predicted by the 'cell assembly' hypothesis (Hebb 1949; Gerstein et al. 1989) and the concept of the 'synfire chain' (Abeles 1982). Moreover, it conforms to a number of related physiological observations (e.g. Eckhorn et al. 1988 and this Volume; Gray and Singer 1989a,b; Aertsen and Gerstein 1991; Vaadia et al. 1991). Finally, the different simultaneous correlation dynamics exhibited by the spiking network model, event coherence and rate coherence, also find their physiological counterpart in observations on cortical recordings (Krüger and Mayer 1990; Vaadia et al. 1991; Aertsen et al. 1992).

One of the salient conclusions of our study was that the task of 'tuning' a feedback network to a stable, low firing rate proved to be quite difficult. This was reflected in the unsolicited experience that, before availing ourselves of the guidance of the stability analysis, we spent impressive amounts of time searching for appropriate parameter settings that would keep the network from oscillating. At this point it should be stressed that none of our network components has any intrinsic tendency to oscillate; the interactions in the network fully suffice to make the network go into oscillation, as anyone who ever tried to build an amplifier will appreciate. In view of this observation, the question how the real cortex, assuming that it works along similar principles, solves this inherent stability problem becomes only more pertinent. It is conceivable that not all parts of the cortex manage this problem equally well, or that the solutions that evolved in different species are not all equally efficient in coping with the unavoidable variations of 'network parameters'. In this respect it is tempting to speculate that experimentally observed oscillations in some physiological cortical networks, e.g. in cat visual cortex (Gray and Singer 1989a,b; Eckhorn et al. 1988 and this Volume) might possibly be instances of systems which failed to solve this stability problem adequately, especially when confronted with effective stimuli and, hence, correspondingly higher levels of input activity. If this were indeed the case, the question might be not so much how the brain functions by virtue of oscillations, as most researchers working on cortical oscillations seem to assume, but rather how it manages to do so in spite of them.

When having to work with a system, which lives on the brink of instability and every once in a while develops partial, transitory 'explosions', another possibility comes to mind. If short, activity-related epochs of instability of portions of the net are apparently unavoidable and bound to occur from time to time, one might as well use them for a convenient purpose. An obvious candidate for such an application, in fact, the one usually put forward in connection with cortical oscillations, is that of 'dynamical linking', in which temporal coherence among active neurons defines their short-lived functional association (e.g. von der Malsburg 1981, 1986). Certainly our finding that networks with strongly nonuniform connectivity exhibit short epochs of synchronized instability, with subgroups of neurons temporarily dissociated from the network (Figs. 6,7) would be consistent with this idea (see also Aertsen and Gerstein 1991; Aertsen and Preissl 1991). Also, the manifestation of two distinct correlation dynamics, event coherence and rate coherence, exhibited both by the spiking network model and in physiological recordings, appears to be relevant in this respect (Neven and Aertsen, in preparation).

Expanding along these lines, one could, in fact, rethink the original goal of striving towards a stable network with fixpoint dynamics and, instead, consider the information processing capabilities of networks with more complex, dynamic attractor states. Clearly the limit cycle attractor is the first one that comes to mind when faced with the oscillating nature of our network dynamics, but obviously there are other, more elaborate possibilities, such as dynamics governed by quasi-periodic 'strange' attractors (e.g. Skarda and Freeman 1987; Preissl and Aertsen, this Volume). Clearly, an essential requirement in this context would be that not the entire net partakes in the instability, since such a trivial global state would not leave any room for a selective coding or computational mechanism to establish itself. Rather, the membership of the 'ignited' subgroups should be selective and transient, preferably determined by the dynamic interplay of connectivity within the net and neural activity feeding into it. In this respect, both the assembly-like activity patterns described above and the rapid, stimulus-dependent modifications of functional connectivity observed earlier (Erb et al. 1986, 1989; Aertsen and Preissl 1991) seem to support this as a viable alternative. A study, specifically aimed to elucidate this dynamic concept of neuronal computation and memory, is currently in progress.

Acknowledgements

We thank Günther Palm, Hubert Preißl and Stefan Rotter for many stimulating discussions. Partial funding for this project was received from the Bundesministerium für Forschung und Technologie (BMFT) and the Stiftung Volkswagenwerk (I/64605).

References

Abeles M. (1982) Local Cortical Circuits. An electrophysiological study. Springer, Berlin Heidelberg New York

Abeles M. (1991) Corticonics. Neural circuits in the cerebral cortex. Cambridge University Press, Cambridge, U.K.

Abeles M, Vaadia E, Bergman H (1990) Firing patterns of single units in the prefrontal cortex and neural network models. Network 1:13-35

Aertsen A, Gerstein G (1991) Dynamic aspects of neuronal cooperativity: Fast stimulus-locked modulations of 'effective connectivity'. In: Krüger J (ed) Neuronal Cooperativity. Springer, Berlin Heidelberg New York, pp 52-67

Aertsen A, Preissl H (1991) Dynamics of activity and connectivity in physiological neuronal networks. In: Schuster H (ed) Nonlinear Dynamics and Neuronal Networks. VHC Verlag, Weinheim, pp 281-301

Aertsen A, Vaadia E, Abeles M, Ahissar E, Bergman H, Karmon B, Lavner Y, Margalit E, Nelken I, Rotter S (1992) Neural interactions in the frontal cortex of a behaving monkey: Signs of dependence on stimulus context and behavioral state. J f Hirnforsch (in press)

Amit DJ, Treves A (1989) Associative memory neural networks with low temporal spiking rates. Proc Natl Acad Sci USA 86:7851-7875

Braitenberg V (1978) Cell assemblies in the cerebral cortex. In: Heim R, Palm G (eds) Theoretical Approaches to Complex Systems. Lecture Notes in Biomathematics, Vol. 21, Springer, Berlin Heidelberg New York, pp 171-188

Braitenberg V, Schüz A (1991) Anatomy of the Cortex. Statistics and Geometry. Springer, Berlin Heidelberg New York

Eckhorn R, Bauer R, Jordan W, Brosch M, Kruse W, Munk M, Reitboeck HJ (1988) Coherent oscillations: a mechanism of feature linking in the visual cortex? Multiple electrode and correlation analysis in the cat. Biol Cybern 60:121-130

Erb M (1985) Computersimulation eines assoziativen Speichers als Modell für die Funktion der Großhirnrinde. MSc Thesis (in German), Eberhard-Karls-Universität Tübingen (FRG)

Erb M, Palm G, Aertsen A, Bonhoeffer T (1986) Functional versus structural connectivity in neuronal nets. In: Strukturbildung und Musteranalyse, Proc. 9th Cybernetics Congress (DGK). Göttingen FRG, p 23

Erb M, Aertsen A, Palm G (1989) Functional connectivity in neuronal systems: context-dependence of effective network organization does not require synaptic plasticity. In: Elsner N, Singer W (eds) Dynamics and plasticity in neuronal systems. Thieme, Stuttgart New York, p 445

Erb M, Aertsen A, Palm G (1990) Stability in physiology-oriented neuronal network models. In: Elsner N, Roth G (eds) Brain - Perception - Cognition. Thieme, Stuttgart New York, p 527

Erb M (1991) Simulation neuronaler Netze: Stabilität, Plastizität und Konnektivität. PhD Thesis (in German), Eberhard-Karls-Universität Tübingen (FRG)

Gerstein GL, Bedenbaugh P, Aertsen AMHJ (1989) Neuronal Assemblies. IEEE Trans Biomed Engin 36:4-14

Golomb D, Rubin N, Sompolinsky H (1990) Willshaw model: Associative memory with sparse coding and low firing rates. Phys Rev A 41:1853-1854

Gray CM, Singer W (1989a) Stimulus-specific neuronal oscillations in orientation columns of cat visual cortex. Proc Natl Acad Sci USA 86:1698-1702

Gray CM, König P, Engel AK, Singer W (1989b) Oscillatory responses in cat visual cortex exhibit inter-columnar synchronization which reflects global stimulus properties. Nature 338:334-337

Hebb DO (1949) The organization of behavior. A neuropsychological theory. Wiley, New York

Krüger J, Mayer M (1990) Two types of neuronal synchrony in monkey striate cortex. Biol Cybern 64:135-140

Marcus CM, Westerveld RM (1989) Stability of analog neural networks with delay. Phys Rev A 39:347-359

Malsburg, C. von der (1981) The correlation theory of brain function. Internal report 81-2. Max-Planck-Institute for Biophysical Chemistry, Göttingen (FRG)

Malsburg, C. von der (1986) Am I thinking assemblies? In: Palm G, Aertsen A (eds) Brain Theory. Springer, Berlin Heidelberg New York, pp 161-176

Palm G (1982) Neural Assemblies. An alternative approach to artificial intelligence. Springer, Berlin Heidelberg New York

Palm G (1986) Associative networks and cell assemblies. In: Palm G, Aertsen A (eds) Brain Theory. Springer, Berlin Heidelberg New York, pp 211-228

Palm G (1987) On associative memories. In: Caianiello ER (ed) Physics of cognitive processes. World Scientific Publishing, Singapore, pp 380-442

Rubin N, Sompolinsky H (1989) Neural networks with low firing rates. Europhys Lett 10:465-470

Skarda CA, Freeman WJ (1987) How brains make chaos to make sense of the world. Brain Behav Sci 10:161-195

Vaadia E, Ahissar E, Bergman H, Lavner Y (1991) Correlated activity of neurons: a neural code for higher brain functions? In: Krüger J (ed) Neuronal Cooperativity. Springer, Berlin Heidelberg New York, pp 249-279

A Theoretical Approach to the Late Components of the Event-Related Brain Potential

Thomas Elbert[1]

Universität Konstanz, Dept. of Psychology, Postfach 5560, 7750 Konstanz, Germany

Introductory examples of late components

In the mid seventies, Brigitte Rockstroh and myself studied avoidance learning in human subjects. We presumed that brain potentials might be a better predictor of resistance to extinction than, for example, autonomic responses. In one experiment, subjects could escape a highly aversive noise by pressing a button fast enough. As it happens in experimental laboratories, a loose connection in the wire which was attached to the button, only randomly transmitted the subject's response to the computer. Consequently the subject experienced a sudden unexpected change in response contingency, which, of course, we completely denied when reported to us. The complaint about the frequent and unpredictable punishment was, at first, answered only with a request to follow adequately the instruction. When we examined the subject's EEG responses we detected a marked negative wave following many of the single motor responses. This was unusual as generally a positive wave accompanies the termination of an overt response. Systematic studies soon revealed that a pronounced negativity develops, whenever expectations of relevant predictions are not fulfilled, whenever there is a need for ongoing processing (Rockstroh et al. 1979; Elbert et al. 1982; Elbert 1986). Controlled experiments soon revealed that such slow negative variations of the EEG-baseline had little to do with the physical properties of the stimulus as such, but were determined by the psychological context the stimuli were put in. Kutas and Hillyard (1980, 1984) extracted a similar finding from an elegant series

---

[1] present address: Institut für Experimentelle Audiologie, WWU Münster, Kardinal-von-Galen-Ring 10, 4400 Münster, Germany

of experiments: word by word they presented sentences to the subject which were either semantically correct or incongruent: "He drank coffee with milk and shoes". When a subject processes such a sentence, word by word, each one will cause a small deflection of the EEG amplifier's needle towards negativity, quickly followed by a positive return. Not so the one quoted last! In our example, the word "shoes" will trigger a huge negativity (Fig. 1, dashed line). The appearance of this brain wave has nothing to do with the physical aspects of the presented words, but depends exclusively on the context the word has been put in. If, for instance, the sentence had been "She put on her high heeled shoes", the very same physical stimulus "shoes" would have triggered a brain wave opposite in polarity, with smaller amplitude, and longer latency (Fig. 1, solid line). And also, the scalp distribution of both waves would be different. This demonstrates that one and the same pattern on the retina may activate completely different neural generators, depending on the context the stimulus is put in. On the other hand, exactly the same EEG pattern can be evoked irrespective of whether the word is presented visually or acoustically. It is not trivial that some of the brain activity accompanying such high-level

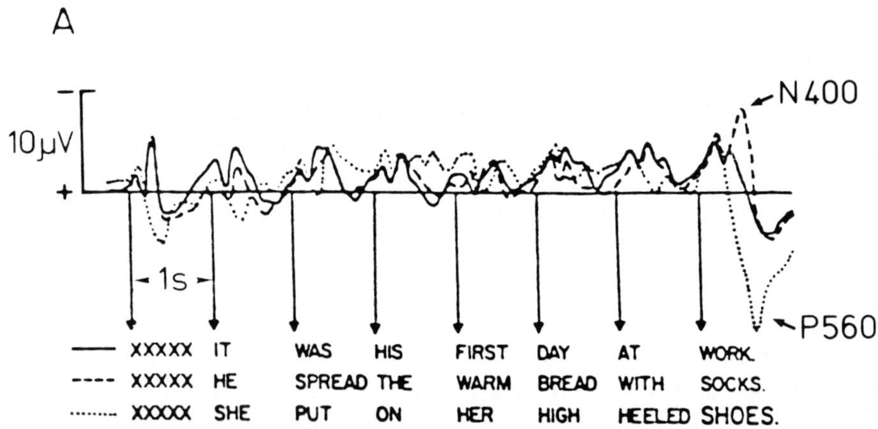

Fig. 1. The EEG averaged over three subjects and a number of presentations of sentences is displayed while subjects process different categories of sentences. The solid line results when the sentences are congruent. A semantically incongruent ending evokes a slow negativity (*dashed line*) while a physical deviation of the stimulus, in this case a change in the letter size, produces a enlarged positivity (P560, *dotted line*). (Extracted from Kutas and Hillyard 1980, with permission)

processing can be recorded from the scalp. Only synchronized neural mass activity generates such large amplitude waves. Information processing should require distinct patterns of neural activity rather than many neurons doing the same thing at the same time.

A physically incongruent stimulus, like in "She put on her high heeled *shoes*" would have produced even another wave. Figure 1 includes several of the components comprising the event-related brain potentials. The N400 is a negative wave, peaking approximately 400 ms after the stimulus, the P560 is a positive wave with 560 ms latency.

Often, the cognitive operations triggering these waves may occur at other latencies than e.g. at 560 ms. It would not, however, be very convenient to give two different names to very similar neural processes. If comparable steps in the information processing trigger brain waves with similar scalp distributions we will give it the same name even if the latency is different.[1]

The concept of a component

Almost any external or internal event may produce a change in the flow of oscillations of the EEG. Patterns which are reproduced with repeated presentation of an event are commonly referred to as *'event-related'* potentials. The term evoked potential is virtually synonymous, but this latter tends to be applied only when the event has little psychological impact, or if relatively short-latency fluctuations are considered. Averaging across repeated trials is commonly assumed to provide a reasonable approximation to the waveform.

Most waveforms are composites of contributions from various functionally separable cerebral processes. It is commonly postulated that the event-related potential results from a sequence of overlapping activities of different assemblies of nerve cells, each such activity representing a component.

The earliest electrical activity a stimulus evokes is the train of exogenous components. It is supposed to reflect the input and transmission of information along the afferent sensory pathway to the primary

---

[1] The reason we often refer to a distinct positive shift as a P300 or simply P3 and not e.g. P560 has to do more with historical development than with its most common latency. If the potential is filtered using a short time constant, the peak latency will be artificially shortened.

projection areas. A different intensity of the tone, a different pitch or location in space of the evoking sound will change these waveforms, but not a different meaning of the signal, not the context the stimulus is put in. After 100 ms the waveforms of the various event-related potentials to different stimuli become more and more alike, even regardless of the modality of the eliciting stimulus. This suggests that these later or slower components are generated by neuronal assemblies that perform operations on the incoming information such as memory or attention-related operations. Such operations are flexible in the sense that they depend on context, task, instructions and so forth; in other words on *internal representations*, even as to whether they are called for or not. Accordingly, the late components are regarded as endogenous.

In the following I will briefly review the most prominent endogenous components, particularly those with relatively long latencies and discuss their relation to psychological processes. Then I will turn to the neural generation of these electrical waves with sources mostly in cerebral cortex and outline a possible theory underlying the generation of these slow cortical potentials.

A brief tour through the zoo of endogenous components:

Fig. 2 represents a schematic overview of those late components which have been investigated most intensely. The N1 or N100-complex refers to a negative half wave with maximal amplitudes over fronto-central regions. Part of it is generated in auditory cortex from where it projects to the frontal scalp. The N1 is a mixture still, of both, exogenous and endogenous subcomponents. One part of it is related to orienting and the arousing aspects of a stimulus, thus it varies with the physical intensity but also with the novelty of the stimulus. This aspect of the N1, the so-called vertex potential or N1/P2 is widespread and seems to be triggered via an unspecific reticular activation. Another subcomponent is more closely linked to selective attention. A subject can suppress responses to incoming stimuli while attending to others, but only if the two stimulus categories can be discriminated on the basis of their physical properties. When hearing a mixture of voices, we can listen to one speaker, and process information from just this one

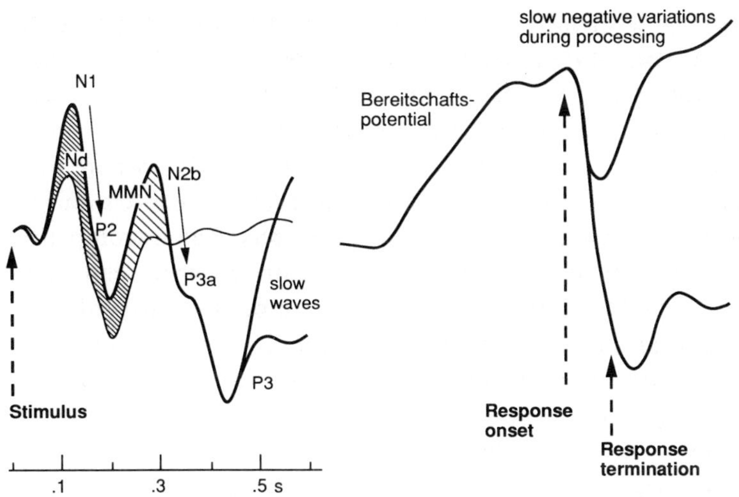

Fig. 2. Schematic categorization of endogenous components of the event-related potential in response to a stimulus (left) and prior to a voluntary response (right)

speaker due to the different frequency characteristics of every voice. Probably, the enhancement of N1-amplitude to stimuli in the attended channel does not originate in an enhanced gain of the attended pathway, but results from an independently generated slow negative shift generated in the secondary sensory areas of the cortex, and superimposed on the faster evoked waveform (Hillyard 1981).

When infrequent, physically deviant stimuli are randomly embedded in a train of standard stimuli, a frontal negative wave is elicited, its scalp distribution being modality-specific. This component which reaches its maximal deflection after 200 ms has been termed N2a or mismatch negativity. (MMN). Unlike the N1-enhancement, the wave is insensitive to the direction of attention: N2a can be recorded whether or not the subject is attempting to detect the deviant stimuli and whether or not that detection is successful. That is to say, the underlying discrimination is a pre-attentive response. Its amplitude increases with decreasing probability of the deviant stimulus. For acoustic stimuli the MMN is generated in the primary auditory cortex, having a dipole moment such that it projects to the fronto-central scalp surface. (A recent theoretical account for the MMN can be found in Näätänen 1990).

The MMN characteristics are contrasted by the N4-properties. After hearing "coffee with milk and ..." a subject probably expects the word sugar. When confronted with "shoes", one might think what's wrong? Is the sentence not yet finished, is the coffee consumed with shoe-fly-pie". All kinds of weird hypotheses are screened in rapid succession with the hope to resolve the ambiguity. Only, when presented in a certain context, the word 'shoe' deserves a second thought. Semantic incongruity triggers the N4, but not physical incongruity. Words are not essential, a sequence of cartoons, for example, can elicit a N4 as well. And the N4 obviously is a member of a family of surface-negative waves, as indicated by the introductory example. When a subject perceives a loss of contingency or control the negativity may be quite long-lasting. The post-processing of the stimulus includes prevailing readiness to accept further information or to generate hypotheses which might resolve the incongruity or ambiguity (Elbert et al. 1982; Birbaumer et al. 1986).

If, in the above sentence the word had been 'sugar', - full-stop - the sentence would have been complete. A subject could have closed that part of information processing. And a positive brain wave, a P3 would appear. More precisely, this component would be a P3b.

Characteristics of the P3b are its positive maximum in the latency range between 280 and 600 ms and its posterior scalp distribution. Its amplitude is inversely related to stimulus probability and also to the subjective outcome probability. The more relevant the task, the higher is the P3 amplitude, thereby task relevance and subjective probability affect P3 in a multiplicative manner. The amplitude is also sensitive to the interval between the events, being inversely proportional to the decay of the representation established by preceding occurrences of the eliciting events. As the P3-amplitude is sensitive to the information value of the stimulus and also related to recall, it is tempting to conclude that "the P3 is a correlate of processes that are invoked whenever there is a need to revise the organism's model of the context. We are assuming that the larger the amplitude of the P3, the larger the change in the model". (Donchin and Coles 1988).[2]

A further example illustrates most clearly that the physical stimulus as such is not important to evoke a P3 but certain steps related to the information processing: Assume you have just purchased an old fashioned Coocoo-Clock from the Black Forest for quite some money

---

[2] Availabe evidence suggests that P3 latency is related to categorization time but unrelated to response execution.

which goes "Tic - tac - tic - tac - tic - - tic - tac - tic ...". Ouups, a tac was missing. A P3b can be recorded each time you are counting such an omitted stimulus.

When the coocoo appears, you are likely to respond with yet another wave, a N2b/P3a followed by a negative afterwave with an amplitude the higher the more crazy you think that these Black Forest people are. Except for its latency around 200 to 300 ms, the N2b/P3a bears close resemblance with the vertex potential. Thus this component also predominates centrally to fronto-centrally. It depends on the attentional set and is sensitive to stimulus novelty. Consequently, it has been associated with a second stage in orienting.

It is interesting to note that we perceive events which arouse a lasting negative brain wave often as positive, they grasp our interest, evoke our curiosity. As sensation seekers we sometimes even look for events which can make our brain potentials more negative.

Slow Cortical Potentials

This leads us to the slow cortical potentials, in particular to the slow negative variations of the EEG-baseline like the Contingent Negative Variation (CNV) and the Bereitschaftspotential (BP) which both are related more to action and output than to input of information (Fig. 2). Although behavior is a continuous process, it can be decomposed into many subunits. Larger subunits are known as 'actions', of which there are many different types. Subunits which uniformly reappear within behavioral sequences are called reactions, with 're'-action indicating that the behavior is elicited as a response to some event. However, reactions can also be emitted without direct relationship to an external event. If the source of action lies within the reacting individual, then the reaction is known as 'voluntary response'.

The onset of a voluntary movement is typically preceded by a ramp-like surface negative shift starting about a second or so prior to the first detectable EMG-response.

Discovered in the sixties by Deecke and Kornhuber, this negative potential became known as the Bereitschaftspotential or readiness potential, referring to the activity of getting ready or becoming prepared for a voluntary response. Psychological parameters largely affect characteristics of the BP. The complexity of the movement enhances BP-amplitude over the motor strip. Visual attention, like spatio-visual tracking will generate negativity over occipital regions, learning and complex task instructions will activate frontal areas (Rockstroh et al. 1989).

The response as such is not important. By means of EEG auto-correlation it has been uncovered that a BP even develops during intended but not executed movements (Keidel 1983).

In a series of elegant experiments Libet (1985, 1982) has asked subjects as to when they became aware of their intention to act. He demonstrated that the increase in scalp-recorded negativity prior to a self-initiated motor response precedes the subjective awareness of the intention to act. The subject will not become aware of his/her will until a distinct amplitude level is reached. Obviously, a certain *threshold* in negativity must be reached before the response will be executed.

The BP is just one representative of a family of slow negativities. Often external rather than internal processes time the response execution. The term contingent negative variation (CNV) refers to those negative shifts which are elicited by a warning signal (S1), indicating to a subject that a certain response is required a few seconds later, with presentation of a second stimulus (S2). The amplitude varies between -10 and -20 μV, reaching extremes of more than 50 μV. It increases with increasing probability of S2-occurrence, with the aversiveness of the expected event (S2) or with the high incentive value of the response. It is also higher when a fast response is required, but decreases with task complexity. It is reduced under CNS-depressants. The scalp distribution, though widespread, indicates maximal excitation in brain regions which will perform the anticipated task.

Selfregulation of slow cortical potentials

We have investigated the modifiability of slow cortical potential in a series of studies, and have attempted to determine its behavioural consequences (Elbert 1978, 1986; Elbert et al. 1980, 1984; Rockstroh et al. 1989).

In these studies the slow cortical potentials fed back to the subject, in other words the subject received information about his own potentials which he or she was about to generate. Subjects were asked to generate increased negativity, or to suppress a shift in the EEG-baseline for intervals of six to eight seconds. Healthy human subjects can quickly learn to control their potentials within two training sessions. They even can learn to regulate the shift in an area-specific manner: After the training subjects are confronted with various task situations. For instance, increased negativity shortens the reaction time and enhances solving of arithmetic problems. In one study subjects held a button in each hand and were asked to press one of the buttons after they had shifted their slow negative potential either to the left or to the right hemisphere. Subjects were instructed to respond with the hand that spontaneously occurred to them. The right hand was preferred more often on trials with increased left-central negativity (63% r.hand vs. 33% l.hand), whereas the choice of hand was equally distributed on trials with pronounced right-hemispheric negativity (Rockstroh et al. 1990); (naturally occurring rate in right handers: 42 vs. 58%). For many tasks, however, there seems to be an optimal level of negativity, sometimes within strict limits. This is best exemplified for signal-detection performance. In one of our experimental arrangements minimal changes in the configuration of a visual stimulus had to be detected. The relationship between slow potential shift and signal detection performance followed an inverted u-shaped function: Subjects detected most signals correctly when they also displayed small negativities. Performance decreased with positive and also with large negative shifts (Elbert 1991).

Closer examination showed that excessive negativities are accompanied by increasing false alarms. Obviously, the negative shift can be too large. Zero or positive shifts, on the other hand, decrease the number of detected signals. This and similar other relationships between behavioural variables and slow potentials led us to the assumption that negativity reflects the degree of excitability of neuronal networks (Elbert 1987; Elbert and Rockstroh 1987). If the threshold for excitation is too high, the incoming signal will be missed. If, on the other hand the networks operate close to firing threshold small fluctuations in the input may ignite the cell assembly leading to false alarms.

Slow surface negativity reflects cortical excitability

Neurophysiological evidence complements the view that slow surface negativity reflects cortical excitability. Depth recordings as well as quantitative considerations about volume conduction show that these slow potentials are primarily cortical in origin. We have set up a spherical model of the head with homogeneous layers, modelling scalp, bone, cerebrospinal fluid and the brain (Lutzenberger et al. 1987; Braun et al. 1991; Elbert 1991).[3] The computations show that the cross section through an active structure is a most important factor in determining the amplitude on the scalp. Closed fields will not result in surface potentials, and polarizations of gyri opposite in space will partially cancel each other. Possible sizes for planar areas of polarization are small in subcortical structures, hence larger potentials (>10 μV, such as P3, CNV) must have their electrical sources distributed mainly (>80%) in extended cortical regions. Subcortical activity may be superimposed but can account for only a small fraction of the potential amplitude. Of course, the generator, triggering synchronous and widespread cortical activity might be located anywhere. The statement that the sources of large-amplitude potentials reside in cortical layers receives support from measurements with electrode arrays in and across the cortex (Mitzdorf 1985; Gemba et al. 1990). Recently electrical activity has been mapped through voltage-sensitive dyes. This method (summarized by Bonhoeffer, this volume) bridges the gap between recordings on a macroscopic and on a microscopic level by staining a section of neuronal tissue with a fluorescent dye. The fluorescence varies with the membrane potential to which the dye attaches and thus the potential can be recorded through optical observation. The results presented by Arieli (this volume) suggest that the macroscopically measured potentials largely result from EPSPs in the den-

---

[3] The following example may demonstrate the conclusion: An active planar area, small in size, with a diameter of 1 cm contributes about 1/25 of an extended layer 10 cm in diameter. Subcortical structures are not only small in size, but also more distant to the surface, diminishing their contributions to surface potentials another 4 to 7 times. Even if a large portion of a subcortical structure is synchronously active and even if we assume that active elements extending over 3 cm^2 have the same orientation in space, their contribution to scalp potentials would still amount to only 1% of that generated by extended cortical sources. Thus an intracranial polarized layer of 1 mV might produce a scalp potential of 200 μm when extensive in the cortex, but only 2 μV when limited in size and in deeper structures (Elbert 1991)

dritic trees of the cortex. Stellate cells do not produce open extracellular far-fields. What we see on the scalp or the surface of the cortex is primarily the summation of post-synaptic potentials at pyramidal cells (see also Mitzdorf 1985, and this volume). Consequently, a surface-negative potential signifies depolarization of the dendritic tree in vast networks of pyramidal cells and hence indicates an increment in excitability of the underlying cortical tissue.

This suggests the apical dendritic tree as a candidate for the regulation of cortical excitability thresholds. Depolarisation of the apical dendrites causes an efflux of negative charges into extracellular space and back into the neuron in the deeper layers. This results in a polarization of the cortex with the negative pole near the surface. A lowering of thresholds for cortical excitability will hence result in an increase in surface negativity, while a positive wave is generated when thresholds are set high, that means, a positive wave - like the P3 - corresponds to an interruption of ongoing activity, to a dysfacilitation of widespread neural activity.

There is also experimental evidence from macroscopic recordings supporting these statements. For instance, drugs which lower cortical excitability lower, in direct proportion, the slow surface negativity. While various anticonvulsant drugs may exhibit quite different effects on earlier components of visual and auditory evoked potentials, as well as on spontaneous EEG-activity (Rockstroh et al. 1987, 1991) they all lower CNV-amplitude and also the negative DC-shifts obtained during hyperventilation (von Bülow et al. 1989; Rockstroh 1991). Certain stimulant drugs may enhance the CNV although there have been several paradoxical results (for a review see McCallum 1988).

Understanding the link between neurophysiology and psychophysiology of slow potentials thus means understanding the regulation of excitability in neuronal networks.

Valentin Braitenberg, Günther Palm and Almut Schüz developed the important bases and ideas regarding this regulation. The following theoretical outline relies on their thoughts, many of them expressed in discussions and personal communications.

The concept of cell assemblies and aspects of memory storage

The concept of cell assemblies (Hebb 1949) has become fundamental to models concerned with the functioning of the brain. Hebb (1949, 1961) postulated that short-term memory is represented in reverberatory circuits as described earlier by Lorento de Nó (1943). Once activated, these circuits can maintain excitation as they are formed by a set of neurons, each of which receives excitation from, and gives excitation to, other members of the same set. If a sufficiently large number of neurons in one such cell assembly is activated, the whole set will become active. The trick to memory storage is that the structure of these cell assemblies is flexible and can be changed rapidly. This requires the strengthening of connections between simultaneously active neurons (Hebb's rule), an assumption which has long been considered the physiological basis of learning and memory storage (Hebb 1949). It is thought that within neural networks the ability of an active synapse to depolarize the postsynaptic membrane is increased, once a certain level of postsynaptic activity is present (based on Hebb's rule, models of the memory have been suggested by Willshaw et al. 1969; Palm 1982, and others). Generally it is assumed that plasticity is realized through NMDA-receptors. (For evidence and models of synaptic plasticity see e.g. Collinridge 1987; Gustafson et al. 1987; Bear et al. 1987). Probably all the synapses on spines are subject to modification in their strength, which would mean that 3 out of four cortical synapses are plastic (Schüz, this volume). Therefore, the build-up and strengthening of a cell assembly requires that a large portion of cells not relevant for the concept of the incoming event be shut off. Otherwise connections would form randomly. From the in vivo experiments with single cells, we can infer that a tetanic burst of say 100 stimulations with 100 Hz frequency is sufficient to alter the strength of synapses. Moreover, even weaker activity will be sufficient, particularly when similar firing patterns are repeated several times. Consequently, cortical excitability must be reduced for a fraction of a second or so before a relevant event can be stored in long-term memory. Based on the considerations of the previous section, we conclude that the widespread reduction in cortical excitability or inhibition respectively will show up in a widespread positive wave on the scalp (Birbaumer and Elbert 1988). There is evidence that the P300, and in part the positive slow wave, reflect exactly this process. P300 has been linked to the updating of memory (Donchin and Coles 1988) and is thought to reflect processes associated with the maintenance of a model of the environment.

The larger the information transmission, the more cells should be involved in the network. As all these must be isolated from background activity, the dysfacilitation must be more widespread, and positivity should increase in expansion and hence in amplitude. An interesting example of the experimental evidence confirming the inhibitory/dysfacilitatory character of the P3 is provided by Woodward et al. (1989). Probe clicks to which subjects had to respond were delivered during the time-course of (an auditory-oddball) P3. Reaction times were significantly slowed during the time course of the P3, a finding which has been recently replicated in our laboratory and which is consistent with the proposed dysfacilitatory process.

Threshold regulation of cortical excitability (TRE-model) and the direction of attention

Pyramidal cells constitute 85% of the cortical neurons (Schüz and Palm 1989; Braitenberg and Schüz 1990)[4]. The connections among them are excitatory and constitute over 70% of all cortical synapses. The strength of synapses between neurons depend to a large extent upon experience. There is, as Braitenberg argued, a danger intrinsic to such interconnected networks that they may become activated beyond control (Braitenberg 1978, 1984). If the number of active networks reaches a certain critical level, there is a high probability that many of the remaining ones will become activated too. A final stage of extreme activation may be seen in an epileptic seizure. Indeed, the few DC-records taken prior to epileptic attacks (summarized in Rockstroh 1991) suggest that extreme negative shifts precede seizure activity. Furthermore, the regulation of slow potentials is impaired in epileptic patients (Elbert et al. 1990). Even sub-epileptic high levels of activation disable information processing, for instance, signal detection.

[4] This figure may seem surprisingly high given the illustrations in many publications. This bias may arise from man's tendency to give greater attention to more exotic animals, i.e. when we see a rare species of interneurons it may evoke a larger P3 than when we are confronted with another illustration of the common pyramidal cell.

Over-activation might be prevented by a threshold control that could rapidly detect an explosive chain reaction among cell assemblies, and that would then regulate cortical excitability by raising thresholds (Braitenberg 1984; Elbert and Rockstroh 1987).

Furthermore, such a threshold control would provide the brain with the ability to interrupt ongoing activity, when relevant information is received. If thresholds are set high consequent upon the presentation of relevant information, ongoing activity will drop to a low level instantaneously, and activity will survive only in the elements pertaining to the concept of the incoming stimulus. Such interruptions will generate positive waves with amplitudes in the microvolt range, like the P300.

If, on the other hand, the total activity were low, further lowering thresholds would encourage circulation of activity throughout the brain. This would avoid the possibility that ongoing subsequent activations become interrupted. One set of cell assemblies would activate the next one and then another in turn, and so forth. As the activation of cell assemblies might correspond to thoughts, such a process would thereby enable a 'train of thoughts', as Braitenberg has put it. In other words, it would enable processing of related information in a sequential manner. Each thought would be related to the next one.

The feedback process inherent in the threshold regulation process will give rise to permanent fluctuations in the depolarization of the dendritic tree and thus will contribute to the fluctuations observed in the EEG.

If thresholds are not adjusted adequately, the process of connected thoughts would be disrupted. Thoughts might be more loosely related which to some extent could contribute to creativity. In more severe cases it may favour thought disorders leading to erroneously activated networks, giving rise to hallucinatory phenomena. False activation of cell assemblies, would result in massive attentional problems, and it is possible that it might favour a schizophrenic breakdown (Elbert et al. 1983). We have tackled this question by investigating the ability to regulate one's own slow potentials in a sample of subjects believed to be at risk for schizophrenic development (Elbert et al. 1983) and more recently in hospitalized patients (Schneider et al. 1991). Compared to the respective controls, we have indeed observed altered or impaired abilities in the regulation of slow potentials in both groups. Too low an activation will bring the train of thoughts to a halt and might make it difficult to initiate it smoothly. While akinesia and rigidity in the motor system are easily observed, corresponding cognitive disruptions

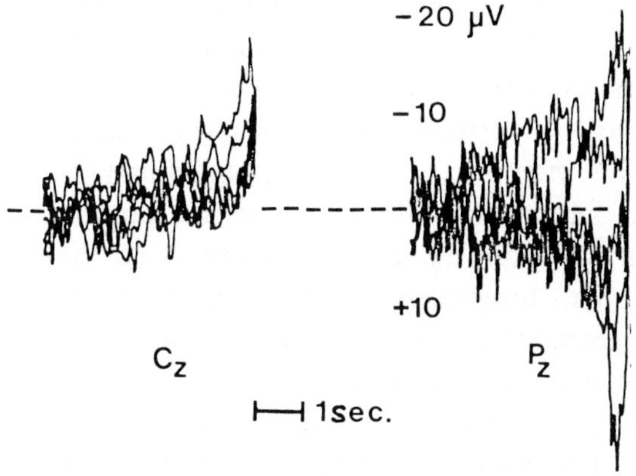

Fig. 3. Superimposed are six single EEG traces recorded prior to a voluntary self-administration of an electric shock. Over central areas, a negative variation of the EEG-baseline occurs prior to the onset of the EMG for every response (From Elbert 1985)

require more sophisticated techniques to be detected (Canavan et al. 1989).

Finally, if the brain were able to adjust thresholds in advance, threshold control could be considered a mechanism for directing attention to future action. Thereby cortical tuning would improve the processing of an expected event. Examination of slow negativities like the CNV or the Bereitschaftspotential (Fig. 2,3) suggest that such processes do indeed exist! As negativity is generated whenever firing thresholds are lowered, a negative shift prior to an expected event might correspond to a state of preparedness in the underlying networks which are to become activated. This view fits well with the one expressed by Deecke (1976) purely on grounds of experimental observation of slow potentials: "We can then interpret the two very slow potentials, BP and CNV, as reflecting a general facilitation process, preactivating those brain regions which will be needed in the special experimental situation under study".

This leads us to the scenario illustrated in Fig. 4, which provides partial explanation for the flow of event-related potentials: Consider an external event or stimulus producing additional input to the cortical networks. Consequently the momentary activity will be changed. Apart from its specific information transmission, the feedback control will also change subsequent firing patterns: The additional activation will call for a compensatory increase in thresholds immediately, generating a transient positive EEG-wave. Indeed, a transient positivity (P2, P3) develops in response to more or less every enhancement of cortical activity. This reflexive limiting of cortical excitability (P2) interrupts weaker ongoing activity, while incoming activity, (particularly, when fed strongly enough through subcortical afferents) is maintained. A pronounced dampening of cortical activity may be required further, if the transmission of information to long-term memory has to be extensive, giving rise to a P3. The scenario is illustrated in Fig. 4. Whenever an event is anticipated - being signalled as in the two-stimulus paradigm - or is self-induced, it is advantageous to the organism to adjust thresholds in advance. Thresholds should be lowered to facilitate processing of the incoming information, but they should not become too low, in order to avoid a 'false start' or premature assumptions.

Support for the functional significance of threshold regulation for attentive behaviour can be derived from the relationship between surface negative slow potentials and behavioural responses. For example,

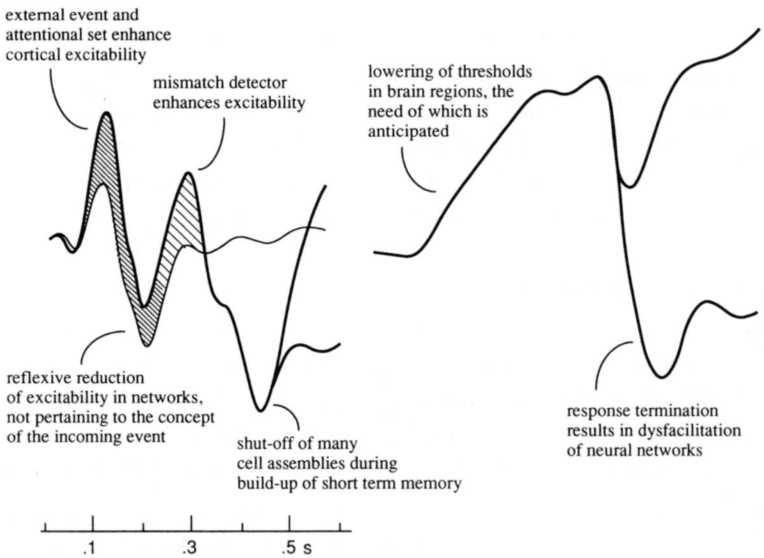

Fig. 4. Explanation of the genesis of the major event-related potential components in the TRE-model. Investigation of these event-related potential components may serve to study threshold regulation and its psychological consequences

response latency is shorter when a reaction time task is presented with high CNV amplitudes than when following decreased negativity (Rockstroh et al. 1982). Spontaneous slow potential shifts have also been found to covary with performance efficiency in various tasks (Stamm 1984; Bauer 1984). When subjects learned to modify their slow potentials systematically within an operant feedback procedure, their performance in various tasks was efficient when negativity was large in those cortical regions related to task processing, whereas subjects performed more poorly if negativity remained suppressed in the 'task-relevant' areas but not elsewhere (Rockstroh et al. 1989).

These data are open to the following interpretation: Tasks presented during increases in negativity are presented when activity was previously low and consequently thresholds have been lowered. Hence, the task is presented to an easily excitable brain region with little ongoing activity, and is consequently processed efficiently.

There is currently no clear evidence which physiological structures participate in the threshold regulation. One candidate is the inhibitory interneurons. About 13% of all cortical synapses are pyramidal synapses which connect to non-pyramidal cells (type I synapses, Schüz, this volume; Braitenberg and Schüz, 1990). There is an equal number of non-pyramidal to pyramidal cell synapses, but they are inhibitory. However, probably less than 2% of all synapses constitute connections among the non-pyramidal cells themselves, and these are type II. It is possible that these inhibitory interneurons help to maintain partial activation but it is unlikely that these cells (with their local range and their limited, inhibitory interconnections) can synchronize larger portions of cortical tissue. Therefore the activity of these cells might not be detectable in surface recordings.

It is more likely that excitability of larger cortical regions can be tuned by non-specific thalamic fibres which synapse on the apical dendrites. This process might be considered a candidate for the regulation of thresholds of neuronal excitability. However such a tuning of nonspecific thalamocortical afferents can only be effective if information about ongoing activity in the networks to be regulated is fed into the system adjusting new thresholds. We must therefore assume the existence of a 'measurement device' that receives information about ongoing cortical activity, and which transmits this information to the thalamus. As suggested by Braitenberg (personal communication) and Palm (1982) the neuroanatomical structures that might fulfill such requirements are the basal ganglia.[5] Their role for the generation of slow potentials has been discussed elsewhere (Elbert and Rockstroh 1987; Rockstroh et al. 1989; Canavan and Sartory 1990; Elbert 1991). Further experimental evidence is needed to elucidate the role of subcortical structures for threshold regulation ad in the TRE-model of event-related potentials as outlined in Fig. 4.

Acknowledgments

Research was supported by the Deutsche Forschungsgemeinschaft (El 101/5 and SFB 307, B1)

References

Arieli A (this volume) Novel strategies to unravel mechanisms of cortical function: From macro- to micro recordings

Bauer H (1984) Regulation of slow potentials affects task performance. In: Elbert T, Rockstroh B, Lutzenberger W, Birbaumer N (eds) Self-Regulation of the Brain and Behavior. Springer, Heidelberg Berlin, pp 216-226

Bear MF, Cooper LN, Ebner FF (1987) A physiological basis of a theory of synapse modification. Science 237:42-48

Bienenstock EL, Cooper LN, Munro, PW (1982) Theory for the development of neuron selectivity: Orientation specificity and binocular interaction in visual cortex. J Neurosci 2:32-48

Birbaumer N, Elbert T, Rockstroh B, Lutzenberger W (1986) On the dynamics of the post-imperative negative variation (PINV). In: McCallum WC, Zappoli R, Denoth F (eds) Cerebral Psychophysiology: Studies in Event-Related Potentials. Journal of Electroenceph. Clin. Neurophysiol. Suppl 38:212-219

Birbaumer N, Elbert T (1988) P3: By-product of a by-product? Behav Brain Sci 11:375-376

Birbaumer N, Elbert T, Canavan A, Rockstroh B (1990) Slow potentials of the cerebral cortex and behaviour. Physiol Rev 70:1-41

---

[5] Every area of the cortex sends projections to the neostriatum where information is preserved in a roughly topographic fashion (Kemp and Powell 1970, 1971; Yeterian and Van Hoesen 1978) thereby 'lateral' inhibition may serve to focus activity.

Braitenberg V (1984) Vehicles - Experiments in Synthetic Psychology. MIT-Press, Cambridge, Mass.

Braitenberg V (1978) Cell assemblies in the cerebral cortex. In: Heim R, Palm G (eds) Theoretical Approach to Complex Systems. Springer, Berlin Heidelberg, pp 171-188

Braitenberg V, Schüz A (1991) Anatomy of the Cortex. Statistics and Geometry. Springer, Berlin Heidelberg

Braun Ch, Lutzenberger W, Miltner W, Elbert T (1990) Can subcortical structures generate potentials large in amplitude? In: Brunia CHM, Gaillard AWK, Kok A (eds) Psychophysiological Brain Research. Tilburg University Press, Tilburg pp 31-35

Canavan AGM, Passingham RE, Marsden CD, Quinn N, Wyke M, Polkey CE (1989) Performance on learning tasks of patients in the early stages of Parkinson's disease. Neuropsychologia 27:141-156

Canavan AGM, Sartory G (1990) Klinische Neuropsychologie. Enke-Verlag, Stuttgart

Collinridge GL, Bliss TVP (1987) NMDA receptors - their role in long term potentiation. TINS 10 (7):288-293

Deecke L (1976) Opening remarks on motor aspects. In: McCallum, Knott (eds) The Responsive Brain. Wright & Sons, Bristol

Donchin E, Coles MGH (1988) Is the P300 component a manifestation of context updating? Behav Brain Sci 11:357-374

Elbert T (1978) Biofeedback langsamer kortikaler Potentiale. Minerva, München

Elbert T (1985) Langsame Hirnpotentiale und Verhalten. Habilitationsschrift, Universität Tübingen

Elbert T (1986) Externally and self-induced CNV patterns of the brain hemispheres - A sign of task-specific preparation. Human Neurobiol 5:67-69

Elbert T (1987) Regulation kortikaler Erregbarkeit: Im EEG ein deterministisches Chaos? In: Weinmann HM (ed) Zugang zum Verständnis höherer Hirnfunktionen durch das EEG. Zuckerschwerdt Verlag, München, pp 93-107

Elbert T (1991) Slow cortical potentials reflect the regulation of cortical excitability. In: McCallum (ed) Plenum Publishing Corp., New York London

Elbert T, Rockstroh B, Lutzenberger W, Birbaumer N (1980) Biofeedback of slow cortical potentials. J Electroenc Clin Neurophysiol 48:293-301

Elbert T, Rockstroh B, Lutzenberger W, Birbaumer N (1982) Slow brain potentials after withdrawal of control. Archiv für Psychiatrie und Nervenkrankheiten 232:201-214

Elbert T, Lutzenberger W, Rockstroh B, Birbaumer N (1983) When regulation of slow brain potentials fails - A contribution to the psychophysiology of perceptual aberration and anhedonia. In: Mendlewicz J, van Praag HM (eds) Advances in Biological Psychiatry, Vol. 13, Karger, Basel, pp 98-106

Elbert T, Rockstroh B (1987) Threshold regulation - a key to the understanding of the combined dynamics of EEG and event-related potentials. J Psychophysiol 4:317-333

Elbert T, Rockstroh B, Canavan A, Birbaumer N, Lutzenberger W, von Bülow I, Linden A (1990) Self-regulation of slow cortical potentials and its role in epileptogenesis. In: Carlson J, Seifert R (eds) Biobehavioral Self-Regulation and Health. Plenum Press, New York pp 65-94

Gemba H, Sasaki K, Tsujimoto T (1990) No-go potential in monkeys and human subjects. In: Brunia CHM, Gaillard AWK, Kok A (eds) Psychophysiological Brain Research, Tilburg University Press, Tilburg pp 133-136

Gustafson B, Wigström H, Abraham WC, Huang YY (1987) Long term potentiation in the hippocampus using depolarizing current pulses as the conditioning stimulus to single volley synaptic potentials. J Neurosci 7 (3):774-780

Hebb DO (1961) Distinctive features of learning in the higher animal. In: Delafresnaye JF (ed) Brain Mechanisms and Learning. Oxford University Press, New York

Hebb DO (1949) The Organization of Behavior. Wiley, New York

Hillyard SA (1981) Selective auditory attention and early event-related potentials: A rejoinder. Canad J Psychol 203-204

Keidel M (1983) The motor intention potential, an electrophysiological correlate to a v(volitional) intention of a non-performed voluntary movement. J Electroenc Clin Neurophysiol 56:1-224

Kemp JM, Powell TP (1970) The cortico-striate projection in the monkey. Brain 93:525-546

Kemp JM, Powell TP (1971) The connections of the striatum and globus pallidus: Synthesis and speculation. Phil Trans Roy Soc Lond B 262:441-457

Kutas M, Hillyard SA (1980) Reading senseless sentences: Brain potentials reflect semantic incongruity. Science 207:203-204

Libet B (1985) Unconscious cerebral initiative and the role of conscious will in voluntary action. Behav Brain Sci 8:529-566

Libet B, Wright E, Gleason C (1982) Readiness-potential preceding unrestricted spontaneous vs. preplanned voluntary acts. Electroenc Clin Physiol 54:322-335

Lorente de Nó, R (1943) Cerebral cortex: Architecture, intracortical connections, motor projections. In: Fulton FJ (ed) Physiology of the Nervous System. Oxford University Press, New York

Lutzenberger W, Elbert T, Rockstroh B (1987) A brief tutorial on the implications of volume conduction for the interpretation of the EEG. J Psychophysiol 1:81-89

McCallum WC (1988) Potentials related to expectancy, preparation and motor activity. In: Picton TW (ed) Human Event-Related Potentials, EEG Handbook (revised series vol. 3) Elsevier, Amsterdam, pp 427-534

Mitzdorf U (1985) Current source-density method and application in cat cerebral cortex: Investigation of evoked potentials and EEG phenomena. Physiol Rev 65:37-99

Näätänen R (1990) The role of attention in auditory information processing as revealed by event-related potentials and other brain measures of cognitive function. Behav Brain Sci 13:201-233

Palm G (1982) Neural assemblies: An alternative approach to artificial intelligence. Springer, Berlin

Rockstroh B (1990) Effects of Clonazepam on Hyperventilation-Induced EEG-Changes in Man. Epilepsy Res 7:146-154

Rockstroh B, Elbert T, Lutzenberger W, Birbaumer N (1979) Slow cortical potentials under conditions of uncontrollability. Psychophysiology 16:374-380. PINV

Rockstroh B, Elbert T, Lutzenberger W, Birbaumer N (1982) The effects of slow cortical potentials on response speed. Psychophysiology 19:211-217

Rockstroh B, Elbert T, Canavan A, Lutzenberger W, Birbaumer N (1989) Slow Brain Potentials and Behaviour. (second, completely revised edition). Urban & Schwarzenberg, München

Rockstroh B, Elbert T, Lutzenberger W, Altenmüller E (1991) Effects of the anticonvulsatory benzodiazepine Clonazepam on event-related brain potentials in humans. J Electroenc Clin Neurophysiol 78:142-149

Rockstroh B, Elbert T, Lutzenberger W, Altenmüller E, Birbaumer N, Diener H-C, Dichgans J (1987) Effects of the anticonvulsant Carbamazepine on event-related brain potentials in humans. In: Barber R, Blum T (eds) Evoked Potentials III. Butterworths, Boston pp 361-369

Rockstroh B, Elbert T, Lutzenberger W, Birbaumer N (1990) Biofeedback produced hemispheric asymmetry of slow cortical potentials and its behavioural effects. Int J Psychophysiol 9:151-165

Schneider F, Rockstroh B, Heimann H, Lutzenberger W, Mattes R, Elbert T, Birbaumer N, Basrtels M (1991) Selfregulation of slow cortical potentials in psychiatric patients I: Schizophrenia. Biofeedback & Selfregulation, (in press)

Schüz A, Palm G (1989) Density of neurons and synapses in the cerebral cortex of the mouse. J Comp Neurol 286:442-455

Schüz A (this volume)

Stamm JS (1984) Performance enhancements with cortical negative slow potential shifts in monkey and man. In: Elbert T, Rockstroh B, Lutzenberger W, Birbaumer N (eds) Self-Regulation of the Brain and Behavior. Springer, Heidelberg Berlin, pp 199-215

von Bülow I, Elbert T, Rockstroh B, Lutzenberger W, Canavan A (1989) Effects of hyperventilation on EEG frequency and slow cortical potentials in relation to an anticonvulsant and epilepsy. J Psychophysiol 3:147-154

Willshaw DJ, Buneman OP, Longuet-Higgins HC (1969) Non-holographic associative memory. Nature 222:960-962

Woodward SH, Brown WS, Marsh JT, Dawson ME Probing P3 with secondary reaction time. (submitted)

Yeterian EH, Van Hoesen GW (1978) Corticostriate projections in the rhesus monkey: The organization of certain cortico-caudate connections. Brain Res 139:43-63

Cortical Information Processing as Viewed from the Mass-Action Domain of Evoked Potentials

Ulla Mitzdorf

Institut für Medizinische Psychologie, Goethestr. 31, 8000 München 2, Germany

The two most fundamental fields concerned with the cortical processing of visual information, anatomy and single-cell physiology, have yielded rather divergent results. Anatomical investigations, on the one hand, have revealed a rather chaotic, dense net of local and widespread interconnections between the cortical neurons. This net of interconnections lacks any apparent spatial order with respect to lengths or densities in the vertical and horizontal directions (Schüz, Braitenberg, this volume). The physiological studies of single cells' response properties, on the other hand, have demonstrated that external information is represented in the visual cortex in a highly specific manner and arranged in a very precise spatial order. The individual cells' receptive fields (RFs) are small; the retinotopic relation is preserved for these RFs between hypercolumns. Moreover, each hypercolumn is further spatially subdifferentiated into ocular dominance- and orientation columns and in the monkey, additionally into color-, motion-, and form-processing subregions (Barlow, this volume). Thus, in contradiction to the results of the intracortical network, RF studies indicate that afferent information is processed in the cortex in a parallel fashion, and in a rather independent manner within each subregion or microcolumn, without strong lateral interactions.

This latter physiologists' standpoint is challenged, however, not only by the conflicting anatomical facts, but also by physiological data if mass activities rather than the individual cells' optimal RF responses are considered. The mass activities of a group of cortical cells can be directly inferred by appropriately adding up the - separately recorded - individual cells' responses. As described in more detail in another chapter (Mitzdorf and Li, this volume), such an averaging of cell responses across a representative cortical cell group yields a view of cortical activity that strongly deviates from the concept of local feature extraction: wide-angle, diffuse-light stimuli cause as strong mass responses as a typical RF-type stimulus. Moreover, visual stimuli do cause significant mass activities also at retinotopically noncorresponding sites in the primary visual cortex.

Another approach to mass activities is the inspection of the macroscopic field potentials. These signals are highly interesting because many of their properties, like amplitudes of certain components of event-related potentials, their temporal correlations at different sites, or the frequency spectrum of the EEG, have been found in humans to correlate with cognitive states and capacities. This suggests that these mass-action signals yield access to the higher stages of intracortical information processing. A severe disadvantage of these signals is that their relation with the underlying, causal neuronal activities is rather obscure. An extensive, detailed study of such evoked potentials in the primary visual cortex of cats and rabbits yielded conclusions about the respective neuronal causes as well as some information about intracortical information processing. The data obtained supplement both the anatomical and the single-cell centered views. These results, published in detail elsewhere (Mitzdorf 1985, 1987, 1991) are briefly outlined here.

In acute experiments with anaesthetized animals, the depth profiles through the visual cortex of potentials evoked by various types of electrical and visual stimuli were recorded. These data were then subjected to current source-density analysis. This procedure allows to localize the physical causes of the potentials: macroscopic sinks and sources in the extracellular space, composed of membrane currents from many individual cells.

By investigating the effects of altering the cortical excitability with pharmacological agents on the evoked sink-and-source patterns, by comparing their spatial and temporal properties with established anatomical and physiological facts, and by taking basic knowledge about the membrane currents into account, the causes of the sinks and sources and thus of the evoked potentials could be revealed. All these correlations lead to the same conclusion, namely that the dominant causes of these mass-action signals are excitatory synaptic activities. A sink, composed mainly of active synaptic inward currents, indicates the site of excitatory synaptic ensemble activity, and the corresponding, simultaneously arising sources are composed of related passive membrane currents indicating the spatial extent of the activated group of neurons. Since the sinks and sources are macroscopic phenomena, they do not reflect all excitatory synaptic activities, but only groups of such events that are focused with respect to time and cortical depth. Metaphorically speaking, they are the iceberg tips of the cortical excitatory synaptic activities. Thus, these signals of intracortical information processing supplement the single-cell results because they reflect input rather than output activity and ensemble rather than individual cells' events. Since these signals imply anatomical and temporal grouping, they also supplement the anatomical findings by emphasizing the importance of certain pathways.

The spatio-temporal pattern of the sinks is the essential mass-action result of afferent information processing within the cortex. This pattern was found to be qualitatively very similar for all types of stimuli applied and is shown schematically in Fig. 1. This pattern of evoked activity does not indicate *what* information is processed. The specific visual information contained in the stimulus is reflected only faintly in slight modulations of this basic pattern. The pattern indicates *how* the information is processed. The afferent activity is relayed through the cortex along three paths, from the input layer IV to the supragranular layers, to the infragranular layers, and within the input layer itself. The speed of processing along these pathways is determined by the strength of the stimuli (see the time-scale range in Fig. 1). The afferent activity is spread tangentially primarily by the layer-IV path to additionally activate retinotopically noncorresponding, dis-

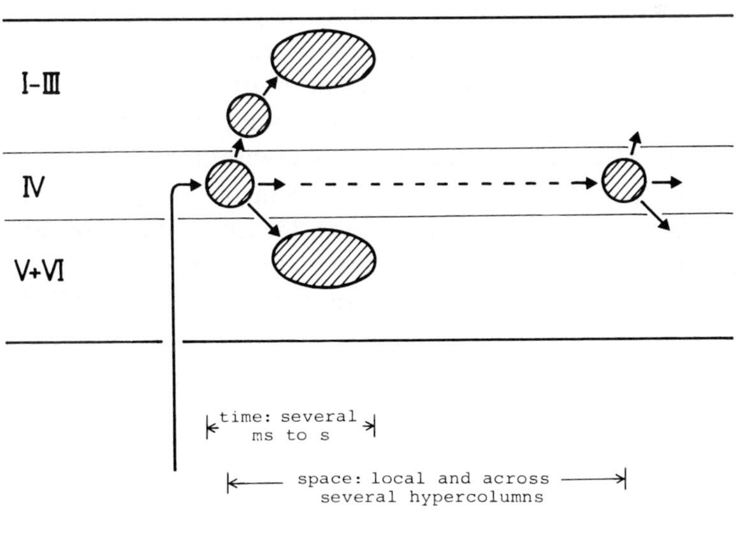

Fig. 1

tant sites (see space-scale range in Fig. 1). At these distant sites, the activity is then processed in the same way as at the retinotopically corresponding site. By the local reactivation of cells in the input layer, this path also causes rhythmic repetitions of the component within layer IV and of the whole pattern throughout all layers. The passage of the activity along the pathways, the relative preponderance of either of the pathways, as well as the number of the oscillatory repetitions depend strongly on nonspecific, central parameters of the global state of the central nervous system. The passage of afferent activity along the paths further depends on the actual state of processing, i.e., the afferent activity and the ongoing activity interfere with one another.

These results from the investigation of physiological mass-action phenomena contradict the single-cell concept of local, parallel processing, but agree with the mass-action view of single-cell responses (Mitzdorf and Li, this volume) because they revealed tangential spread of activity within the cortex. They further throw the dense net of anatomical connections into relief by emphasizing certain pathways as the main processing routes. Finally, they stress the influence of central parameters and the temporal aspects of the cortical processing. They thus relate the intracortical processing of afferent information with those parameters which were found to correlate with cognitive states and capacities.

A general conclusion from these results allows neither a specific spatial nor a specific temporal resolution to be identified as specifically relevant. The information contents appear to be encoded by the spatial pattern of activity. The structure of this pattern appears to be relevant at all levels of resolution, from the dimension of the microcolumns to the dimension of the coarsest subdivisions of the brain. The processing, i.e., the brain-specific decoding of this information, appears to rely strongly on temporal relations of the activities within and between brain regions. In this time domain - as judged from the frequencies of the above described recurrences of the layer-IV component or the whole cortical activation pattern and in agreement with others (Eckhorn, this volume) - the whole range of all the characteristic EEG bands appears to be relevant.

Acknowledgements

This work has been supported by Deutsche Forschungsgemeinschaft, grants SFB 220/D 3 and Po 121/13. I thank Dr. U. Engler for secretarial help and Dr. B. Herzberger for English corrections.

References

Mitzdorf U (1985) Current source-density method and application in cat cerebral cortex: investigation of evoked potentials and EEG phenomena. Phys Rev 65:37-100

Mitzdorf U (1987) Properties of the evoked potential generators: current source density analysis of visually evoked potentials in the cat cortex. Int J Neuroscience 33:33-59

Mitzdorf U (1991) Physiological sources of evoked potentials. Suppl. of EEG Journal, in press

Current Source Density Analysis of Spatio-Temporal Fluorescence Maps in Organotypical Slice Cultures

Dietmar Plenz and Ad Aertsen[1]

Max-Planck-Institut für biologische Kybernetik, Spemannstrasse 38, 7400 Tübingen, Germany

Spatio-temporal spreading of activity in the CA3 region of organotypical slice cultures from the rat hippocampus was studied by measuring the intracellular potential distributions, using the optical recording technique. To enhance the spatial resolution, a specifically developed CSD-like transformation was applied to the fluorescence maps, enabling to calculate the locations of the transmembrane current generators (iCSD).

The iCSD-profiles provided a surprisingly good basis for the interpretation of spatio-temporal activity in the organotypical cultures, moreover, at a much higher spatial resolution than the original amplitude-latency fluorescence profiles. On the basis of these iCSD-profiles, the existence of aberrant projections between the CA1 and CA3 regions was revealed.

Introduction

Over the last years, organotypical slice cultures (Gähwiler 1989) gained considerable attention as a preparation to study the dynamics in nervous tissue under physiological, pharmacological and developmental considerations. Such quasi two-dimensional tissue preparations particularly provide a convenient possibility for studying the reorganization of intrinsic and/or the development of new fibre systems by mapping the spatio-temporal dynamics of the electrical activity. One of the

---

[1] present address: Institut für Neuroinformatik, Ruhr-Universität, P.O. Box 102 148, 4630 Bochum, Germany

methods to do this, the calculation of Current-Source Density profiles on the basis of the extracellular field potential distribution (*CSD*, Freeman and Nicholson 1975; Mitzdorf 1985), however, is particularly difficult in cultures. The main reason for this is the problem of assuring stable field potential measurements in such thin, quasi-monolayered tissue preparations.

Recently, another technique was developed to map the spatio-temporal dynamics of electrical activity in nervous tissue. This new technique of 'optical recording' consists of measuring the changes in optical properties of the tissue during neural activity (Grinvald et al. 1988; Salzberg 1989). Optical recording, particularly by application of voltage-sensitive fluorescent dyes to the nervous tissue, provides the opportunity to measure the summated intracellular activity of neuronal populations as well as the glia activity involved. It can be easily used to assess the spatio-temporal patterns of activity in *in vivo* (e.g. Grinvald et al. 1986) and *in vitro* (e.g. Bonhoeffer and Staiger 1988) preparations. The interpretation of these optical signals on the basis of their latency and amplitude distributions, however, does not achieve the spatial resolution obtained with classical CSD-analysis of field potential distributions from similar vertebrate tissue preparations.

In order to improve the spatial resolution and, hence, the interpretability of the fluorescence activity maps, we adopted the following approach. After rigorously identifying the fluorescence signals with the intracellular population activity integrated over a number of nerve cells or nerve cell circuits per unit tissue volume, we calculated from these signals the transmembrane current densities as viewed from the intracellular space (iCSD, Plenz and Aertsen 1991a,b). Thus, we combined the convenient method of optical recording with the high spatial resolution of the Current Source Density approach.

Here we used this newly developed transformation to study the various fibre projection areas in the CA3 region in organotypical slice cultures from the rat hippocampus.

Methods

Transverse organotypical hippocampal cultures from 4 to 7 days old rats were prepared by using the roller tube technique (Gähwiler 1989;

Caeser and Aertsen 1991). For recording, cultures were transferred to the recording chamber, which was mounted on an inverted microscope (Zeiss, IM35), equipped with an epifluorescence filter set (Zeiss, BP 546, FT 580, LP 590). The chamber was continuously perfused with HBSS (Gibco), to which were added 350 mg/l $NaHCO_3$ and 294 mg/l $CaCl_2x2H_20$. The latter was not added in case of calcium-free conditions. The flow rate was set to 0.5 ml/min and the temperature kept at 33.0 ± 0.1 °C. Slice cultures were lying submerged on thin coverslips. The voltage-sensitive styryl dye RH237 was applied to the bathing medium for 15 minutes before each experiment. Monopolar tungsten micro-electrodes were used for electrical double-pulse stimulation (ISI 40 ms) of the mossy fibres (first stimulus) and the alveus of the CA1 region (second stimulus).

For optical recording, cultures were illuminated by a mercury lamp (Zeiss, HWO 100 W/2, duration of trials 96 ms). The image of the nervous tissue was projected with an objective (Leitz, 25x NPL Fluotar, 0.75 oil immersion) onto a 12x12 photodiode array (Centronics, M144-5). The photodiode currents were amplified, multiplexed and fed into a microcomputer (DEC LSI 11/73) at a sample rate of 2 kHz per channel. The data were transferred to a VAX 750 (DEC) for further processing (Bonhoeffer and Staiger 1988). Each photodiode integrated the fluorescence over an area of 60x60 μm^2. In order to cover the entire depth of the CA3 region, a montage of two 12x12 fields with a spatial overlap of 33% was made, thus simulating an 20x12 photodiode array (cf. Fig. 2b). From the photodiode matrix a one-dimensional array of photodiodes was selected for the calculation of one-dimensional iCSD-profiles.

The fluorescence change dF was calculated for each separate location by taking the difference in fluorescence between successive trials with and without a stimulus (Procedure I; Bonhoeffer and Staiger 1988), or alternatively, as the difference between the response to a stimulus and a linear approximation of the non-stimulus sweep, based on the start and end points of the corresponding stimulus sweep (Procedure II). The relative fluorescence change dF/F was obtained by dividing this difference by the absolute fluorescence at that same location. Generally, we averaged the responses over 6 to 8 trials.

Under the assumptions of a quasi-static electric field and an extracellular space which behaves as an ohmic conductor with approximately constant conductivity, the CSD-profile is proportional to the second-order spatial derivative of the extracellular field potential distribution (eCSD). In addition, if the field potentials change predominantly along one-dimension only, the true eCSD-distribution can be approximated by applying the one-dimensional eCSD-analysis (Mitzdorf 1985) according to the formula:

$$-I_m(z,t) \sim \frac{U(z-n\Delta h,t) - 2U(z,t) + U(z+n\Delta h,t)}{(n\Delta h)^2} \tag{1}$$

where $I_m(z,t)$ indicates the transmembrane current, $U(z,t)$ is the field potential at position z and time t, Dh denotes the sampling interval between adjacent recording locations, and nDh is the differentiation grid size.

For the calculation of 1-dimensional CSD-profiles on the basis of relative fluorescence changes, we developed a very similar transformation (iCSD, Plenz and Aertsen 1991b). In short, we made the following main assumptions: (1) the orientation of the linear photodiode array is parallel to the main orientation of the recorded cells in the nervous tissue, (2) the distance between two photodiodes is much smaller than the extent of the activated cells seen by each photodiode, and (3) the intracellular space can be approximated by a purely ohmic resistance R_i. Then, for any point in time, the distribution of relative fluorescence change dF/F over the photodiode array is linearly related to the distribution of the intracellular membrane potential U_i along the dendrosomatic axis:

$$U_i(k,t) = K\,(dF/F)(k,t) \tag{2}$$

with the proportionality constant K and compartment number k. The current i(k) in the intracellular space between two adjacent compartments k-1 and k, measured by the corresponding photodiodes, is described by

$$i_{(k)} = KR_i^{-1}{}_{(k)} \frac{(dF/F)_{(k)} - (dF/F)_{(k+1)}}{\Delta z} \qquad k \in [1,\ldots,m-1] \tag{3}$$

where m represents the total number of compartments, and Dz is the width of a single compartment. From Equations (2) and (3), and assuming (4) a constant intracellular resistance along the dendrosomatic axis, it follows that the current density $i_m(k)$ is proportional to the second spatial derivative of the fluorescence signal distribution:

$$I_m(z,t) \sim - \frac{(dF/F)(z-nDz,t) - 2\,(dF/F)(z,t) + (dF/F)(z+nDz,t)}{(n\Delta z)^2} \qquad (4)$$

where z indicates the spatial dimension along the photodiode array and t denotes time. Finally, since sinks/sources in the intracellular space are seen as sources/sinks from the extracellular space, a sign inversion has to be made. The integer n was set equal to one. This then defines the transformation which was applied to the fluorescence distribution in order to calculate the iCSD-profiles. Notice the strong similarity between Equ. (4) and the classical one-dimensional CSD-analysis described by Equ. (1): the role of the extracellular field potential distribution U has simply been taken by the relative fluorescence distribution dF/F.

Results

A sketch of the recording situation is given in Fig. 1. The dashed frame indicates the area from which the optical recordings were made. Fig. 2a shows a photomontage of the CA3 region, with the pyramidal cell body layer clearly visible. The entire 20x12 matrix of photodiode responses, together with an indication of the anatomical borders, can be seen in Fig. 2b. Each trace in this plot represents the time course of the relative fluorescence change under high calcium condition, measured by a photodiode at the corresponding matrix location. From this matrix we selected the indicated row of photodiode responses for calculation of the iCSD-profile; this row was oriented in parallel to the main axis of the CA3 pyramidal cells.

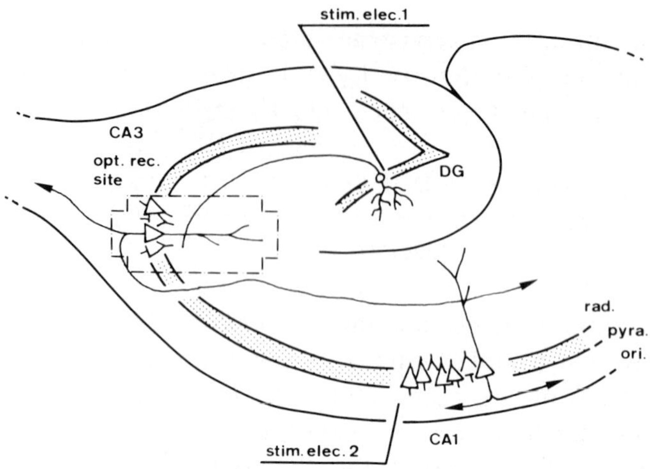

Fig. 1. Sketch of the anatomical and experimental situation in hippocampal organotypical slice cultures. *DG* gyrus dentatus; *rad.* stratum radiatum; *pyra.* stratum pyramidale; *ori.* stratum oriens; *stim.elec.1* stimulus electrode in the mossy fibres; *stim.elec.2* stimulus electrode in the alveus of the CA1 region; *opt.rec.site* location of photodiode matrix

Fluorescence maps and iCSD-profiles from the CA3 region of organotypical slice cultures

The following Figures 3 to 6 show typical results for the fluorescence maps and the calculated iCSD-profiles under different calcium levels. Negative deflections in the relative fluorescence changes, indicating intracellular depolarisations, are drawn upwards. In the iCSD-profiles, sinks are drawn upwards and sources downwards, as viewed from the extracellular space.

The fluorescence map under high calcium concentration (3.5 mM), calculated according to correction procedure I (see Methods), and the corresponding iCSD-profile are presented in Fig. 3. In the fluorescence map (Fig. 3a) we observe that a few milliseconds after the stimulus in the mossy fibres (i.e. the first stimulus), depolarisations occur in the entire CA3 region. The shortlasting peak at the beginning of the depolarization in the stratum pyramidale indicates the presence of action potentials (* in Fig. 3a). The response to stimulation of the alveus (second stimulus) looks nearly the same as the response to the mossy fiber stimulus, the only difference being that the initial peak in the stratum pyramidale is missing.

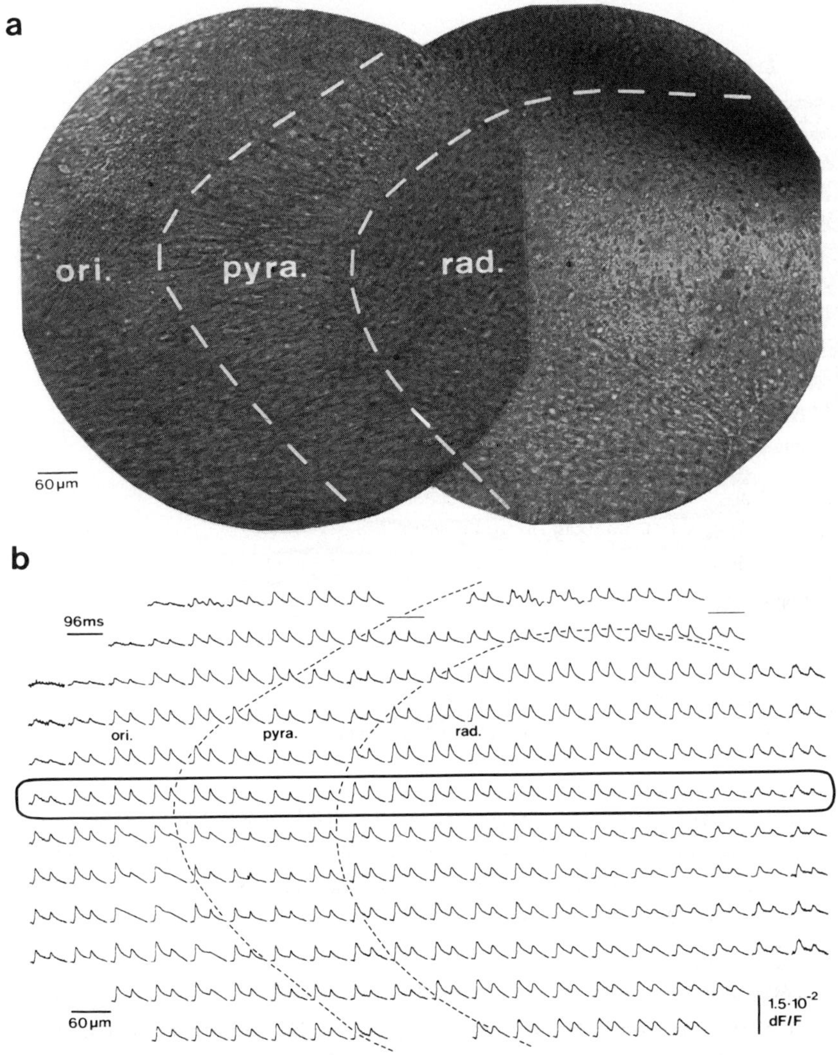

Fig. 2. Optical recording from the CA3 region of organotypical hippocampal slice cultures. **a**: Photographic view of the CA3 area, monitored by the optical recording; **b**: Optical recording of the activity in the CA3 region under high calcium conditions (3.5 mM). Each trace (duration 96 ms) displays the averaged activity (6 stimuli) recorded by a single photodiode from the corresponding tissue location. The encircled row of photodiodes was selected for calculation of the iCSD-profile (Fig. 3). *rad.* stratum radiatum; *pyra.* stratum pyramidale; *ori.* stratum oriens

From anatomical considerations on organotypical hippocampal cultures (Zimmer and Gähwiler 1984; Caeser and Aertsen 1991), we propose

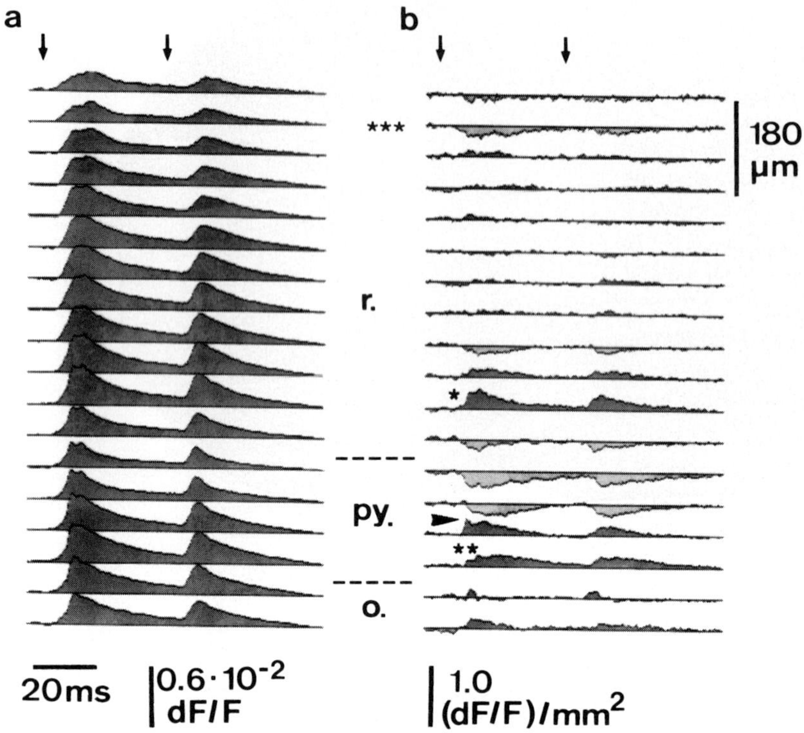

Fig. 3. Distribution of relative fluorescence change (**a**) under high calcium conditions (3.5 mM; encircled row of fluorescence signals in Fig 2b) and associated iCSD-profile (**b**). In this case correction procedure I (Methods) was applied to determine the relative fluorescence change

that the response to the first stimulus is mainly due to synaptic activation by the mossy fibres, resulting in spike activity in the CA3 pyramidal cells. It is well known, however, that the anatomical termination area of mossy fibres on CA3 pyramidal cells is on the proximal dendritic tree. Consequently, one would expect the synaptic depolarisations to arise mainly in the vicinity of the pyramidale/radiatum border, rather than being distributed over the whole stratum radiatum (comp. Figs. 2a,b and 3a). At least two reasons may account for this discrepancy: either the course of the mossy fibre bundle is less well preserved in hippocampal slice cultures, or the location of the synaptic input cannot be judged with enough precision from the relative fluorescence maps.

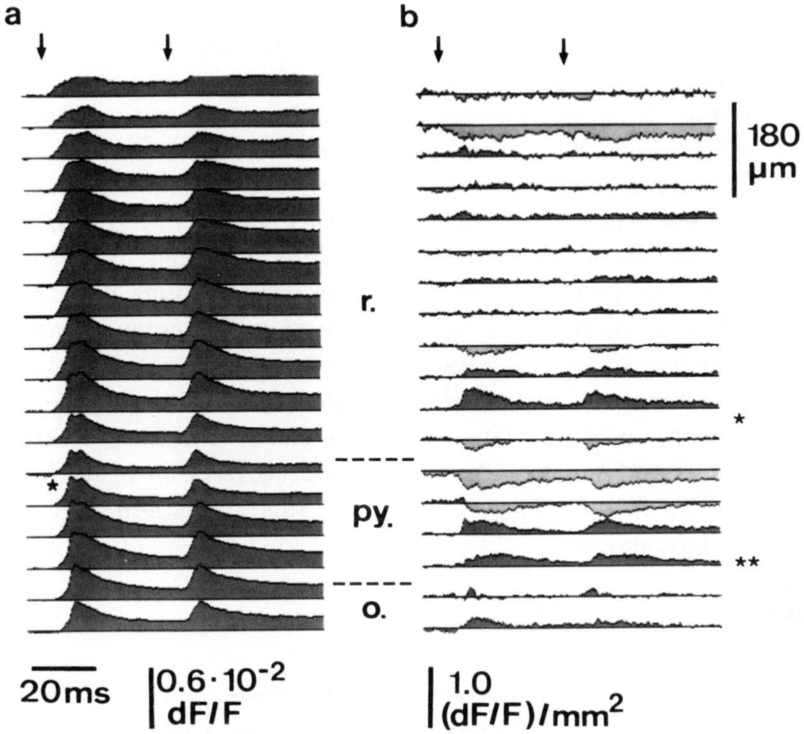

Fig. 4. Distribution of relative fluorescence change (**a**) unter high calcium conditions (3.5 mM) and associated iCSD-profiles (**b**) of the same experimental data as in Fig. 3. In this as well as in all following cases correction procedure II (Methods) was applied

Similarly, for the response to stimulation of the alveus one would expect mainly antidromically induced spike activity in the stratum pyramidale, together with synaptic or spike activity in the outer region of stratum pyramidale due to axonal collaterals. Hence, the two large depolarisation areas, particularly the large and early depolarisation in the stratum radiatum, are somewhat unexpected.

Faced with these differences, it would be highly beneficial to apply a transformation, which increases the spatial resolution. This can indeed be achieved, as witnessed by the iCSD-profiles shown in Figs. 3b and 4b. In these plots, sinks (i.e. positive ions flowing into the cell) are indicated as upwards deflections and, likewise, sources as downward deflections. Hence, areas which mark excitatory synaptic influx show up as sinks with a monophasic time course, joined by similar adjacent sources. Using this criterion, the analysis of the responses to both the mossy fibre stimulus and the alveus stimulus, reveals two synaptic input areas (* and ** in Figs. 3b and 4b). In addition, however, the iCSD-profile in Fig. 3b shows longlasting, negative and positive ramps at a number of locations. We presume that these longlasting events in the iCSD-profiles are artefacts, due to an incorrect normalization for bleaching and inhomogeneities in the fluorescence plots, and amplified by the CSD-analysis. As an alternative, therefore, we used procedure II (see Methods). The results from the same experimental data are shown in Fig. 4. The differences achieved in the fluorescence maps can be recognized by comparing Figs. 3a and 4a: the overall depolarization in the fluorescence distribution is strongly diminished. As a result, the associated iCSD-profile (Fig. 4b) shows a much clearer distribution of sinks and sources. We will use this correction procedure II for all profiles to follow. The adequacy of this correction will be elaborated in the Discussion.

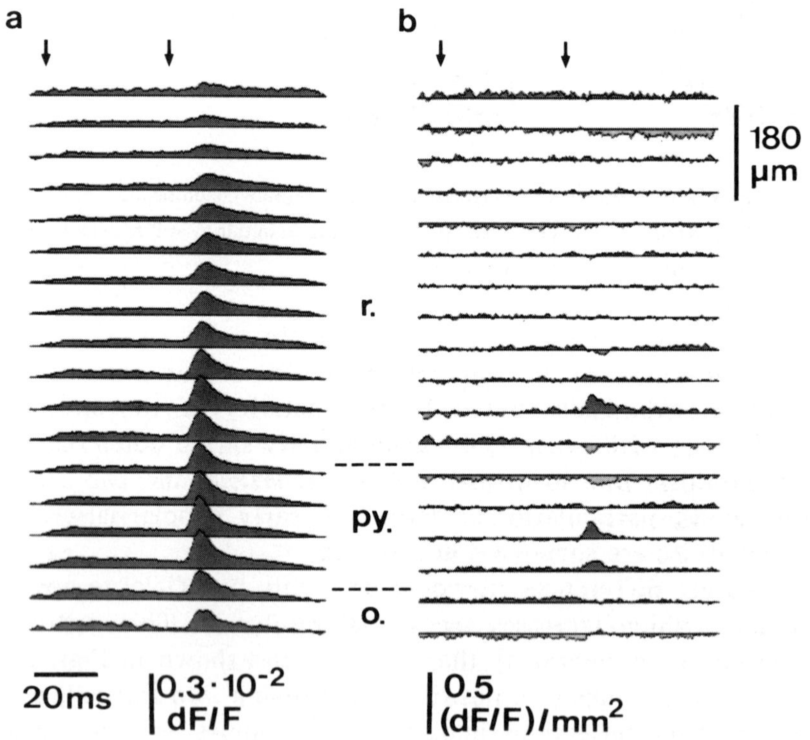

Fig. 5. (**a**) Relative fluorescence change unter calcium-free conditions; (**b**) associated iCSD-profile.

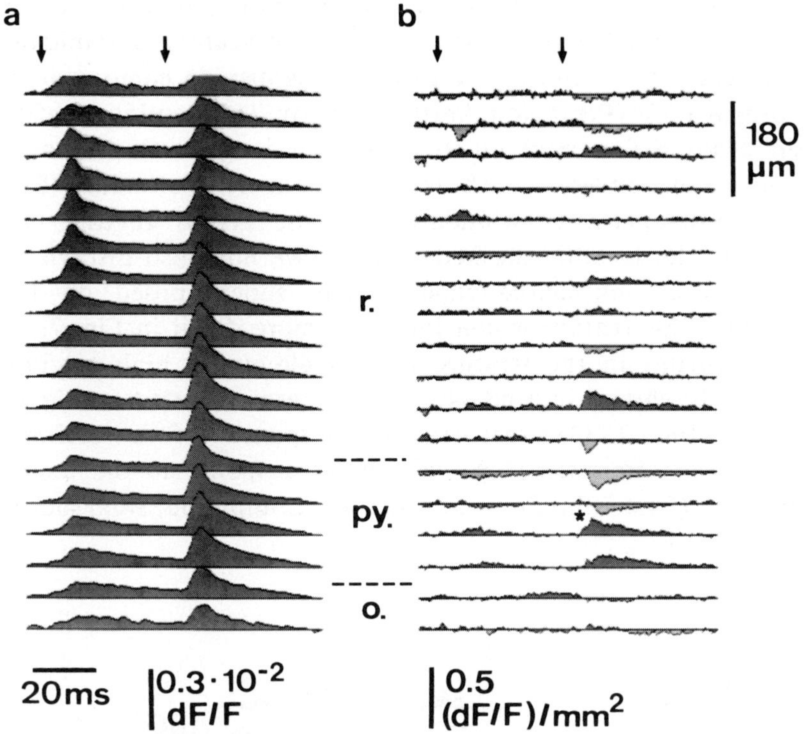

Fig. 6. Recovery of responses 30 min after the change from calcium-free to high calcium conditions. Distribution of relative fluorescence change (**a**) and associated iCSD-profile (**b**)

The first response in the iCSD-profile in Fig. 4b shows a clear sink with adjacent sources in the stratum radiatum and stratum pyramidale (*). This sink is now situated close to the pyramidale/radiatum border, as was expected from the mossy fiber termination area. A second sink, appearing in the outer region of the stratum pyramidale (**), indicates the presence of additional synaptic input. This latter feature occurs in both responses. Additional sinks show up in the distal dendritic region (***). These reflect activity in the dendate gyrus. Finally, the small action potential pattern in the stratum pyramidale (arrowhead) will be shown and discussed in greater detail later (cf. Fig. 7a).

In order to separate synaptically and antidromically evoked responses, we performed the same experiment under calcium-free conditions. The results are shown in Fig. 5. In this case, the fluorescence map and the iCSD-profile only reveal responses to stimulation of the alveus.

The iCSD-profile (Fig. 5b) shows the composite sink/source profile of antidromically generated action potentials in the stratum pyramidale. The adjacent sinks above and below reflect both passive compensation and active propagation (Plenz and Aertsen 1991b). Thirty minutes after changing the calcium-free medium to high calcium again, the response recovered, albeit incompletely with respect to the first stimulus (Fig. 6b). Again, the response to stimulation of the alveus reveals two distinct sinks. At the location marked with (*) we now also discern an additional, biphasic sink/source time course, superimposed on the monophasic sink. This feature is considered in more detail in Fig. 7.

The iCSD-profiles in the stratum pyramidale under high calcium conditions, already shown in Figs. 4b and 6b, are replotted at higher magnification in Fig. 7. Consider first the response before calcium-free conditions were imposed (Fig. 7a). In the response to the mossy fibre stimulation (first stimulus) we discern a biphasic sink/source

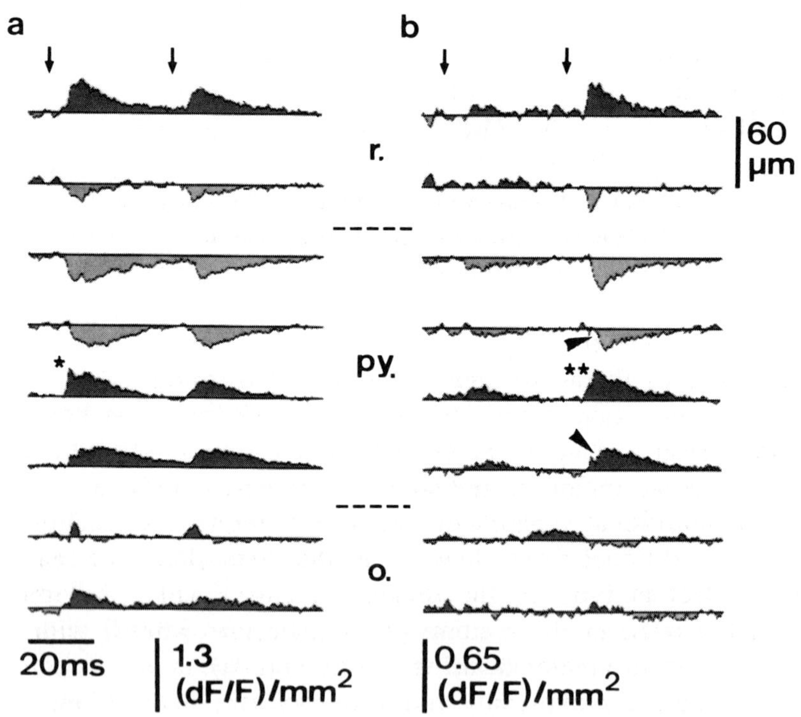

Fig. 7. Enlarged view of the iCSD-profiles in the stratum pyramidale from Fig. 3b (**a**) and Fig 5b (**b**)

waveform, superimposed on a sink (*). Such a biphasic waveform does not arise in the response to stimulation via the alveus (second stimulus), indicating that no pyramidal cell body action potentials arise in this case. The latter can be explained by the phenomenon of double-pulse inhibition. In contrast to this, Fig. 7b shows that under the condition of partial recovery from calcium-free medium, when mossy fiber stimulation failed to elicit action potentials in the pyramidal cell body layer, stimulation in the alveus does succeed to evoke action potentials. This is indicated by the sharp sink riding on the basal sink (**), the corresponding short-lasting source in the lower trace (arrowhead) and the steepening of the source in the upper trace (arrowhead).

Discussion

The purpose of the present study was to investigate the flow of neural activity in area CA3 of organotypical slice cultures of the rat hippocampus. In particular, we focussed on the question of orderly development of fibre bundle projections in such slice cultures. We approached these issues by studying CSD-profiles obtained from relative fluorescence maps (iCSD). Before turning to the results, we will first discuss a number of methodological aspects of the optical recording technique.

Methodological aspects of fluorescence maps in organotypical slice cultures

In general, it is nearly impossible to determine the precise origin of the fluorescence signal, collected by a single photodetector (Grinvald et al. 1988). However, in the organotypical hippocampal slice culture, because of its orderly topography, we made the assumption that each photodiode is collecting the activity from a tissue area which is dominated by a particular type of cell elements: we measure mainly dendritic activity in the stratum radiatum, cell body activity in the stratum pyramidale, and axonal. activity in the stratum oriens/alveus region.

We used two different procedures to calculate the relative fluorescence dF/F. From theoretical considerations, subtraction of the non-stimulus sweep from the stimulus sweep (procedure I) should be the most adequate approach. In our experiments we observed, however, that the light source may undergo slow, but considerable amplitude changes from trial to trial. Clearly this leads to residual terms when subtracting successive stimulus and non-stimulus sweeps. Although these residues tend to cancel when averaging over many trials, they give rise to distinct artefacts when working with low numbers of stimuli, as demonstrated by the long-lasting positive or negative dilatations in the iCSD-profile in Fig. 3b. The spurious nature of these features is underlined by the lack of correlation with location within the tissue when comparing across experiments. As a simple alternative, we chose to apply correction procedure II, which uses a linear approximation of the non-stimulus sweep and, thus, avoids the nonstationarity problem altogether.

CSD-profiles of relative fluorescence distributions (iCSD)

Several assumptions had to be made in the calculation of the iCSD-profile (see Methods and extensive discussion in Plenz and Aertsen 1991b). For the orderly arranged CA3 pyramidal cells in organotypical hippocampal slice cultures, the first assumption is fulfilled by properly orienting the photodiode array in parallel to the cells' main axis (Fig. 2a,b). Assumption (2), high spatial resolution, is implicit in the reasoning on different cell compartments. In addition, the required distance between neighboring photodiodes should be based upon a spatial Fourier analysis of the fluorescence distribution (Plenz and Aertsen 1991b). Assumption (3) stating that the intracellular resistance can be considered as purely ohmic, is based on the ionic nature of the intracellular medium.

Finally, some special attention should be given to assumption (4): constant intracellular resistance along the dendrosomatic axis. This assumption clearly contradicts the observation that this resistance is, amongst others, a function of the diameter of the different cell compartments, and is regarded to be highest in the axonal branches and lowest in the cell body region. Consequently, this assumption introduces a systematic error in the iCSD-profiles, calculated on the basis of Equ. (4): the cell body region compartments receive less weight than the dendritic and axonal compartments. As a result, iCSD-profiles preferentially reveal their activity in the strata radiatum and oriens, at the expense of activity in the stratum pyramidale (for a discussion on additional procedures we refer to Plenz and Aertsen 1991b).

Abberrant projections in the organotypical slice culture of rat hippocampus

We found that any attempt to unravel the underlying processes in the CA3 region on the basis of amplitude-latency distributions of the fluorescence maps is seriously hampered by the lack of adequate spatial resolution. This refers to the problem of determining the location of synaptic input as well as the differentiation between active and passive events. In this respect, the introduction of iCSD-profiles presents a significant improvement when interpreting the spatio-temporal activity patterns. For instance, the position of the synaptic sink in the stratum radiatum matches the location one would expect from the neuroanatomy.

In addition, it could be shown that the activity in the stratum pyramidale and in the border region of stratum pyramidale and stratum oriens consists of a mixture of action potentials and a second synaptic sink. The slight time delay between the first and second sink suggests that the latter is due to the activation of inhibitory interneurons via recurrent axon collaterals from the CA3 pyramidal cells (Schwartzkroin and Knowles 1983). This interpretation of recurrent inhibition is in accordance with the finding that an action potential pattern is lacking in the response to the second stimulus, if action potentials were elicited in the first response (Fig. 4b). Such double-pulse inhibition has, in fact, been observed in organotypical cell cultures (Cornish and Wheal 1989; Caeser et al. 1990), and is to be expected because of the presence of GABAergic neurons in such cultures (Caeser and Aertsen 1991). The synaptic sink in the stratum oriens of the CA3 region, however, could also result from sprouting of the mossy fibres. This phenomenon was reported for kindled rats (Ben-Ar and Represa 1990) and could therefore also be expected in cultures, which are known to have a tendency for epileptic behaviour (Furshpan and Potter 1989; Koroshetz and Furshpan 1990).

The presence of antidromically evoked action potentials in the iCSD-profiles under calcium-free conditions clearly reveals the presence of abberant axonal projections in organotypical hippocampal slice cultures. In the case of alveus stimulation under high calcium conditions, this AP-pattern is lacking and, instead, a synaptic sink shows up in the stratum radiatum and a second one in the stratum oriens (Fig. 4b). Whereas the former sink can again be attributed to the activation of inhibitory interneurons, two explanations may account for the second sink. It could either result from (not *in vivo* occurring) axonal projections of CA1 pyramidal cells into the CA3 region (Caeser and Aertsen 1991) or, alternatively, from aberrant projections of the Schaffer collaterals and their profound recurrent axon collaterals (Miles and Wong 1986; Ben-Ari and Represa 1990; Caeser and Aertsen 1991). The former possibility of an unusual target projection of the CA1 region in organotypical slice cultures is supported by findings of Zimmer and Gähwiler (1984) of an increased autoinnervation of the CA1 region.

Acknowledgements

We thank Volker Staiger for skillful assistance throughout the experiments and in the preparation of the Figures. In addition, we thank Ulla Mitzdorf for helpful discussions during the early stages of this work. Partial funding for this study was received from the Bundesministerium für Forschung und Technologie (BMFT).

References

Ben-Ari Y, Represa A (1990) Brief seizure episodes induce long-term potentiation and mossy fibre sprouting in the hippocampus. TINS 13:312-318

Bonhoeffer T, Staiger V (1988) Optical recording with single cell resolution from monolayered slice cultures of rat hippocampus. Neurosci Lett 92:259-264

Caeser M, Aertsen A (1991) Morphological organization of rat hippocampal slice cultures. J Comp Neurol 307:87-106

Caeser M, Plenz D, Aertsen A (1990) Spatio-temporal spreading of electrical activity in rat hippocampus slices and cell cultures. In: Elsner N, Roth G (eds) Brain - Perception - Cognition. Georg Thieme Verlag, Stuttgart New York

Cornish SM, Wheal HV (1989) Long-term loss of paired pulse inhibition in the kainic acid lesioned hippocampus of the rat. Neurosci 28:563-571

Freeman JA, Nicholson C (1975) Experimental organisation of current source density technique for anuran cerebellum. J Neurophysiol 38:369-382

Furshpan EJ, Potter DD (1989) Seizure-like activity and cellular damage in rat hippocampal neurons in cell culture. Neuron 3:199-207

Gähwiler BH (1989) Organotypic cultures of neural tissue. TINS 11:484-489

Grinvald A, Frostig RD, Lieke E, Hildesheim R (1988) Optical imaging of neuronal activity. Physiol Rev 68:1285-1366

Grinvald A, Lieke E, Frostig RD, Gilbert CD, Wiesel TN (1986) Functional architecture of cortex revealed by optical imaging of intrinsic signals. Nature 324:361-364

Koroshetz WJ, Furshpan EJ (1990) Seizure-like activity and glutamate receptors in hippocampal neurons in culture. Neurosci Res 8 Suppl. 13:S65-S74

Miles R, Wong RKS (1986) Excitatory synaptic interactions between CA3 Neurones in the Guinea-pig hippocampus. J Physiol (Lond) 373:397-418

Mitzdorf U (1985) Current source density method and application in cat cerebral cortex: Investigation of evoked potentials and EEG phenomena. Physiol Rev 65:37-100

Plenz D, Aertsen A (1991a) On the correspondance of intra- and extracellullar space: Convergence of classical field potential measurements and optical recording with voltage-sensitive dyes at the level of current source density analysis. In: Penzlin H, Elsner N (eds) Synapse - Transmission - Modulation. Thieme Verlag, Stuttgart, p 312

Plenz D, Aertsen A (1991b) Current Source Density profiles of optical recording maps: a new approach to the analysis of spatio-temporal neural activity patterns. (submitted)

Salzberg BM (1989) Optical recording of voltage changes in nerve terminals and in fine neuronal processes. Ann Rev Physiol 51:507-526

Schwartzkroin PA, Knowles WD (1983) Local interaction in the hippocampus. TINS 3:88-92

Zimmer J, Gähwiler BH (1984) Cellular and connective organization of slice cultures of the rat hippocampus and fascia dentata. J Comp Neurol 228:432-446

The Contribution of the Striatum to Cortical Function

Jeff Wickens

Anatomy Department, Otago University Medical School, Box 913, Dunedin, New Zealand

Introduction

In the struggle for survival the ability to learn to associate temporally contiguous events is clearly advantageous. By forming such associations it becomes possible to reconstruct the external world from the fragments of information impinging on the senses. Equally so, it is important to be able to learn from the effects of actions directed outward upon the external world. Only then does it becomes possible to learn how to act upon the world in order to obtain a desired result. Thus, there appear to be at least two different types of learning. The distinction between these two types of learning is logical as well as psychological. This has been pointed out in various terms by a number of authors (Hirsh 1974; Mishkin et al. 1984; Miller 1988).

The distinction between these two types of learning is reminiscent of a split between two schools of psychological learning theory in the first half of this century. One side reduced everything to instrumental conditioning, in which the essential feature of learning is the modification, by reinforcement, of connections between a stimulus and a response (Thorndike 1911; Hull 1943). The other side maintained that reinforcement is not at all necessary, but that animals learn "what leads to what" by temporal contiguity, and thus acquire a map which leads them to the objects they desire (Tolman 1932).

However, although each type of learning described in this paper has some common features with one side or other of the learning theory debate, the parallel should not be taken any further. The learning theory debate was a matter of rivalry between competing theories, each attempting to account for all learning. In this paper, animal learning is treated as a combination of at least two types which may each contribute in many situations. The learning theory debate may then be seen as partly due to the tendency of each school to concentrate on situations which called for only one or other type of learning. The territorial boundaries between the different theories thus differ from the distinctions between the two types of learning.

The distinction advocated here is based on a neurobiological argument. It was suggested by Miller (1981; 1988) that learning can be dissected along anatomical lines, into two different types, each dealt with by a different part of the brain. This division is difficult to see from psychological evidence alone, because the two types of learning usually work together. The validity of the split proposed depends on the identification of the two types of learning with separate anatomical substrates in the brain.

In the following discussion the argument that each of the two types of learning has a corresponding substrate in the brain will be briefly reviewed. The structural features of each substrate, which suit it to deal with its learning task, will be described. In particular, it will be argued that the cerebral cortex deals primarily with learning on the basis of temporal contiguity, while the striatum deals primarily with learning from the results of acting upon the external world.

The way in which these two structures interact will then be considered, with a view to understanding how the two types of learning may combine in situations which involve both. Finally, the possible implications of these interactions for theoretical approaches to cortical function will be discussed.

Learning on the basis of temporal contiguity

Learning by temporal contiguity involves the detection of coincidences (unexpected conjunctions of events). The registration of such conjunctions presumably involves synaptic modifications, which may establish associative links between corresponding brain states. The most widely recognized mechanism for the detection of a conjunction appears to be localized near to synapses on dendritic spines. Here, a conjunction of presynaptic activity and postsynaptic excitation may activate mechanisms (reviewed by Wickens 1988) which trigger long-lasting synaptic modification, such as long-term potentiation (LTP) or depression (LTD).

The modifiable synapses on dendritic spines provide a mechanism by which the statistics of coincidences of events may be transformed into changes in the connections between the elements of a network. According to Braitenberg (1989) and Palm (1982), the cerebral cortex is a favourable substrate for the growth of cell assemblies in the manner envisaged by Hebb (1949). The argument is that the majority of synapses in the cortex are between pyramidal cells and end on dendritic spines (and are therefore probably modifiable). The individual synapses are weakly excitatory, so that when a sufficiently large number of connected cells are coactivated, they may ignite a self-sustaining assembly. The strength of the connections is a function of the past history of conjunctions. This provides a substrate for learning by temporal contiguity.

Learning on the basis of temporal contiguity does not require any action on the part of the learner. An illustration of this is provided by McNamara et al (1956). These authors wheeled ten rats (one at a time) through a T-maze on a little cart, to a goal box where they obtained a reward. Another group of rats had to run through the maze to get the reward. The investigators found that, when each group was tested in extinction, there was no reliable difference between the groups in their tendency to choose the arm of the maze which held the reward.

In terms of learning by temporal contiguity, we can imagine that the rats in the cart experienced the ride as a series of snapshots of the surrounding view. These they may piece together into a "motion picture" sequence of associated images. Such an associative memory could be used to "look ahead" and guide the approach to the goal box. Clearly, under these conditions, learning can occur without performance.

The same experiment also provided a valuable insight into the second type of learning, which involves learning from the effects of actions performed on the external world. If the cues from outside the maze were reduced, so that all the rats could see was the inside of the maze, then the animals that actually ran the maze did much better than the ones that had only been taken for a ride. This illustrates the second type of learning, in which an action performed by the organism is required to produce an effect which may then modify subsequent choices.

Learning from the effects of actions

In contrast to learning on the basis of contiguity, a mechanism for learning from the effects of acting upon the environment requires something additional to an associative rule based on coactivation. Such a mechanism must include a way for the outcome of past actions to be incorporated into future actions. The outcome must retroactively modify the action that brought it about. This must be done selectively, in order to ensure that the modifications only affect the action in appropriate situations. Thus, the mechanism must combine three factors: situation, action and an outcome (which is known only after a time delay).

The time delay is of some importance. A delay in outcome is obligatory whenever action on the external world is involved. This is because it takes time for neural activity to produce a muscular action, and the effect of the action in the physical world cannot be instantaneous. By the time it is known the situation may have changed or some other action initiated. The time delay between the antecedent neural activity and the outcome means that synaptic modification must occur at the subset of synapses that were active some time before it occurred.

But, if the outcome of an action is delayed for even a second, Hebbian learning as we currently know it (in the form of LTP) will not be sufficient for this type of learning. The reason is simply that in order to produce LTP, the interval within which a conjunction of activity must occur is of the order of tens of milliseconds and certainly much less than a second (see Levy and Steward 1979; Kelso et al. 1983; Gustafsson et al. 1987). Although this data is from the hippocampus, it is the best estimate we can make of this interval in neocortical LTP.

This problem cannot solved by postulating reverberating circuits to hold the situation in memory until the outcome is known. Additional mechanisms would be needed to distinguish the actual situation from the reverberating situation. These would be very problematic, if not logically impossible. Some means would also be required to transfer the effects of outcome on the reverberating situation to the connections where the actual situation would be processed.

Thus, it would appear from what we know of the mechanism of LTP, which is our best animal model for Hebbian synaptic modification, that this mechanism is not sufficient for learning from the delayed effects of acting on the world. Some additional mechanism is required, which has been called a "state of readiness" by Miller (1981), and an "eligibility trace" by Barto et al. (1981). Such a mechanism could bridge the delay until the outcome by maintaining a kind of synaptic "after-image" of the action and its antecedents. It has been suggested by Wickens (1990a) that elevations of spine calcium at corticostriatal synapses may be the physical basis of the state of readiness. Once elevated by a conjunction of pre- and postsynaptic activity, spine calcium may persist for a second or so. This could bridge the temporal gap between the antecedents of an action and the outcome.

The proposed state of readiness is a short-lasting trace of a conjunction of pre- and postsynaptic activity. To complete the synaptic modification rule, this must interact with a third factor mediating the outcome. There is considerable evidence that striatal dopamine is involved in feedback of results from the environment, at the very least as a reward signal. Lesions of dopaminergic afferents to the striatum block the rewarding effects of food and water. These same afferents are a powerful substrate for rewarding intracranial stimulation, which may be preferred to natural reward. The literature on reward functions of dopamine is vast and a number of reviews exist (Stellar and Stellar 1985; Wickens 1990b; Miller et al. 1990). There is also considerable evidence that dopaminergic afferents to the striatum are necessary for the acquisition of open-loop control (Viallet et al. 1986), which can only be acquired on the basis of knowledge of the outcome of actions.

If dopamine mediates some kind of feedback of results, it may function as a third, necessary factor for synaptic modification in the striatum. There is a morphological argument to support this idea. In the striatum, the corticostriatal inputs often terminate on a dendritic spine which also has a dopaminergic terminal of midbrain origin. Perhaps as many as 39% of striatal spines are contacted by two boutons: one of probable cortical origin which makes an asymmetrical synapse, and another one staining positively for markers of dopaminergic synapses (Freund et al. 1984). A dendritic spine receiving one cortical input and one dopaminergic input is a likely site for a three factor synaptic modification rule in which dopamine is the third factor, because it is a site at which the three factors may combine in biochemical reactions.

In the cortex or hippocampus (where most of the synapses between pyramidal cells are on dendritic spines which have only one presynaptic terminal per spine) a conjunction of pre- and postsynaptic activity produces an elevation of spine calcium which may be sufficient to produce LTP. In the striatum, it is possible that elevated spine calcium may be necessary, but not sufficient, for synaptic modification to occur. Activation of the dopamine input while the spine calcium is still elevated may also be necessary, perhaps to cause a calcium and dopamine-dependent reaction to proceed. Although speculative, the biochemical machinery for such an interaction between spine calcium and dopamine receptor activation certainly exists in the spines of the relevant neurons of the striatum (Hemmings et al. 1987; see also Wickens 1990a).

Interactions between the cortex and striatum

In order to relate a rule for synaptic modification in the corticostriatal pathway to the problem of learning on the basis of results of actions, it is necessary to consider what sort of information might be stored in the corticostriatal synapses. This question requires some reflection upon the interactions between the cortex and the striatum.

The striatum is part of a loop from cortex to striatum and back to cortex via the thalamus (Alexander et al. 1986). The shortest path around this loop involves two excitatory and two inhibitory synapses. The cortical afferents are excitatory and synapse directly upon the striatal output neurons (Somogyi et al. 1981). The striatal output neurons are inhibitory to the pallidal neurons, which are in turn inhibitory to thalamic neurons. The net effect of the striatum upon the cortex is excitation brought about by disinhibition (Deniau and Chevalier 1985). This is an important source of activation of the motor areas of the cortex (Passingham 1987).

Braitenberg (1978) first suggested that such a loop through the striatum could regulate the threshold of cortical neurons. Such a regulator could integrate over a wide area of cortex and control, by negative feedback, the number of active neurons. The progression from one cortical cell assembly to another might then be controlled by a nonspecific effect of the striatum. This could help to hold a given pattern or be withdrawn to induce a change in cortical activation to a new pattern (Palm 1987). However, the evidence cited above suggests the shortest path around this loop is excitatory, and therefore has the wrong sign for a negative-feedback mechanism. On the other hand, all the loops which involve an odd number of inhibitory synapses will be inhibitory, and there will be a greater number of these, as explained in the following paragraph.

The interactions which occur between the striatal output neurons are mutually inhibitory (Aronin et al. 1986; Pasik et al. 1988). This arrangement suggests that the prevailing dynamic within the striatum should be one of competition. A "winner-takes-all" situation may prevail within striatal "domains" defined by the distance over which mutually inhibitory interactions occur. This means that while the most active neuron in a domain is exciting certain cortical neurons by disinhibition, excitation would be withdrawn from other cortical neurons, because the striatal neurons projecting to them (via the thalamus) will be inhibited. Thus, the striatum is a very special kind of regulator, acting as a kind of lens in the feedback loop, producing activation at an excitatory focus surrounded by a zone of non-specific inhibition (see Tremblay and Filion 1989).

The neocortical afferents to the striatum originate from all major areas of both sides of the cortex (McGeorge and Faull 1989). The afferents from different cortical areas are drawn together and laid out side by side (Selemon and Goldman-Rakic 1985). The importance of this is that activity from a wide area of cortex may converge on striatal neurons which lie within the same domain of mutual inhibition.

There are some advantages in bringing afferents from a wide area of cortex into a striatal domain in which competition can occur. Although competition mediated by inhibitory interneurons may occur in the cortex, it probably has a limited spatial extent, because the inhibitory neurons tend to have shorter axons than the pyramidal cells. Thus, in order for competition to occur between cortical cell assemblies extending beyond the range of inhibitory interneurons, something external to the cortex is required. A striatal domain may serve this function, by acting as a focal point at which competition between different cortical cell assemblies can occur. This assumes that striatal neurons are in some way selective for cortical cell assemblies, and leads to the question of what determines the selectivity of striatal neurons.

Despite integrating over a wide area, the striatal neurons preserve a high degree of specificity in their responses (Rolls et al. 1983). This specificity is partly attributable to the pattern of efficacy of the corticostriatal synapses. This will be determined by the rules for synaptic modification in this pathway. The action of these rules may be expected to produce striatal neurons that respond selectively to particular cortical cell assemblies, as outlined in the following arguments.

The corticostriatal positive feedback loop is intersected at the corticostriatal synapses by a dopaminergic input from the midbrain (as described in the previous section). This is one route by which dopaminergic influence may be felt in the cortex. The influence of dopamine is to increase the excitatory responses of a subset of striatal neurons to cortical inputs (Schneider et al. 1984; Hirata et al. 1984) and bring about an increase in variability of striatal output (Waszczak et al. 1984).

A cortical cell assembly which produces an action which leads to a favourable result will increase the dopaminergic input to the striatum. The effect of dopamine, by the rules proposed in the previous section, will be to strengthen the corticostriatal synapses that were put into a state of readiness by a recent conjunction of presynaptic cortical activity and postsynaptic striatal outputs. The synapses to be strengthened will be the ones on striatal neurons that were activated by the most recently active cortical cell assemblies.

After many repetitions, a striatal neuron may come to be highly selective for a particular cortical cell assembly. Moreover, the vigour with which it responds will represent the expectation (in a statistical sense) that the particular cortical cell assembly will lead to a favourable result. Thus, striatal output neurons may acquire, on the basis of an outcome signal mediated by dopamine, a selectivity for certain cortical activation patterns.

What effect does this have on the cortical cell assemblies? The influence of the striatum upon the cortex, via the thalamus, is weakly excitatory and widely distributed. The relevant thalamocortical fibres run tangential to the cortical surface, as if trying to contact as many different assemblies as possible (Arbuthnott et al. 1986). A particular cortical cell assembly which increased the activity of some set of striatal neurons would receive increased activation by positive feedback (provided the increased activity did not change which striatal neurons were active).

The effect increasing the selectivity of a set of striatal neurons for some cortical cell assembly would be to make it more "attractive". A cortical cell assembly which had frequently been active before a dopaminergic reward would thus become increasingly likely to occur in the future. In figurative terms, it may be imagined that a cell assembly which had acquired a striatal representation would take on a kind of "hue", or "dopamine aura". A striatal response to such an attractive cell assembly would be like a nod of the head, in affirmation of an appealing idea.

The effect of striatal dynamics on cortical function

Competition within striatal domains may ensure that only the most attractive cortical cell assemblies will be amplified in the corticostriatal feedback loop. Cortical cell assemblies which have less frequently been associated with a favourable outcome will be suppressed by inhibition from their more successful neighbours in the striatum. Thus, the contrast between two otherwise similar cortical cell assemblies may be increased by their past track record.

This fast dynamic effect will have cumulative structural effects on the development of cortical cell assemblies. Active striato-thalamo-cortical inputs to active cortical cell assemblies may show LTP (Iriki et al. 1989). At the same time, it is likely that inactive striato-thalamo-cortical inputs may show long-term depression similar to the heterosynaptic depression reported in the hippocampus (Abraham and Goddard 1983). Thus, cortical cell assemblies which are recognized by striatal neurons may become more strongly attached to the active striatal neurons, and disconnected from the inactive ones. This will bring about a partitioning of the cortical assemblies, based on the selectivity of the striatal neurons.

Such partitioning would be ideal for the representation of mutually exclusive propositions. A simple case where this could be useful is the representation of muscular antagonism. For example, it is not possible to simultaneously flex and extend the elbow joint. Although it is possible to coactivate both flexor and extensor groups of muscles (such as biceps and triceps), to do so would in many cases be a waste of energy. There is some advantage, perhaps, in such actions having a mutually exclusive representation.

How can such a representation be acquired? For sensory areas of the cortex, the problem of representation is largely one of extracting statistical structure that is already present in the inputs. However, for areas of the brain concerned with action there is an added difficulty. The logic of action which describes the external world cannot be grasped passively. An action must first be performed before its effects can be known. The resistance of the world will not be felt until force is applied.

The interactions between the cortex and striatum suggest a mechanism by which this "logic of action" may be incorporated into the brain. In the example of the agonist-antagonist pair of muscles, attempting to contract both groups of muscles would be unrewarding, but contracting one without the other would produce movement, which might be regarded as relatively rewarding. When flexion or extension occur separately, the relatively rewarding effect would cause separate striatal neurons to acquire strong selectivity for the corresponding cortical assemblies. Coactivation of both cortical assemblies, however, would be unrewarding, and in this event the synapses activating striatal neurons would be weakened.

Significance for theories of cortical function

Important progress has been made in recent years, towards an understanding of coding schemes that do not assume a complete partition into mutually exclusive possibilities as is normally assumed in information theory (see Palm 1987). A sparse coding scheme is efficient for storing many patterns and makes it possible to represent similar things by similar codes. Much of this derives from the observation that if detectors are tuned to unlikely features, then the presence of a feature is far more significant than its absence. However, while in sensory processing, "the complement of something interesting is not generally interesting", the motor system is always balanced between opposing tendencies. The complement of flexion (extension) may also be interesting. This perhaps reflects the tight coupling in the mechanics of the musculoskeletal system.

This touches on a fundamental issue. In sensory processing classification on the basis of temporal contiguity may adequately reflect the relations between the parts of the surrounding world. But consider this question. Why do we see a pile of books on the desk and not an uneven surface? Is it because the parts of a given book are more similar to other parts of the same book than they are to the parts of other books? This would seem to be the implication of a purely conjunctive model of learning.

An alternative suggestion is that we see a pile of books because each book can be held and moved about independently of the other. Each book is a detachable object, which can be manipulated independently of other objects. It is not only the relation between elements, in terms of groupings, arrangement, correspondence that is important. A way to operate upon these elements must also be acquired. This ability is produced by interactions with the external world.

Conclusion

Activity in a positive feedback loop which includes the cortex and striatum may be amplified according to the selectivity of striatal neurons for particular cortical cell assemblies. The strength of the corticostriatal synapses may depend on the accumulated history of results of previous activity in this loop, and come to represent the expectation that a particular cortical cell assembly will lead to a favourable result. Competition within the striatum will ensure that the action with the greatest expectation of a favourable outcome will be selected. These mechanisms are necessary for learning on the basis of results of actions upon the external world, which cannot be accomplished by the cortex alone.

Acknowledgements

I wish to thank the organizers of the meeting for generous support for travel and accommodation. I thank Dr R. Miller, Prof V. Braitenberg and Prof G. Palm for helpful discussions, suggestions and encouragement. I thank Ruth Nuttall for a helpful discussion at a critical point in the preparation of this paper.

References

Alexander GE, DeLong MR, Strick PL (1986) Parallel organization of functionally segregated circuits linking basal ganglia and cortex. Ann Rev Neurosci 9:357-381

Abraham WC, Goddard GV (1983) Asymmetric relations between homosynaptic long-term potentiation and heterosynaptic long-term depression. Nature 305:717-719

Arbuthnott GW, MacLeod NK, Maxwell DJ, Wright AK (1986) The detailed morphology of the cortical terminals of the thalamocorticl fibres from the ventromedial nucleus in the rat. In: The Basal Ganglia II, International Basal Ganglia Society, Victoria B.C. pp 283-291

Aronin N, Chase K, Difiglia M (1986) Glutamic acid decarboxylase and enkephalin immunoreactive axon terminals in the rat neostriatum synapse with striatonigral neurons. Brain Res 365:151-158

Barto AG, Sutton RS, Brouwer PS (1981) Associative search network: A reinforcement learning associative memory. Biol Cybern 40:201-211

Braitenberg V (1978) Cell assemblies in the cerebral cortex. In: Heim R, Palm, G (eds) Theoretical Approaches to Complex Systems. Springer, Berlin Heidelberg New York, pp 171-188

Braitenberg V (1989) Some arguments for a theory of cell assemblies in the cerebral cortex. In: Nadel L, Cooper LA, Culicover P, Harnish RM (eds) Neural Connections, Mental Computation. MIT-Press, pp 137-145

Deniau JM, Chevalier G (1985) Disinhibition as a basic process in the expression of striatal functions II. The striatonigral influence on thalamocortical cells of the ventromedial thalamic nucleus. Brain Res 334:227-233

Fox CA, Andrade AN, LuQui IJ, Rafols JA (1974) The primate globus pallidus: A Golgi and electron microscopic study. J Hirnforsch 15:75-93

Freund TF, Powell JF, Smith AD (1984) Tyrosine hydroxylase-immunoreactive boutons in synaptic contact with identified striatonigral neurons, with particular reference to dendritic spines. Neuroscience 13:1189-1215

Gustafsson B, Wigstron H, Abraham WC, Huang YY (1987) Long-term potentiation in the hippocampus using depolarizing current pulses as the conditioning stimulus to single volley synaptic potentials. J Neurosci 7:744-780

Hebb DO (1943) The organization of behaviour. Wiley, New York.

Hemmings HC, Walaas SI, Ouimet CC, Greengard P (1987) Dopamine regulation of protein phosphorylation in the striatum: DARPP-32. TINS 10:377-383

Hirata K, Yim CY, Mogenson GJ (1984) Excitatory input from sensory motor cortex to neostriatum and its modification by conditioning stimulation of the substantia nigra. Brain Res 321:1-8

Hirsh R (1974) The hippocampus and contextual retrieval of information from memory: a theory. Behavioural Biology 12:421-444

Hull CL (1943) Principles of Behavior. Appleton-Century-Crofts, New York

Iriki A, Pavlides C, Keller A, Asanuma H (1989) Long-term potentiation in the motor cortex. Science 245:1385-1387

Kelso SR, Ganong AH, Brown TH (1983) Hebbian synapses in the hippocampus. Proc Natl Acad Sci (USA) 83:5326-5330

Levy WB, Steward O (1979) Synapses as associative memory elements in the hippocampal formation. Brain Res 175:233-245

McGeorge AJ, Faull RLM (1989) The organization of the projections from the cerebral cortex to the striatum in the rat. Neuroscience 29:503-537

McNamara HJ, Long JB, Wike EL (1956) Learning without response under two conditions of external cues. J Comp Physiol Psychol 49:477-480

Miller R (1981) Meaning and Purpose in the Intact Brain. Oxford.

Miller R (1988) Cortico-striatal and cortico-limbic circuits: a two-tiered model of learning and memory function. In: Markowitsch H (ed) Information Processing by the Brain: Views and hypotheses from a cognitive-physiological perspective. Hans Huber Press, Bern, pp 179-198

Miller R, Wickens JR, Beninger RJ (1990) Dopamine D-1 and D-2 receptors in relation to reward and performance: A case for the D-1 receptor as a primary site of therapeutic action of neuroleptic drugs. Prog Neurobiol 34:143-183

Mishkin M, Malamut B, Bachevalier J (1984) Memories and habits: Two neural systems. In: Lynch G, McGaugh JL, Weinberger NM (eds) Neurobiology of Learning and Memory. Guilford Press, New York, pp 65-77

Palm G (1982) Neural assemblies: An alternative approach to artificial intelligence. Springer, Berlin Heidelberg New York

Palm G (1987) Associative memory and threshold control in neural networks. In: Casti JL, Kalqvist A (eds) Real Brains, Artificial Minds. North-Holland, New York Amsterdam London, pp 165-179

Pasik P, Pasik T, Holstein G, Hamori J, (1988) GABAergic elements in the neuronal circuits of the monkey neostriatum: A light and electron microscopic immunocytochemical study. J Comp Neurol 270:157-170

Passingham RE (1987) From where does the motor cortex get its instructions. In: Wise SP (ed) Higher Brain Functions: Recent explorations of the brain's emergent properties. Wiley, New York, pp 67-97

Rebec GV, Curtis SD (1988) Reciprocal zones of excitation and inhibition in the neostriatum. Synapse 2:633-635

Rolls ET, Thorpe SJ, Maddison J (1983) Responses of striatal neurons in the behaving monkey. 1 Head of the caudate nucleus. Behav Brain Res 7:179-210

Schneider JS, Levine MS, Hull CD, Buchwald NA (1984) Effects of amphetamine on intracellular responses of caudate neurons in the cat. J Neurosci 4:930-937

Selemon LD, Goldman-Rakic PS (1985) Longitudinal topography and interdigitation of cortico-striatal projections in the rhesus monkey. J Neurosci 5:776-794

Somogyi JP, Bolam JP, Smith AD (1981) Monosynaptic cortical input and local axon collaterals of identified striatonigral neurons. A light and electron microscopic study using the Golgi-peroxidase transport degeneration procedure. J Comp Neurol 195:567-584

Stellar JR, Stellar E (1985) The Neurobiology of Motivation and Reward. Springer, Berlin Heidelberg New York Tokyo

Strick P (1985) How do the basal ganglia and cerebellum gain access to the cortical motor areas? Behav Brain Res 18:107-124

Thorndike E (1911) Animal Intelligence. Macmillan, New York

Tolman E (1932) Purposive Behavior in Animals and Man. Century, New York London

Tremblay L, Filion M (1989) Responses of pallidal neurons to striatal stimulation in intact waking monkeys. Brain Res 498:1-16

Viallet F, Trouche E, Beaubaton D, Legallet E, Khalil R (1986) Visual feedback and motor performance in human and animal basal ganglia dysfunction. In: Basal Ganglia and Behaviour: Sensory aspects of motor functioning. Hans Huber, Toronto Lewiston New York Bern Stuttgart, pp 71-82

Waszczak BL, Lee EK, Ferraro T, Hare TA, Walters JR (1984) Single unit responses of substantia nigra pars reticulata neurons to apomorphine: Effects of striatal lesions and anesthesia. Brain Res 306:307-318

Wickens J (1988) Electrically couple but chemically isolated synapses: Dendritic spines and calcium in a rule for synaptic modification. Prog Neurobiol 31:507-528

Wickens J. (1990a) Striatal dopamine in motor activation and reward-mediated learning: Steps towards a unifying model. J Neural Transm 80:9-31

Wickens J (1990b) A Theory of the Mammalian Striatum. Unpublished Ph.D. Thesis. University of Otago, Dunedin, New Zealand.

Wickens JR, Alexander ME, Miller R (1991) Two dynamic modes of striatal function under dopaminergic-cholinergic control: simulation and analysis of a model. Synapse 8:1-13

Reconstruction and Characterisation of Neuronal Dynamics: How Attractive is Chaos?

Hubert Preißl and Ad Aertsen[1]

Max-Planck-Institut für biologische Kybernetik, Spemannstrasse 38, 7400 Tübingen, Germany

During the last years there has been a great emphasis on the possibility of characterising neuronal dynamics with methods from non-linear dynamical system theory. These new methods, especially the determination of the correlation dimension of time series, were applied to continuous activity as measured by the EEG and also to pulse train activity of single neurons. We could show that the calculation of the correlation dimension leads to incompatible results for a continuous process and for a pulse train generated from that process. This result has implications not only for neuronal data but also for other fields in biology and physics, where one deals with these two types of data.

Recent years have shown a growing interest in the description of dynamics in complex systems, both at a theoretical and experimental level. It was shown that one can distinguish between stochastic and deterministic, non-periodic ('chaotic') processes; various measures for the characterisation were developed and applied in such different fields as ecology, climatology, fluid dynamics, quantum physics and life sciences (for example see the contributions in Mayer-Kress 1986; and Pool 1989).

One goal of electrophysiology and theoretical neuroscience is a better understanding of the dynamics of processes taking place in brain during information processing. In the context of our studies of the dynamics of activity and connectivity in the Neocortex (Preißl and Aertsen 1991), we decided to investigate the applicability of methods for dynamical system theory, in particular the dimension analysis, to the characterisation of these physiological processes. As we will

---

[1] present address: Institut für Neuroinformatik, Ruhr-Universität, P.O. Box 102 148, 4630 Bochum, Germany

demonstrate, one has to be aware of severe limitation when interpreting results of this approach.

Non-linear dynamics and chaos

A dynamical system can be defined by a set of differential equations

$$\dot{x} = F_\mu(x) \tag{1}$$

where x is in general an n-dimensional vector $(x_1,...,x_n)$ The components of this vector are functions of an independent variable, usually of the time t. The vector $(x_1,...,x_n)$ is called state vector and F_μ is a function of it. In the context of deterministic, dynamical systems this function only contains non-stochastic elements. The parameter μ usually stands for another vector $(\mu_1,...,\mu_m)$, the components of which are called control parameters; these parameters determine the dynamic behaviour. One can distinguish two main classes of functions F_μ:

- F_μ is linear in each component of the state vector, these systems are called *linear*
- F_μ contains non-linear combinations of the single components of the state vector, e.g. squares or products, these systems are called *non-linear*.

Up to now we have described systems which are continuous in time, but there are also many dynamical systems which evolve in discrete time steps. In that case Equation (1) changes to $x_{t+1} = F_\mu(x_t)$, where the variable x_t is the state vector at time t. The concepts which will be presented below are also applicable to such discrete dynamical systems.

The main interest in the investigation of a single dynamical system is the determination of the *trajectories*. These are the curves in the n-dimensional state space which the system traverse in the course of time, i.e. which specify the value of the state vector for a time $t = t_1$, if the system was in the state $(x_1(0),...,x_n(0))$ at time $t = 0$. For linear systems there is a well-established theory on how to go about to solve such equations and describe the dynamical behaviour (Hirsch and

Smale 1974). In the non-linear case, however, it is more difficult to get the solutions. In general, it is not possible to solve a non-linear system and get explicit formulas $x_i(t) = f_\mu(t,(x_1,...,x_n)$ for all $i \in \{1,...,n\}$, from which one could calculate the state vector $(x_1,...,x_n)$ for an arbitrary time t. For the characterisation of the dynamics, one has to calculate the trajectories for that system with specified control parameters.

A special class of dynamical systems are the *dissipative* systems. These are characterised by the fact that the volume of an arbitrary cell in state space goes to 0 as time proceeds. These systems have a so-called *attractor* which is reached for t approaching infinity, i.e. the attractor is the asymptotically reached state of the dynamical system, and all trajectories are drawn to this attractor after a transient time. The simplest example is the damped pendulum which has its resting point as the attractor, but there are systems with more complex attractors e.g. limit cycles. By definition, dissipative systems have an attractor with a dimension lower than that of the state space.

In the study of non-linear systems special interest was given to this kind of systems. An important observation was made by Lorenz (1963) when he calculated the trajectories of a non-linear 3-dimensional system as a simple model for the dynamics in the atmosphere. The system is definded by the following differential equation:

$$\frac{d}{dt}\begin{pmatrix} x \\ y \\ z \end{pmatrix} = \begin{pmatrix} -\sigma x + \sigma y \\ -zx + Rx - y \\ xy - bz \end{pmatrix} \qquad (2)$$

For the control parameter he chose the following values $\sigma = 10$, b = 8/3 and $R = 28$. In that case the system is dissipative and, hence, the asymptotic dynamics are restricted to an attractor. This attractor looks like a two-dimensional surface. However it is impossible that the dimension is two or lower, since in a deterministic system two trajectories can never intersect. It also can not be three, because the system is dissipative. This leads to a new concept for the description of attractors by a non-integer dimension, called *fractal* dimension. This term goes back to the work of Mandelbrot (for an introduction to this concept see Mandelbrot 1983; and Falconer 1990). An attractor with a fractal dimension is called a *strange attractor*.

Another finding was the effect of *sensitive dependence on initial conditions*. In some non-linear dynamical systems the following observation can be made: if we follow the time development of two vectors

x and x' that were initially lying within a small disc of radius ϵ it turns out that their distance will grow exponentially with time. This dynamic behaviour can be characterised by the so called Lyapunov exponents. A system with at least one positive Lyapunov exponent is called *chaotic*.

The resume of Lorenz was the following:
'A finite set of ordinary differential equations representing forced dissipative flow often has the property that all of its solutions are ultimately confined within some bounds. [...] Our principal results concern the instability of nonperiodic solutions. A nonperiodic solution with no transient component must be unstable, in the sense that solutions approximating it do not continue to do so.'

It is obvious that these two measures reflect two different aspects of a system: the fractal dimension of the attractor characterises the asymptotic state, while Lyapunov exponents describe the dynamics. It was, however, shown that these two measures are not independent, and that one can, in fact, calculate the fractal dimension if one knows the Lyapunov exponents. After all, one has to distinguish between chaotic systems and systems with a strange attractor, in most cases these two properties go hand in hand. For a more extensive discussion on these topics see Eckmann and Ruelle (1985) and Bergé et al. (1984).

In view of this theoretical background, there are some important questions regarding the applicability of these concepts:

1. What can be said about an experimental system of which not all state vector components are known and not all components can be observed at the same time?
2. How can the fractal dimension and Lyapunov exponents actually be measured?

Reconstruction and correlation dimension

In most experimental situations the differential equations for the system under investigation and, consequently, the state variables are unknown. The experimenter usually has only access to consecutive measurements of a single scalar observable $z(t)$. A considerable step forward was made when it was shown that the attractor of the underlying system can be reconstructed from such a time series by a procedure known as *embedding* (Packard et al. 1980; Takens 1981). A vector in an m-dimensional *pseudo state space* is defined from the measurements by taking an appropriately spaced comb of values ($z(t)$, $z(t+\tau),\ldots,z(t+(m-1)\tau)$); different values of t correspond to different vectors in that space. For the two-dimensional case this means that the time series: ($z(t),z(t+\tau),\ldots,z(t+(m-1)\tau)$) is represented by the following vectors for reconstruction in a two-dimensional pseudo state space: $\{(z(t),z(t+\tau)\},\{(z(t+\tau),z(t+2\tau)\},\{(z(t+2\tau),z(t+3\tau)\}$.

The *embedding theorem* (Takens 1981) states that if z is the result of a smooth function, mapping the original attractor to the space of real numbers, and if $m \geq 2n+1$ (where n is the dimension of the attractor), the reconstructed attractor in pseudo state space is diffeomorphic to the original attractor: both have the *same dimension.*

This finding gave a possible way for a sufficient reconstruction of an attractor. Grassberger and Procaccia (1983a, b), building on considerations of Renyi (1962), developed an algorithm for determining one special kind of fractal dimension, the so-called *correlation dimension* (G-P algorithm). This dimension measures the density of sample points in the state space by calculating the *correlation integral* $C(\epsilon)$, which determines the number of state vectors x which fall in a region with size smaller than ϵ:

$$C(\epsilon) = \lim_{N\to\infty} \left(\frac{1}{N^2}\right) \sum_{i=1}^{N} \sum_{j\neq i=0}^{N} \theta(\epsilon - |x_i - x_j|) \tag{3}$$

In this formula θ is the so-called Heaviside function, which is 1 if the argument is larger than 0 and 0 otherwise. The indices i and j mark state vectors at different time steps. For small ϵ, $C(\epsilon)$ behaves like a power of ϵ: $C(\epsilon) \sim \epsilon^{\sigma}$, where σ is called the *correlation dimension.* From the correlation integral (3) one can obtain the correlation dimension very simply:

$$\sigma = \lim_{\epsilon\to 0} \frac{\log C(\epsilon)}{\log \epsilon} \tag{4}$$

Thus the correlation dimension can be determined as the slope of the log $C(\epsilon)$ vs. log ϵ curve in the so called *scaling region* (sr), i.e. where this curve is linear.

The embedding theorem and the G-P algorithm now provide the means to analyse the dynamics of a system under experimental observation: a time series is recorded, the data are embedded in an m-dimensional space (usually starting with $m = 1$) and a dimension d is determined with the G-P algorithm. This procedure is then repeated with increasing m. Initially the dimension d will increase with embedding dimension m. However if the underlying system has a low-dimensional attractor with a correlation dimension σ, the dimension d will saturate at this value for increasing m. In the scaling region the log $C(\epsilon)$ vs. log ϵ curves for different m will consequently become parallel.

It is important to realize that the correlation dimension is a geometric characterisation of the attractor. If the observed trajectory is long enough the attractor will be densely covered by it and the exact value of the correlation dimension can be calculated.

However, serious problems may arise when using this procedure. The first is the determination of the time delay τ from a certain time series. If the time delay is too short, the correlation integral is dominated by the data points which are too close to the reference point, which leads to so-called 'spurious dimensions' (Theiler 1986). If, on the other hand, the time delay is too large, consecutive data points are independent. In the experimental situation there are basically two methods to determine an appropriate time delay: the first is based on the auto-correlation function, the second, and the one to be preferred, is based on mutual information (e.g. Fraser and Swinney 1986).

The second problem is the *number of data points*, which should be taken for the calculation. One method is to vary the number of data points and to compare the results of different runs (for example see Dvorak and Siska 1986; Layne at al. (1986). From such studies it was concluded that it is necessary to use only stationary time series, the length of which can be determined experimentally. In addition, theoretical analysis considering the length of the time series required to obtain reliable results provided the following rule of thumb (Smith 1988): for a dynamical system with a correlation dimension of κ one should have at least $42^{\kappa_{int}}$ data points, where κ_{int} is the largest integer less than the correlation dimension.

The product of these two parameters, the time delay and the number of data points, determines the duration of the time series, necessary to obtain a reliable estimate of the correlation dimension.

Correlation dimension and neuronal signals

During the last years there have been several attempts by different groups applying the G-P algorithm to neuronal signals. It was shown, that finite correlation dimensions can indeed be calculated from this data (for example, see Rapp et al. 1985 and the papers in Basar 1990). These studies were done on single neuron spike trains as well as on more global electrophysiological measurements such as the EEG. Since, however, it is not obvious how to apply these methods to the analysis of a distributed system like the brain, we decided to focus on the description of single neuron dynamics.

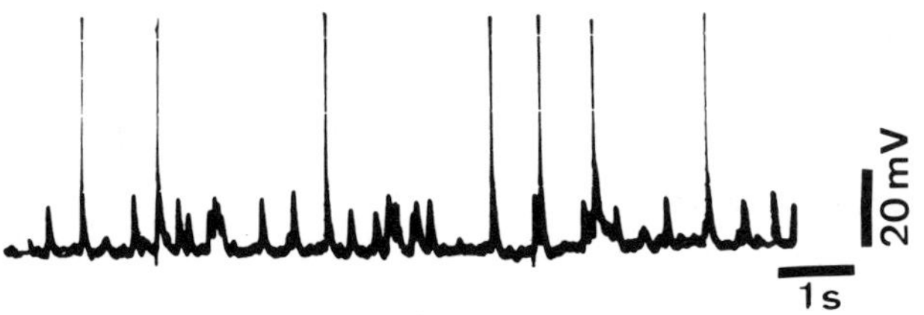

Fig. 1. The membrane potential of a single cell with clearly visible action potentials. Two types of data can be obtained from such a measurement: the continuous time course of membrane potential, and a point process, specified by the time intervals between successive action potentials

The dynamics of a single neuron can in principle be determined from two different experimental observations: the membrane potential, which is a *continuous* signal, and the train of action potentials (spikes), described as a *point process* (c.f. Fig 1). It is not clear beforehand whether a choice of either the continuous signal or the pulse train might possibly influence the outcome of the analysis. Therefore we decided to investigate this question in more detail (Preißl et al. 1990). To this end we analysed several well-known dynamical systems (Lorenz, Rössler, Henon), each one with a strange attractor and chaotic dynamics. In addition we studied the membrane potentials and spike trains derived from a neural network simulator which employs a pseudo-random generator (Boven and Aertsen 1990). In each case we focused on the issue of continuous versus discrete time series observations.

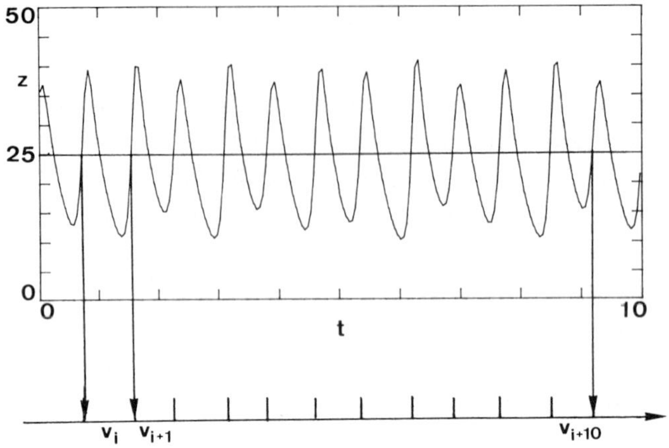

Fig. 2. Generation of the pulse train observations from the z-component of the Lorenz system: the dynamic variable for the reconstruction procedure is the sequence of time intervals between successive, positive-going level crossings at a fixed threshold value Z=25. Note that in this case the vectors are defined by taking sequences of adjacent intervals

In order to obtain the two types of data for each of the various systems, we recorded the time course of one of the system variables (continuous signal) as well as the series of time intervals between successive, positive-going level-crossings of a fixed amplitude threshold (pulse train) (c.f. Fig 2). In the latter case these time intervals were regarded as the variable of the dynamical system.

Here we present results obtained for the Lorenz system (simulation parameters as in Caputo and Atten 1987). We recorded the *z* component of the Lorenz system, and used 5000 data points with an time delay of 0.2. We embedded these data points in a pseudo state space with a dimension ranging from 1 to 6, and calculated the correlation integral (for the algorithm see Parker and Chua 1989; Grassberger and Procaccia 1983a). From the continuous measurement we obtained the correct correlation dimension of 2.06.

In the case of pulse-train measurements, we used a time series v_i, where v_i is the time between two i^{th} and $(i+1)^{th}$ positive going level-crossings of the z-component with a certain threshold. This time series was regarded as a discrete dynamical system, e.g. the $(i+1)^{th}$-interval is a function of one or more preceeding intervals. The length of this time series was again taken to be 5000. The embedding-dimension ranges

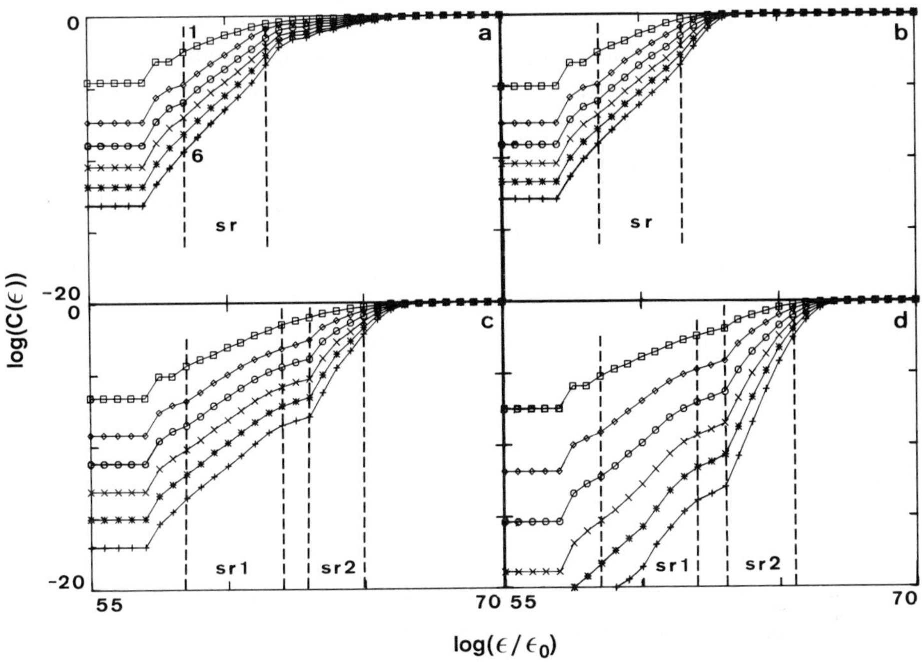

Fig. 3. Results of dimension analysis for pulse trains obtained with different thresholds Z on the z-component of the Lorenz system: Z=35 (a), Z=25 (b), Z=15 (c) and Z=12 (d). In each case the reconstruction was performed with 5000 intervals; the embedding ranges from 1 to 6.

from 1 to 6. In neurophysiology the embedding in the two-dimensional pseudo-state space is usually called scatter plot (Rodieck et al. 1962).

Rather to our surprise, however, the pulse train measurements gave quite different results as compared to the continuous signals. Moreover, the results depended on the threshold level Z used to generate the pulse trains (c.f. Fig 3). For Z=35 and Z=25 we were indeed able to determine a correlation dimension: for Z=35 it was 1.92, whereas for Z=25 it amounted to 1.79. Clearly these two values differ from each other as well as from the correlation dimension of the continuous system. With a threshold at Z=15 or at Z=12 one obtains two scaling regions (sr1, sr2). For Z=15 the correlation dimension equals 1.52 in sr1, whereas in sr2 it could not be determined at all; for Z=12 neither of the two scaling regions allowed to determine a correlation dimension. We made similar observations on the other (x and y) components of the Lorenz-system, as well as for the Rössler- and the Henon-system. In addition, we considered other types of pulse train generation mechanisms, e.g. the sequence of intervals between maxima in a selected component, and the sequence of intervals between consecutive points of entry into an arbitrarily selected box in pseudo state space. In *none* of these cases was it possible to obtain the correct correlation dimension of the attractor from an analysis of pulse train measurements. Finally we analysed both the continuous membrane potential and the simultaneously recorded spike train from a neuronal network simulator. Again, the two different types of measurements gave different results for the correlation dimension.

Discussion

From our observations on the behaviour of the correlation dimension for different types of measurements we are forced to conclude that there exists a fundamental discrepancy between the outcome of an analysis of a continuous process and of pulse trains generated from the same process. Consequently, correlation dimension analysis in its present form is not an appropriate tool for the characterisation of the dynamics underlying spike sequences. The reason is that the pulse train measurement is not the result of a smooth mapping of the underlying continuous process, as is required in the embedding theorem (Takens 1981). This fact also influences other methods for determining dynamical system parameters, such as the Lyapunov exponents. All these methods essentially rely on the assumption that the reconstruction process results in a diffeomorphic attractor. In addition, a point process, by its very nature, induces a description in terms of intervals between events. This dynamical variable does not generate a proper Poincare map of the underlying system. Consequently, this approach of making qualitative statements regarding the systems dynamics seem to be precluded too.

In addition to the above described problems, the concept of correlation dimension faces further, as yet unsolved questions in the field of neurophysiology. The first was already mentioned: the question of stationarity of time series with an very large number of data points. Adopting the boundary of Smith (1988), this implies that an attractor with a correlation dimension between 3 and 4 one needs some ten thousands of data points. This, of course, is not a trivial requirement to be met, especially in a working brain with continuously changing levels of activity.

However there is a second, even more fundamental problem. In the last years it was recognized that spatially extended systems with many interacting components, of which the brain surely is an example, may exhibit dominating long transients (Crutchfield and Kanenko 1988). This makes it impossible for the system to reach the attractor during a reasonable observation interval. Moreover, such systems may have multiple, coexisting attractors (Mayer-Kress and Kaneko 1989). This means that the spatio-temporal dynamics of a spatially extended system cannot possibly be characterised by means of an attractor reconstructed from the measurement of a single variable, irrespective of it concerns a single-neuron pulse train or a continuous signal such as a membrane potential or some other form of spatio-temporal summation like the EEG. Consequently, attractor characteristics such as fractal dimensions and Lyapunov exponents would be of little value here (see also Chate and Manneville 1987; and Lorenz 1991).

This, obviously, directly affects the question whether the concept of attractors, be they fractal or not, may be useful in the study of information processing in the brain. In our opinion, cortical information processing is not governed by attractors. Rather it seems more plausible to us that the dynamics are governed by transient state transduction, perhaps between different attractor states (Skarda and Freeman 1987). Consequently, although the calculation of a correlation dimension can be done on any time series, one has to be very careful in interpreting the results functionally.

Methods from dynamical system theory may possibly lead to new insights in various fields, including neuroscience. However, one should be aware of the fact that fractal dimension analysis is not an appropriate tool for the characterisation of pulse train (or interval) measurements, nor does it seem to be an adequate descriptor for the dynamics of a distributed system like the brain. In this context, concepts that are currently being developed for measuring complexity and prediction of time series seem to be more promising (see e.g. various contributions in Atmanspacher and Scheingraber 1991).

References

Aertsen A, Preißl H (1991) Dynamics of activity and connectivity in physiological neuronal networks. In: Schuster HG (ed) Nonlinear dynamics and neuronal networks. VHC-Verlag, New York

Atmanspacher H, Scheingraber H (1991) Information Dynamics. Plenum Press, New York, London

Basar E (1990) Chaos in Brain Function. Springer-Verlag, Heidelberg, New York

Bergé P, Pomeau Y, Vidal C (1986) Order within chaos. Wiley, New York

Boven K-H, Aertsen A (1990) Dynamics of activity in neuronal networks give rise to fast modulation of functional connectivity. In: Eckmiller et al. (eds) Parallel processing in neural systems and computers. Elsevier Science Publisher, Amsterdam, pp 53-56

Caputo JG, Atten P (1987) Metric entropy: An experimental means for characterizing and quantifying chaos. Phys Rev A 35:1311-1316

Chate H, Manneville P (1987) Transition to tubulence via spatiotemporal intermittency. Phys Rev Lett 58:112-115

Cruchtfield JP, Kaneko K (1988) Are attractors relevant to turbulence. Phys Rev Lett 26:2715-2718

Eckmann J, Ruelle D (1986) Ergodic theory of chaos and strange attractors. Rev Mod Phys 57:617-656

Falconer K (1990) Fractal Geometry. John Wiley and Sons, Chichester

Fraser AM, Swinney HL Independent coordinates for strange attractors from mutual information. Phys Rev A 33:1134-1140

Grassberger P, Procaccia I (1983 a) Characterisation of strange attractors. Phys Rev Lett 50:346-349

Grassberger, P., Procaccia, I.: Measuring the strangeness of strange attractors. Physica 9D: 189-208 (1983 b)

Hirsch MW, Smale S (1974) Differential equations, dynamic systems and linear algebra. Acadamic Press, New York

Layne SP, Mayer-Kress G, Holzfuss P (1986) Problems associated with dimensional analysis of encephalogram data. In: Mayer-Kress G (ed) Dimensions and entropies in chaotic systems. Springer-Verlag, Berlin

Lorenz EN (1963) Deterministic nonperiodic flow. J Atmos Sci 20:130-141

Lorenz EN (1991) Dimension of weather and climate attractors. Nature 353:241-244

Mandelbrot B (1983) The fractal geometry of nature. W.H. Freeman and Company, New York

Mayer-Kress G (1986) Dimensions and entropies in chaotic systems. Springer-Verlag, Berlin

Mayer-Kress G, Kaneko K (1989) Spatiotemporal chaos and noise. J Stat Phys 54:1589-1508

Parker TS, Chua LO (1989) Practical algorithms for chaotic systems. Springer-Verlag, Berlin

Pool R (1989) Science 234:25; 310; 604; 893; 1290

Preißl H, Aertsen A, Palm G (1990) Are fractal dimensions a good measure for neuronal activity? In: Eckmiller et al. (eds) Parallel processing in neural systems and computers. Elsevier Science Publisher, Amsterdam pp 83-86

Rapp PE et al. (1985) Dynamics of spontaneous neural activity in the simian motor cortex: The dimension of chaotic neurons. Phys Lett 110A:335-338

Renyi A (1962) Wahrscheinlichkeitsrechnung. VEB Verlag, Berlin

Rodieck RW, Kiang NY-S, Gerstein GL (1962) Some quantitative methods for the study of spontaneous activity of single neurons. Biophys J 2:351-368

Skarda CA, Freeman WJ (1987) How brains make chaos in order to make sense of the world. Behav Br Sci 10:161-173

Smith LA (1988) Intrinsic limits on dimension calculations. Phys Lett A 133:283-288

Theiler J (1986) Spurious dimensions from correlation algorithms applied to limited time series data. Phys Rev A 34:2427

Part Three
Visual Cortex

Horizontal Intracortical Contributions to Functional Specificity in Cat Visual Cortex

Ulf T. Eysel and F. Wörgötter

Abt. für Neurophysiologie, Ruhr-Universität Bochum, Universitätsstr. 150, 4630 Bochum, Germany

Introduction

Topographical and functional specificity of lateral cortical interactions

Intracortical lateral connections have initially been shown in anatomical studies by degeneration methods in monkey (Fisken et al. 1975) and cat (Creutzfeldt et al. 1977). However, only the use of modern tracer techniques has disclosed details like the periodic spatial pattern of such intracortical connections (Rockland and Lund 1982, 1983; Gilbert and Wiesel 1983; Gilbert 1985) or the axonal and dendritic distribution of single excitatory or inhibitory cells (Gilbert and Wiesel 1979; Somogyi et al. 1983; Kisvárday et al. 1985). Intracortical excitation can be laterally transmitted by a long-range axonal network of excitatory connections between pyramidal cells spanning up to about 5 mm in the adult cat visual cortex (Kisvárday and Eysel 1991; see also the contribution of Kisvárday in this volume). Intracortical inhibition can be mediated by GABAergic cells which comprise on the average 20% of the cortical neurons in rat, cat and monkey (Ribak 1978; Hendrickson et al. 1981; Gabbott and Somogyi 1986; Fitzpatrick et al. 1987; Hendry et al. 1987). These nonpyramidal cells are a heterogenous group which show a variety of morphological specializations (Somogyi 1986). Some of the GABAergic cells give rise to locally restricted axonal systems (Kisvárday et al. 1985), others send axons over distances from 0.5 to 2 mm (Somogyi et al. 1983; Matsubara et al. 1987b).

Although the morphology of the different systems of inhibitory and excitatory connections have been well established, their functional significance is just beginning to be understood. Without doubt intracortical inhibition is involved in the generation or at least the sharpening of specificities such as orientation and direction tuning of visual cortical cells. With the $GABA_A$ antagonist bicuculline direction as well as orientation selectivity could be abolished in a high proportion of visual cortical cells (Sillito 1975, 1977, 1979; Tsumoto et al. 1979; Wolf et al. 1986). These observations led to the assumption of cross-orientation inhibition being involved in orientation tuning (Sillito 1979; Sillito et al. 1980). This hypothesis is supported by a number of findings which showed inhibition from a broader range of orientations including iso- and cross-orientation with respect to the target cell (Blakemore and Tobin 1972; Morrone et al. 1982; Ramoa et al. 1986; Matsubara et al. 1987a; Hata et al. 1988). On the other hand, intracellular recordings failed to demonstrate the corresponding inhibitory potentials except for iso-orientation excitation and inhibition (Ferster 1986). Different studies using similar techniques obtained divergent results concerning the possible functional properties of horizontal connections in the visual cortex. Retrograde tracing of cells labelled from a horseradish peroxidase (HRP) injection site in area 18 was combined with mapping of orientation preferences and led to the conclusion that connections between cells with non-corresponding orientation preferences predominate in area 18 ("cross-orientation" connectivity, Matsubara et al. 1985, 1987a). Accordingly these authors favoured the hypothesis that horizontal connectivity is involved in inhibitory phenomena useful for sharpening of orientation tuning. However, similar studies performed in area 17 of the cat with 2-deoxyglucose labelling combined with local injections of rhodamine latex beads showed that regions with iso-orientation properties were connected (Gilbert and Wiesel 1989). Excitatory connections are the main candidates for this connectivity (Nelson and Frost 1985). This is also supported by electron microscopy of the patchy connections visualized by HRP injections in area 18 (LeVay 1988). However, with cross-correlation analysis iso-orientation excitation (T'so et al. 1986) as well as non-iso-orientation inhibition (Hata et al. 1988) have been demonstrated.

In terms of functional significance, it is quite obvious that iso-orientation connectivity can play a major role in intracortical mechanisms for linking different cell groups with similar properties (Gray et al. 1989) or in generating direction selectivity (Bishop et al. 1971; Creutzfeldt et al. 1974; Innocenti and Fiore 1974). Even inhibition between non-oriented cells can introduce orientation specificity (Heggelund 1981). Cross-orientation inhibition can sharpen orientation preferences (Ferster and Koch 1987) which might be primarily introduced by aligned geniculate inputs (Hubel and Wiesel 1962), an orientational bias already present in retina (Levick and Thibos 1982; Leventhal and Schall 1983; Thibos and Levick 1985) and LGN (Daniels et al. 1977; Vidyasagar and Urbas 1982; Soodak et al. 1987; Shou and Leventhal 1989) or the mechanism suggested by the Heggelund model described above.

Without doubt there is still considerable debate on the possible role of lateral excitation and inhibition in shaping cellular specificities in the visual cortex. For the last five years we have employed different methods to functionally dissect the visual cortex of the cat. Following studies in which we applied mainly local lesions and cooling (Eysel et al. 1987), we more specifically continued with microiontophoresis of the potent inhibitory transmitter gamma-aminobutyric acid (GABA) to locally and reversibly inactivate cortical cells remote from the recording sites in area 17 (Eysel et al. 1987, 1988). The method has been further elaborated to inactivate larger groups of cells at a fixed distance for a study of orientation specificity in area 17 (Eysel et al. 1990), and a quantitative comparison of areas 17 and 18 of the cat was performed (Crook et al. 1991). From the obtained data a picture of the functional contributions of medium range excitatory and inhibitory horizontal interactions (1-2 mm) is emerging that also fits independently conducted experiments on the orientational and axial responses of striate cortex cells (Wörgötter and Eysel 1989, 1991; Wörgötter et al. 1990a, 1991) and theoretical work concerning the possible role of inhibition in the generation of orientation selectivity (Wörgötter et al. 1990b; Wörgötter and Koch 1991). Some of the basic results and a model of horizontal cortical interactions based on these findings will be described and shortly discussed in the following.

Methods

Our experiments were performed under standard neurophysiological conditions in lightly anesthetized cats (Eysel et al. 1988, 1990; Wörgötter et al. 1990a; Crook et al. 1991). Single cells were recorded with glass-coated tungsten electrodes (Wörgötter and Eysel 1988) or with single or multi-barrel glass pipettes. Visual stimuli (light bars moving through the receptive field) were presented on a computer controlled display. Responses were stored and peri-stimulus-time histograms

(PSTHs) computed. From the PSTHs polar diagrams were derived in which the response peaks in impulses per second are represented as vector length and the direction of stimulus motion as vector angle. The cells were conventionally classified as belonging to the S- or C- family (Henry 1977; Henry et al. 1979). During continuous recording of a single cell remote cortical cell clusters were locally inactivated by special methods elaborated in detail in our laboratory.

Methodical considerations concerning remote local cortical inactivation

The common rational of our experiments is based on the assumption that horizontal interactions in the visual cortex are specific in terms of topographical origin and in terms of synaptic action at the target cell; projections of the visual field with certain response specificities interact with others according to given spatio-temporal rules. Inactivation of a cluster of cortical cells at some horizontal distance from a target cell should accordingly result in specific losses of functions based on intracortical interactions originating from the silenced cortical cells.

Inactivation was achieved by remote microiontophoresis of GABA in the supragranular layers of the visual cortex. GABA is known to silence all cortical cells in the vicinity of an injection site (Bolz and Gilbert 1986). This was also controlled in our own experiments; in addition we have recorded at different horizontal and vertical distances from the inactivation site and found - in analogy to Bolz and Gilbert's finding that there was no direct influence in layer IV when inactivating in layer VI - no direct GABA effects in layer VI when inactivating in layer III above (Eysel et al. 1988). Quite differently, direct inhibition of cells was observed over considerable horizontal distances like 1.4 mm after 30 minutes of GABA microiontophoresis with 160 nA. It can be assumed that the GABA effects decline with increasing distance and that they are limited by metabolism and uptake so that in most cases the affected cortical volume remains rather close to the tip of the inactivation pipette.

One problem inherent to remote GABA application is the necessity to discriminate between effects due to silencing of inputs to a given cell on the one hand and direct effects of GABA at the cell under study on the other hand. Increased responses observed during GABA iontophoresis are most likely due to a loss of inhibition converging onto the studied cell. Decreased responses, however, can always be due to reduced excitatory input or to direct action of the applied inhibitory transmitter GABA at the investigated cell.

Results

Directional specificity of striate cortical cells

Experiments with bicuculline blockade of $GABA_A$ receptors at the target cells have clearly shown that the underlying mechanism of cortical direction selectivity is GABAergic inhibition (Sillito 1975, 1977). Quite similarly, in our experiments direction selectivity of cells in area 17 was changed during remote inactivation with GABA (Fig. 2). In addition to showing this effect, our approach also allows conclusions concerning the topography of the involved intracortical connectivity. Thus, the projection of the visual field to the cat visual cortex (Fig. 1 A,B) and the related topographical arrangement of recording electrode and inactivation site (Fig. 1C) are important for further consideration of the remote inactivation effects.

From 143 simple and complex cells recorded from layers II to VI in area 17 of the cat only 7% showed no effect during remote GABA inactivation, 36% showed increased responses in the preferred or non-preferred direction and 57% decreased responses to stimulation in the preferred direction. Reduction of responses to stimulation with optimal orientation could be found as well in the just described as in all other relations between recording and inactivation site (Fig. 2C). Increased responses (interpreted as losses of lateral inhibition) were only observed if the local inactivation was applied along the path taken by the response-wave in the cortex during stimulation with optimal orientation, and only when the stimulus-evoked response moved on the cortical map in direction from the GABA pipette towards the recorded cell (Fig. 1C, Fig. 2A,B). From 66 S-cells and 29 C-cells recorded under such conditions S-cells showed predominantly changes due to losses of inhibition (61%) while C-cells displayed more excitatory convergence (62%). The observed changes in direction specificity led us to the conclusion that lateral inhibition from both sides of a cell but with asymmetrical strength might be involved in the generation of direction selectivity in the cat striate cortex. Furthermore, we gained the impression that direction selectivity was organized "on top" of orientation specificity. We could increase or decrease direction specificity by remote local inactivation in the surrounding of a recorded cell without influencing orientational tuning significantly (Fig. 2 A,B; see also Eysel et al. 1988).

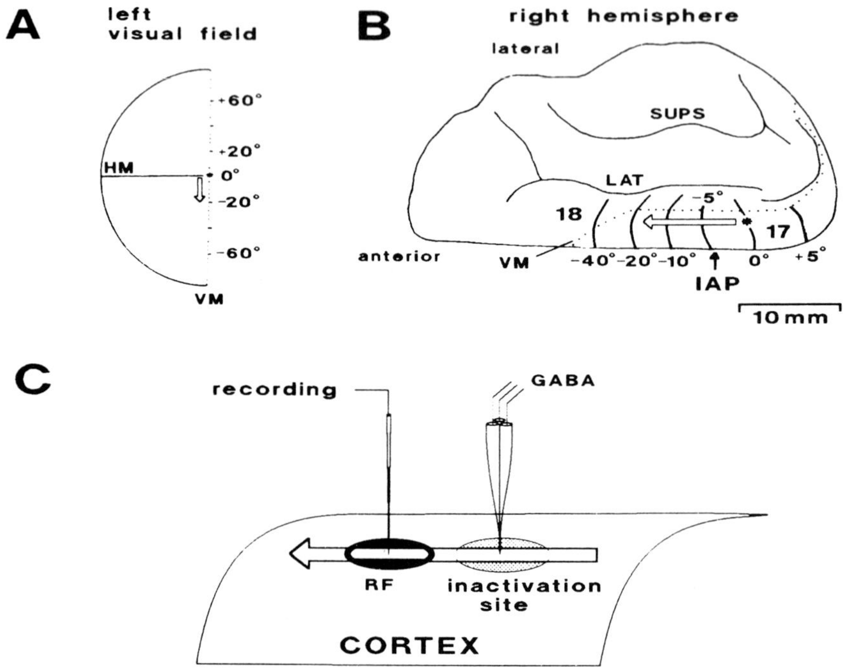

Fig. 1. Projection of the visual field (**A**) to the cat visual cortex (**B**) and schematic drawing of recording and inactivation sites (**C**). A. Left visual field with vertical (*VM*) and horizontal (*HM*) meridian. **B**: Projection of left visual field to right hemisphere of the cat. The arrow corresponds to the arrow in (**A**). The zero reference of the Horsley-Clarke coordinate system is indicated (interaural plane - *IAP*). Suprasylvian sulcus (*SUPS*), lateral sulcus (*LAT*). **C**: Schematic drawing of inactivation site (GABA) silencing cortical tissue involved in signal processing during downwards movement of a stimulus towards the receptive field of a cell under investigation (recording)

Orientation specificity of cortical cells

Figure 3 shows a complex and a simple cell from cat area 17 with strong orientation specificity which is abolished by remote GABA

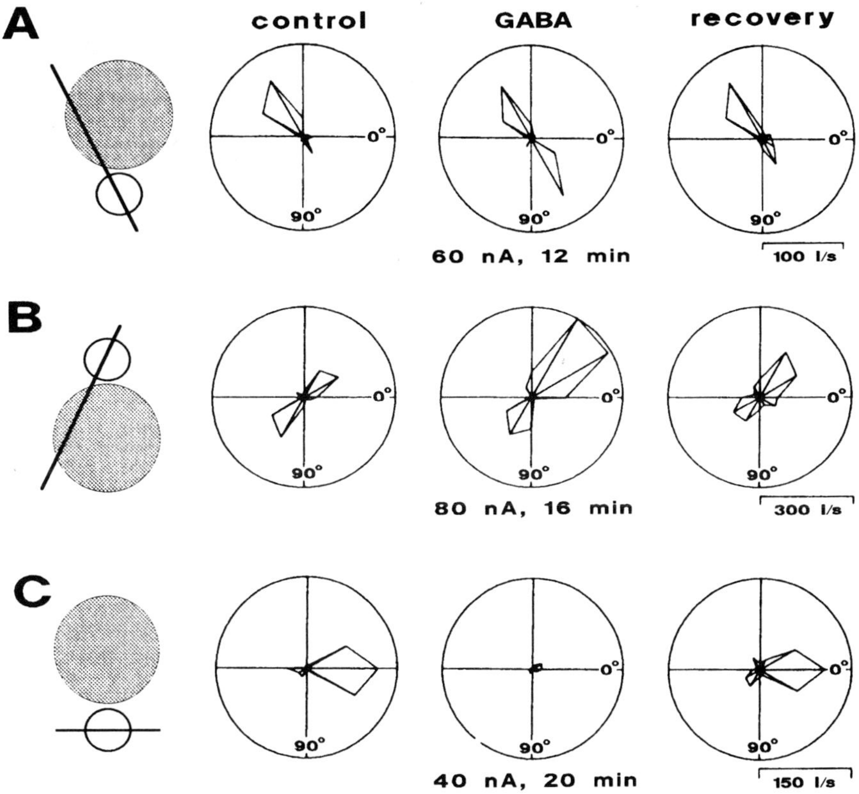

Fig. 2. Influence of remote inactivation on direction selectivity. Three simple cells in area 17 with different arrangement of recording sites (circle) and inactivation sites (shaded) as indicated left of the polar diagrams. **A**: Direction selective cell with inactivation posterior to the recording site. **B**: Cell not direction selective before GABA develops direction selectivity during inactivation anterior to the recording site. **C**: Cell with preferred axis of motion outside posterior inactivation site displays only direct inhibition. Control shown to the left, GABA ejection current and time indicated in middle row, recovery to the right

inactivation. The changes have been quantified by Fourier analysis of polar plots (SDO-analysis, Wörgötter and Eysel 1987) which seems to be equivalent or superior to the methods of quantification conventionally applied to visual cortical cells (Wörgötter et al. 1990a). For the simple cell the distance between recording and inactivation site was 900 μm (Fig. 3A) and the effect was associated with a decrease of the response to the preferred orientation and a concomitant increase of responsiveness in the non-preferred orientations. Quite differently, the complex cell selected as second example (Fig. 3B, distance of inactivation site 700 μm) showed a broadening of orientation tuning by an overall increase in responsiveness which was, however, much stronger in the non-preferred orientations. The cell lost its direction selectivity at the same time.

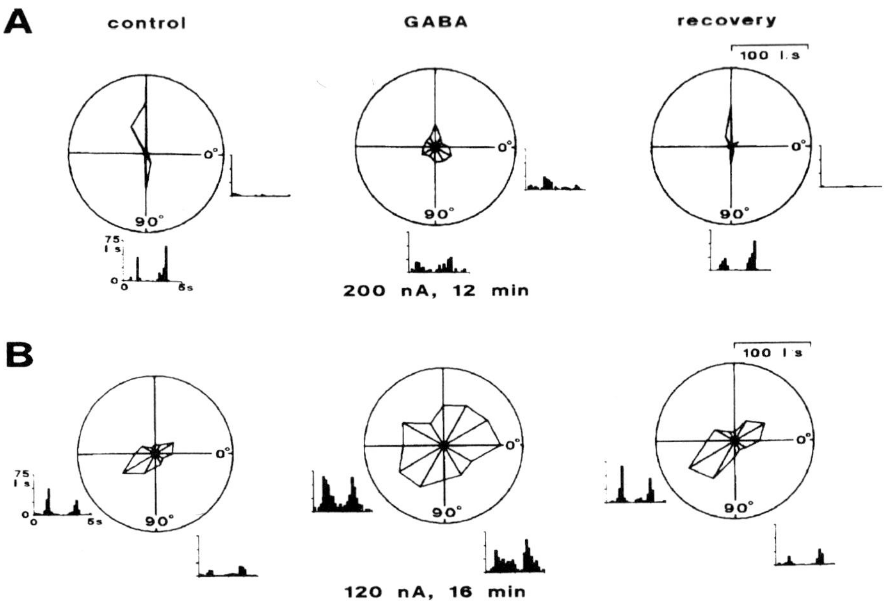

Fig. 3. Changes of orientation selectivity during remote cortical inactivation. **A**: Simple cell with inactivation 900 μm distant from the recording site. The small histograms indicate responses to optimal (decreasing during GABA application) and non-optimal orientations (increasing with remote inactivation). **B**: Inactivation at a distance of 700 μm. Facilitation is stronger in the originally non-optimal orientations and leads to reduced orientation tuning

45% of 145 cells subjected to remote GABA inactivation displayed no effect on orientation tuning. The majority of the remaining cells (36%) displayed broadening of tuning width due to increased responses to non-optimal orientations while 19% showed reductions of orientation tuning due to decreased responses to the optimal orientation. A broadening of orientation tuning width by more than 25% was considered significantly different from chance. The standard deviation of spontaneous changes observed in a control group of 50 cells with the GABA pipette in situ but with the GABA retaining current switched on was 12.9%, and twice the standard deviation was set as significance level. 48 S- and 32 C-cells showed significantly broader orientation tuning during remote inactivation with GABA; the effect was due to a net increase of responses in 63% of the S-cells and 69% of the C-cells. Remote inactivation can lead to changes of orientation specificity due to losses of excitation or inhibition or combinations of both effects at the target cell.

Differential effects elicited from different distances

Sequences of effects observed during long lasting periods of inactivation raised the question whether certain influences could be associated with certain average distances between recording and inactivation sites. Figure 4 shows a sequence of different inactivation effects elicited during continuous GABA microiontophoresis at a distance of 1.35 mm with increasing time (t) and current (I). With the growing product of $I \cdot t$ an increase of responses along the preferred axis of motion was followed by a decrease in responsiveness along that axis and increased responses to non-optimal orientations. Thus, firstly the directional bias of the cell was changed and secondly the orientation selectivity reduced. This was followed by an overall suppression of spontaneous activity and responses at the cell under study. Following termination of GABA application the cell recovered. The observation of such sequences of effects during continuous GABA inactivation (Fig. 5A) triggered a more detailed analysis of the effect of distance on remote inactivation. For different distances between inactivation and recording sites we determined the value of GABA units (ejection current multiplied by ejecting time, $I \cdot t$) that was necessary to elicit one of the typical remote inactivation effects described above. Increments of responses leading to changed direction selectivity were most easily elicited from a distance of 1 mm and above while at 0.5 mm most GABA units were necessary to elicit this effect (Fig. 5B). Increased responses to non-optimal orientations leading to a reduction in orientation tuning were most readily obtained when inactivation was applied at distances of around 0.5 mm and many more GABA units were needed to elicit the same effect from 1.0, 2.0 or 2.5 mm (Fig. 5C). Quite differently, the reduction of orientation specificity associated

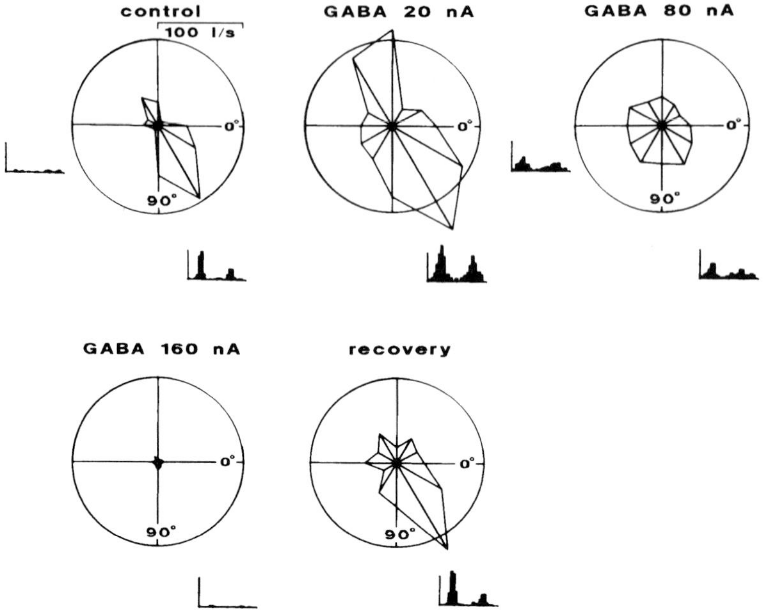

Fig. 4. Sequence of effects during remote inactivation observed in a simple cell. The histograms show responses in optimal and non-optimal orientations where necessary. A loss of directional tuning is followed by a loss of orientation selectivity and general inhibition of the cell. Complete recovery after termination of GABA application

with reduced responses to the optimal orientation showed a minimum in terms of GABA units again at 1.0 mm (Fig. 5D). These results showed that orientation specificity and direction specificity can be influenced differentially dependent on the distance of the inactivation site. From given distances predominantly excitatory or predominantly inhibitory inputs or a combination of both were reduced by local inactivation.

Orientation tuning investigated with a circular 4-electrode array

Figure 6 shows the array of 4 electrodes used to optimize the effects on orientation specificity (Eysel et al. 1990; Crook et al. 1991). The geometry of the electrode was based on the results from the preceding experiments that had shown that 0.5 mm was the distance at which in

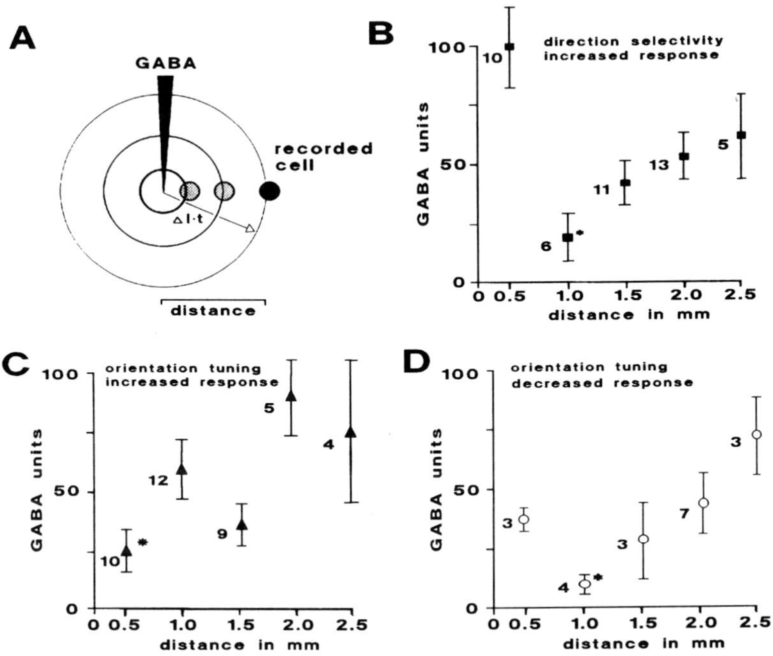

Fig. 5. A: Increasing release of GABA units (I · t) leads to an increasing diameter of inhibitory action. **B**: Direction selectivity is most easily affected by iontophoresis from 1.0 mm. **C**: Lateral inhibition involved in orientation is most effective from 500 μm but as well from 1.5 mm. **D**: Lateral excitation from 1.0 mm also seems to affect orientation selectivity

activation would change orientation tuning of a cell with the lowest threshold in terms of GABA ejecting current and time.

Indeed, with this array faster and more isolated effects on orientation selectivity have been observed (Eysel et al. 1990). This is exemplified by a simple cell in area 17 (Fig. 7). Responses in non-optimal orientations appear shortly after commencing inactivation with GABA from all four surrounding inactivation sites. Some of the newly arising responses even surpassed in peak rate the response to the originally optimal orientation. A surprising observation was made in about 20 percent of the cells that displayed a clear loss of orientation specificity due to increases in responsiveness to non-optimal orientations: a vigorous and quite isolated response occurred to the orientation approximately orthogonal to the optimal orientation (Fig. 8).

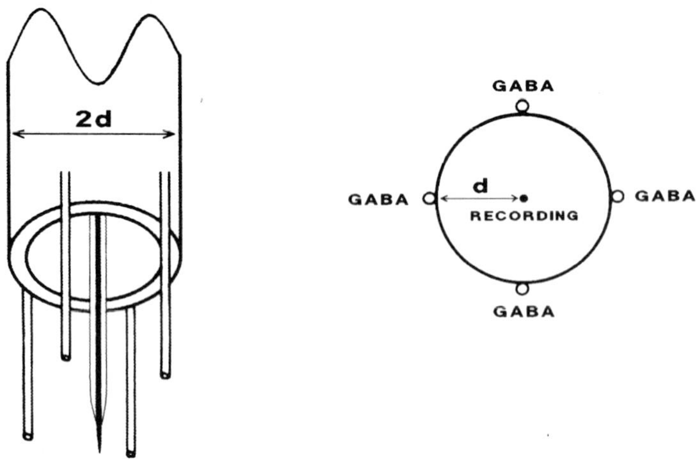

Fig. 6. A circular array of 4 electrodes was constructed to most effectively influence orientation tuning. The array provided an average distance of d (500 μm in area 17 and 600 μm in area 18) between recording and inactivation sites. While recording from the central electrode, GABA could be released from the surrounding pipettes

Investigations into the properties of area 17 cells have shown that an orientational component and an axial component orthogonal to the orientational component can be discriminated with bar and spot stimuli (Wörgötter and Eysel 1989, 1991). The isolated appearance of such an orthogonal response during remote inactivation might indicate the loss of a normally present suppression of the axial response during stimulation with a long bar.

Comparison of effects in Area 17 and 18

When subjected to the remote inactivation paradigm with the 4-electrode array the distribution of effects was similar for areas 17 and 18 (Crook et al. 1991) and the tuning widths prior to GABA application confirmed those reported earlier for the different cell classes in area 17 and 18 of the cat (Crook 1990).

Again, the significance level for broadening of tuning was set to an increase of tuning width by more than 25%. 61% of 74 cells tested in area 18 showed a significant broadening of orientation tuning (half-width at half height) due to increased responses in non-optimal orien-

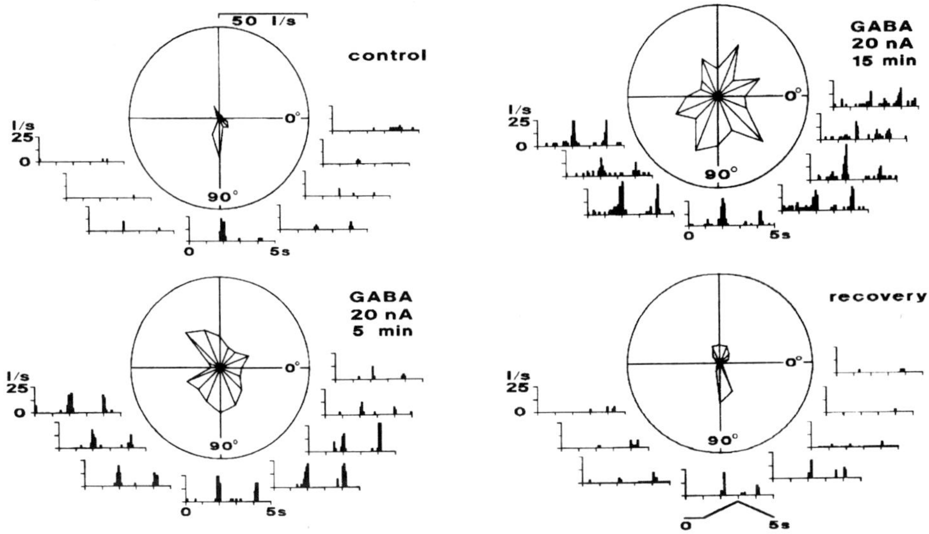

Fig. 7. Loss of orientation selectivity of an S-cell in area 17 during remote inactivation. Peri-stimulus time histograms are shown for each orientation and both directions of motion respectively. The cell was sharply tuned for horizontal orientation and downwards movement. After 5 minutes of GABA release from all four surrounding pipettes the cell responded to all orientations and had lost most of its direction selectivity. Following 10 more minutes of GABA release spontaneous activity increased and some previously non-optimal orientations now evoked responses larger than the original optimum. Recovery was nearly complete 12 minutes after termination of GABA microiontophoresis

tations. 70% of 54 cells tested in area 17 showed a significant broadening of orientation tuning, 4% of which were, however, due to a decline of the response to the optimal orientation and 66% due to increased responses in the non-optimal orientations. The average increase was slightly larger in area 17 than in area 18 (90% and 79% respectively). The stronger effects in area 17 are also reflected by the fact that about 6% of the area 17 cells completely lost their orientation tuning while a residual bias remained in all area 18 cells. The differences between area 17 and 18 effects were statistically not significant (Crook et al. 1991).

GABA effects were not dependent on stimulus motion. On the contrary, the originally narrower tuning width obtained with stationary flashing bars broadened more strongly during remote GABA application and showed an average increase in tuning width by 132%. In 3 cells the responses to moving and stationary stimuli and the changes associated with remote GABA inactivation could be directly compared. A 55% increase of tuning width during GABA application with the moving bar was clearly surpassed by a 147% increase during testing with a stationary flashing bar (Crook et al. 1991).

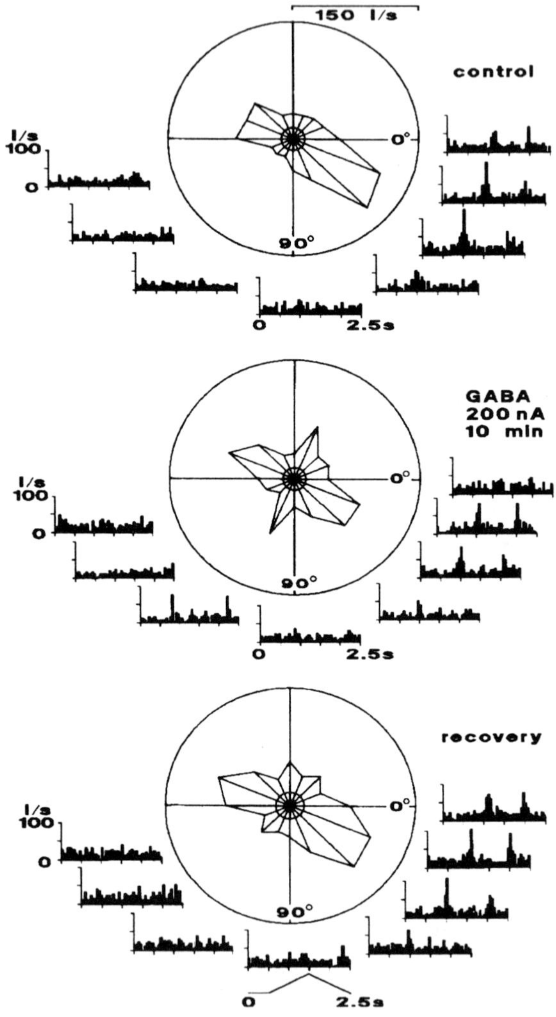

Fig. 8. C-cell from area 17 shows a vigorous response to the orientation approximately orthogonal to the optimum after 10 minutes of remote GABA inactivation. The polar plot showing recovery was sampled 4 minutes after termination of GABA release

Discussion

Functional specificity of horizontal intracortical connections in the visual cortex

Intracellular injections of different excitatory and inhibitory cell types have shown specific morphological features of the different cell classes in cat visual cortex (Gilbert and Wiesel 1979, 1983; Somogyi et al. 1983; Martin and Whitteridge 1984; Kisvárday et al. 1985, 1986, 1987). It has been demonstrated that the horizontal long-ranging connections are made by axons of pyramidal cells (Gilbert and Wiesel 1973; Martin and Whitteridge 1984; Kisvárday et al. 1986) with a high percentage of synapses at other excitatory and a comparatively low percentage at inhibitory cells (Kisvárday et al. 1986; LeVay 1988). The excitatory system spans several millimeters (up to 5 mm, Kisvárday and Eysel 1991; see also Kisvárday in this volume). The longest ranging horizontal connections in the inhibitory system are made by large basket cell axons (Somogyi et al. 1983) and are restricted to distances of about 2 mm. This suggests that the excitatory and inhibitory systems of the visual cortex operate on a different spatial scale. Extracellular tracer injections have revealed a periodic, patchy system of connections (Gilbert and Wiesel 1983; Rockland and Lund 1982, 1983) with a periodicity around 1 mm. The excitatory connections seem to be made with cells possessing iso-orientation properties (Gilbert and Wiesel 1989). Similar experiments in area 18 of the cat suggested horizontal connections over shorter distances with non-iso-oriented cells, including cross-orientation columns (Matsubara et al. 1985, 1987a). There is so far no clear explanation for the divergent results. Our data seem to support both anatomical findings on the basis of different functional effects during remote GABA inactivation. Figure 9 shows a schematic representation of excitatory and inhibitory regions surrounding a given target cell in the visual cortex as derived from our inactivation experiments. The central core with a radius of about 250 μm (containing the orientation column with the recorded cell) cannot be assessed with our method that does not allow to study this region because the cell under study is inactivated concomitantly during GABA microiontophoresis. A ring surrounding the cell with an inner radius of roughly 250 μm and an outer radius of 750 μm exerts predominantly inhibitory influences while the adjacent ring with radii of 750 μm and 1250 μm, respectively, gives rise to predominantly excitatory horizontal inputs. This was derived from the differential effects of inactivation at different

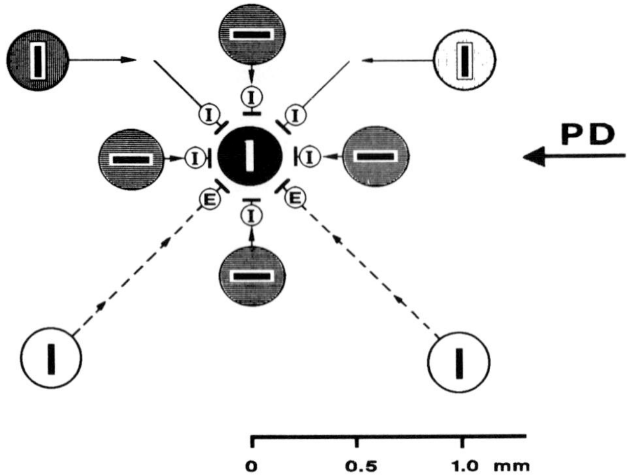

Fig. 9. Simple diagram of possible horizontal connections that could explain the experimental results of our studies. A cell with vertical orientation preference and preferred direction of motion (*PD*) to the right is shown in the center. The close vicinity of the cell (black) cannot be investigated with our method (see text). Clusters of cells with broadly tuned cross-orientation inhibition surround the cell and contribute to orientational tuning. The long-range iso-orientation inhibition in the upper half of the diagram is stronger from the left leading to a preferred direction of motion from the right. Iso-orientation excitation is indicated with broken lines in the lower part of the diagram. The interrupted pathways and arrows indicate the uncertainty concerning the anatomical substrate for the functional mechanisms (i.e. direct connections vs. interneuronal chains)

distances. The clear effects exerted on inhibitory mechanisms with the 4 electrode array placed at an average distance of 500 or 600 μm from the recorded cells strongly supports the interpretation of the inner ring of inhibition. There are good reasons to assume that the inner ring of inhibitory effects is associated with non-iso-orientations, while the more distant excitatory influences come from iso-orientation columns. The direct evidence of Gilbert and Wiesel (1989) supports the latter while the former follows indirectly from the spatial organization of the orientation domain in the cat striate cortex (Albus 1975). Furthermore, the spatial autocorrelation computed from mapping experiments showed the highest statistical probability to meet cross-orientation properties at a distance of 600 μm in area 18 of the cat (Swindale et al. 1987). Our model also includes a spatially more specific long-range inhibition which only acts in a relatively narrow sector around the preferred axis of motion. This type of inhibition is derived from the inactivation experiments that showed changes of direction selectivity due to loss of inhibition only when the GABA pipette was placed along the projection of the preferred axis of motion in area 17 of the cat (Eysel et al. 1988).

The diagram in Figure 9 is entirely based on functional data. Although it is supported by anatomical data, such data were not used to construct the scheme. With some precautions predictions can be made which connectivity might underlie the effects observed during horizontally distant remote inactivation. Inhibitory connections - directly or indirectly acting via interneurons - should originate predominantly from intermediate distances between 250-750 μm. Excitatory convergence should be found from longer horizontal distances, mainly from an average distance of about 1 mm. This in fact corresponds to the excitatory connectivity pattern and the known axonal lengths of excitatory and inhibitory cell types in the visual cortex.

The inhibitory effects from the surrounding of a cell seem to strongly sharpen orientation selectivity, since their removal by inactivation in this study led to a severe loss of orientation tuning up to a complete abolition in a number of cases. The inhibition from longer distances might be involved in directional tuning. At least inactivation of such inputs affected directional tuning in a way that the original direction bias could be eliminated or even inverted without changes in orientation selectivity (Eysel et al. 1988). This further supports the hypothesis that directional and orientational tuning in the visual cortex might depend on distinctly different mechanisms (Hammond 1978). Interestingly, this seems to suggest that direction specificity might be added to orientation specificity in a hierarchical manner. A statistical analysis of the dependence of orientation and direction tuning in a large number of cat visual cortical cells came to the conclusion that the two properties are not completely independent. A low but significant correlation was found between direction and orientation tuning (Wörgötter et al. 1991). According to the inactivation experiments the cells that are involved in sharpening of orientational tuning seem to be situated in the vicinity of their target cell and might partially overlap with the population of cells contributing to direction specificity. It cannot be ruled out that one cell group is involved in shaping both specificities: while influences on directionality elicited from a longer distance were not intermingled with but superimposed on orientation tuning, inactivation of the inhibitory elements closer to the target cell decreased orientation tuning and eliminated directionality at the same time. This might be due to a common final path. The inhibition observed in direction selectivity could be elicited by excitation of a subpopulation of the inhibitory cells close to the target cell. Direct inactivation of these inhibitory cells would consequently result in a loss of both properties. However, the lower threshold to influence directionality from 1 mm than closer to the cell strongly supports the hypothesis that long-range GABAergic connections are involved between iso-orientation columns.

The axial response of cells in area 17 is normally only elicited by small spots or very short bars (Wörgötter and Eysel 1989, 1991) while long bars evoke the orientational component of the response which is orthogonal to the axial response. During local inactivation at an average distance of 500 μm with the 4-electrode array in area 17 the axial response component appeared in addition to the orientational component when stimulating with the same long bar that did not evoke the axial response before. It can be concluded that the axial response is normally suppressed by an intracortical mechanism which is eliminated by local inactivation lateral to the recording site. A loss of side-band inhibition (Hubel and Wiesel 1962; Palmer and Davis 1981; Ferster 1988) would be a straightforward explanation, however, in that case the effect of inactivation should result in a significant broadening of the RF width. As can be seen in Figure 8 such a broadening was not observed when the axial response appeared. Alternatively not a loss of iso-orientation side bands but the release from a quite specific cross-orientation inhibition could underlie the phenomenon.

Quite recently a model of inhibitory connectivity in the visual cortex was independently developed that closely relates to our findings (Wörgötter et al. 1990b; Wörgötter and Koch 1991). In this model circular inhibition with a broad non-iso-orientation tuning in a way similar to that derived from our inactivation results was shown to create strong orientational tuning in computer simulations of visual cortical circuitry when slightly orientation biased subcortical inputs as present in LGN cells (Daniels et al. 1977; Vidyasagar and Urbas 1982; Soodak et al. 1987; Shou and Leventhal 1989) were assumed.

Acknowledgements

We gratefully acknowledge the contributions and discussions of Drs. J.M. Crook and Z.F. Kisvárday. We are indebted to the Deutsche Forschungsgemeinschaft [SFB200/A4; Ey 8/17-1] and the European Communities [0329-c(MB)] for financial support.

References

Albus K (1975) A quantitative study of the projection area of the central and the paracentral visual field in area 17 of the cat. II. The spatial organization of the orientation domain. Exp Brain Res 24:181-202

Bishop PO, Coombs JS, Henry GH (1971) Interaction effects of visual contours on the discharge frequency of simple striate neurones. J Physiol 219:659-687

Blakemore C, Tobin EA (1972) Lateral Inhibition Between Orientation Detectors in the Cat's Visual Cortex. Exp Brain Res 15:439-440

Bolz J, Gilbert CD (1986) Generation of end-inhibition in the visual cortex via interlaminar connections. Nature 320:362-365

Creutzfeldt OD, Kuhnt U, Benevento LA (1974) An intracellular analysis of visual cortical neurones to moving stimuli: Responses in a cooperative neuronal network. Exp Brain Res 21:251-274

Creutzfeldt OD, Garey LJ, Kuroda R, Wolff JR (1977) The distribution of degenerating axons after small lesions in the intact and isolated visual cortex of the cat. Exp Brain Res 27:419-440

Crook JM (1990) Directional tuning of cells in area 18 of the feline visual cortex for visual noise, bar and spot stimuli: a comparison with area 17. Exp Brain Res 80:545-561

Crook JM, Eysel UT, Machemer HF (1991) Influence of GABA-induced remote inactivation on the orientation tuning of cells in area 18 of feline visual cortex: a comparison with area 17. Neurosci 40:1-12

Daniels JD, Norman, JL, Pettigrew, JD (1977) Biases for oriented moving bars in lateral geniculate nucleus neurons of normal and stripe-reared cats. Exp Brain Res 29:155-172

Eysel UT, Crook JM, Machemer HF (1990) GABA-induced remote inactivation reveals cross-orientation inhibition in the cat striate cortex. Exp Brain Res 80:626-630

Eysel UT, Wörgötter F, Pape HC (1987) Local cortical lesions abolish lateral inhibition at direction selective cells in cat visual cortex. Exp Brain Res 68:606-612

Eysel UT, Muche T, Wörgötter F (1988) Lateral interactions at direction selective striate neurones in the cat demonstrated by local cortical inactivation. J Physiol (Lond) 399:657-675

Ferster D (1986) Orientation selectivity of synaptic potentials in neurons of cat primary visual cortex. J Neurosci 6:1284-1301

Ferster D (1988) Spatially opponent excitation and inhibition in simple cells of the cat visual cortex. J Neurosci 8:1172-1180

Ferster D, Koch Ch (1987) Neuronal connections underlying orientation selectivity in cat visual cortex. TINS 10:487-492

Fisken RA, Garey LJ, Powell TPS (1975) The Intrinsic, Association and Commissural Connections of Area 17 of the Visual Cortex. Phil Trans R Soc Lond B 272:487-536

FitzPatrick D, Lund JS, Schmechel DE, Towles AC (1987) Distribution of GABAergic Neurons and Axon Terminals in the Macaque Striate Cortex. J Comp Neurol 264:3-91

Gabbott PLA, Somogyi P (1986) Quantitative distribution of GABA-immunoreactive neurons in the visual cortex (area 17) of the cat. Exp Brain Res 61:323-331

Gilbert CD (1985) Horizontal integration in the neocortex. TINS 8:160-165

Gilbert CD, Wiesel TN (1979) Morphology and intracortical projections of functionally characterized neurones in the cat visual cortex. Nature 280:120-125

Gilbert CD, Wiesel TN (1983) Clustered intrinsic connections in cat visual cortex. J Neurosci 3:1116-1133

Gilbert CD, Wiesel TN (1989) Columnar specificity of intrinsic horizontal and corticocortical connections in cat visual cortex. J Neurosci 9:2432-2442

Gray CM, König P, Engel AK, Singer W (1989) Oscillatory responses in cat visual cortex exhibit inter-columnar synchronization which reflects global stimulus properties. Nature 338:334-337

Hammond P (1978) Directional tuning of complex cells in area 17 of the feline visual cortex. J Physiol 285:479-491

Hata Y, Tsumoto T, Sato H, Hagihara K, Tamura H (1988) Inhibition contributes to orientation selectivity in visual cortex of cat. Nature 335:815-817

Heggelund P (1981) Receptive field organization of simple cells in cat striate cortex. Exp Brain Res 42:89-98

Hendrickson AE, Hunt SP, Wu J-Y (1981) Immunocytochemical localization of glutamic acid decarboxylase in monkey striate cortex. Nature 292:605-607

Hendry SHC, Schwark HD, Jones EG, Yan J (1987) Numbers and proportions of GABA-immunoreactive neurons in different areas of monkey cerebral cortex. J Neurosci 7:1503-1519

Henry GH (1977) Receptive field classes of cells in the striate cortex of the cat. Brain Research 133:1-28

Henry GH, Harvey AR, Lund JS (1979) The afferent connections and laminar distributions of cells in the cat striate cortex. J comp Neurol 187:725-744

Hubel DH, Wiesel TN (1962) Receptive fields, binocular interaction and functional architecture in the cat's visual cortex. J Physiol (Lond) 160:106-154

Innocenti GM, Fiore L (1974) Post-synaptic inhibitory components of the responses to moving stimuli in area 17. Brain Res 80:122-126

Kisvárday ZF, Eysel UT (1991) Cellular organization of reciprocal patchy networks in cat visual cortex (Area 17). Neuroscience, in press

Kisvárday ZF, Martin KAC, Freund TF, Maglóczky Zs, Whitteridge D, Somogyi P (1986) Synaptic targets of HRP-filled layer III pyramidal cell in the cat striate cortex. Exp Brain Res 64:541-552

Kisvárday ZF, Martin KAC, Friedlander MJ, Somogyi P (1987) Evidence for interlaminar inhibitory circuits in the striate cortex of the cat. J Comp Neurol 260:1-19

Kisvárday ZF, Martin KAC, Whitteridge D, Somogyi P (1985) Synaptic connections of intracellularly filled clutch cells: a type of small basket cell in the visual cortex of the cat. J Comp Neurol 241:111-137

LeVay S (1988) Patchy intrinsic projections in visual cortex, area 18, of the cat: Morphological and immunocytochemical evidence for an excitatory function J Comp Neurol 269:265-274

Leventhal AG, Schall JD (1983) Structural basis of orientation sensitivity of cat retinal ganglion cells. J Comp Neurol 220:465-475

Levick WR, Thibos LN (1982) Analysis of orientation bias in cat retina. J Physiol (Lond) 237:49-74

Martin KAC, Whitteridge D (1984) Form, function and intracortical projections of spiny neurones in the striate visual cortex of the cat. J Physiol (Lond) 353:463-504

Matsubara JA, Cynader MS, Swindale NV (1987a) Anatomical properties and physiological correlates of the intrinsic connections in cat area 18. J Neurosci 7:1428-1446

Matsubara J, Cynader M, Swindale NV, Stryker MP (1985) Intrinsic projections within visual cortex: Evidence for orientation- specific local connections. Proc Natl Acad Sci USA 82:935-939

Matsubara JA, Nance DM, Cynader MS (1987b) Laminar Distribution of GABA-Immunoreactive Neurons and Processes In Area 18 of the Cat. Brain Res Bull 18:121-126

Morrone MC, Burr DC, Maffei L (1982) Functional implications of cross-orientation inhibition of cortical visual cells. I. Neurophysiological evidence. Proc Roy Soc Lond 216:335-354

Nelson JI, Frost BJ (1985) Intracortical facilitation among co-oriented, co-axially aligned simple cells in cat striate cortex. Exp Brain Res 61:54-61

Orban GA (1984) Neuronal operations in the visual cortex. In: Braitenberg V (ed) Studies of Brain Function, Vol 11. Springer, Berlin Heidelberg New York Tokyo

Palmer LA, Davis TL (1981) Comparison of responses to moving and stationary stimuli in cat striate cortex. J Neurophysiol 46:277-295

Ramoa AS, Shadlen M, Skottun BC, Freeman RD (1986) A comparison of inhibition in orientation and spatial frequency selectivity of cat visual cortex. Nature 321:237-239

Ribak CE (1978) Aspinous and sparsely-spinous stellate neurons in the visual cortex of rats contain glutamic acid decarboxylase. J Neurocytol 7:461-478

Rockland K, Lund JS (1982) Widespread periodic intrinsic connections in the tree shrew visual cortex. Science 215:1532-1534

Rockland K, Lund JS (1983) Intrinsic laminar lattice connections in primate visual cortex. J Comp Neurol 216:303-318

Shou T, Leventhal AG (1989) Organized arrangement of orientation-sensitive relay cells in the cat's dorsal lateral geniculate nucleus. J Neurosci 9:4287-4302

Sillito AM (1975) The contribution of inhibitory mechanisms to the receptive field properties of neurones in the striate cortex of the cat. J Physiol (Lond) 250:305-329

Sillito AM (1977) Inhibitory processes underlying the directional specificity of simple, complex and hypercomplex cells in the cat's visual cortex. J Physiol (Lond) 271:699-720

Sillito AM (1979) Inhibitory mechanisms influencing complex cells orientation selectivity and their modification at high resting discharge levels. J Physiol (Lond) 289:33-53

Sillito AM, Kemp JA, Milson JA, Berardi N (1980) A re- evaluation of the mechanisms underlying simple cell orientation selectivity. Brain Res 194:517-520

Somogyi P (1986) Seven distinct types of GABA-immunoreactive neurons in the visual cortex of cat. Soc Neurosci Abstr 12:583

Somogyi P, Kisvárday ZF, Martin KAC, Whitteridge D (1983) Synaptic connexions of morphologically identified and physiologically characterized large basket cells in the striate cortex of the cat. Neurosci 10:261-294

Soodak RE, Shapley RM, Kaplan E (1987) Linear mechanisms of orientation tuning in the retina and lateral geniculate nucleus of the cat. J Neurophysiol 58:267-275

Swindale NV, Matsubara JA, Cynader MS (1987) Surface organization of orientation and direction selectivity in cat area 18. J Neurosci 7:1414-1427

Thibos LN, Levick WR (1985) Orientation bias of brisk transient Y-cells of the cat retina for drifting and alternating gratings. Exp Brain Res 58:1-10

Ts'o DY, Gilbert CD, Wiesel TN (1986) Relationships between horizontal interactions and functional architecture in cat striate cortex as revealed by cross correlation analysis. J Neurosci 6:1160-1170

Tsumoto T, Eckart W, Creutzfeldt OD (1979) Modification of orientation sensitivity of cat visual cortex neurons by removal of GABA-mediated inhibition. Exp Brain Res 34:351-363

Vidyasagar TR, Urbas JV (1982) Orientation sensitivity of cat lgn neurones with and without inputs from visual cortical areas 17 and 18. Exp Brain Res 46:157-169

Wolf W, Hicks TP, Albus K (1986) The contribution of GABA-mediated inhibitory mechanisms to visual response properties of neurones in the kitten's striate cortex. J Neurosci 6:2779-2795

Wörgötter F, Eysel UT (1987) Quantitative determination of orientational and directional components in the response of visual cortical cells to moving stimuli. Biol Cybern 57:349-355

Wörgötter F, Eysel UT (1988) A simple glass-coated, fire-polished tungsten electrode with conductance adjustment using hydrofluoric acid. J Neurosci Meth 25:135-138

Wörgötter F, Eysel UT (1989) Axis of preferred motion is a function of bar length in visual cortical receptive fields. Exp Brain Res 76:307-314

Wörgötter F, Gründel O, Eysel UT (1990a) Quantification and comparison of cell properties in cat's striate cortex determined by different types of stimuli. Europ J Neurosci 2:928-941

Wörgötter F, Niebur E, Koch C (1990b) Modeling visual cortex: Hidden anisotropies in an isotropic connection scheme. In: R Eckmiller (ed) Advanced Neural Computers. Elsevier, Amsterdam p 87-95

Wörgötter F, Eysel UT (1991) Axial responses in visual cortical cells: Spatio-temporal mechanisms quantified by Fourier components of cortical tuning curves. Exp Brain Res 83:656-664

Wörgötter F, Koch C (1991) A detailed model of the primary visual pathway in the cat: comparison of afferent excitatory and intracortical inhibitory connection schemes for orientation selectivity. J Neurosci, in press

Wörgötter F, Muche T, Eysel UT (1991) Correlations between directional and orientational tuning of cells in cat striate cortex. Exp Brain Res 83:665-669

Excitatory, Inhibitory and Neuromodulatory Influences in Central Visual Function

A. M. Sillito

Dept. of Visual Science, Institute of Ophthalmology, Judd Street, London WC1H 9QS, U.K.

Introduction

Attempts to relate function to synaptic organisation in the central visual system seem at first sight to have made surprisingly little progress since the early sequential processing model of Hubel and Wiesel (1962). This in part reflects a growing awareness of the complexity of the circuitry in terms both of its interconnectivity and the subtlety of the transmitter mediated events pertaining at the synapses making the connections in the system. Equally it is clear that our procedures for assessing system function in the sense of the way we categorise and monitor receptive field properties may greatly underestimate the range of influences that shape and integrate the responses of cells. Paradoxically there is still substantial controversy about the basic logic of the mechanisms establishing the elemental response properties of orientation, direction and length tuning. For example there is far from a consensus regarding the extent, if at all, that inhibitory mechanisms contribute to orientation tuning in visual cortical cells. Intriguingly, contradictions in the data used to support alternate explanations for the generation of specific types of response selectivity often seem to identify limitations in the analytical capacity of the different experimental approaches better than they tackle the problems of the circuitry they seek to unravel. It is highly likely that several overlapping mechanisms contribute to any one response property and that the mix of mechanisms can vary for different cells. A major conceptual difficulty underlying the neurophysiological approaches has been a failure to recognise that the neuronal elements are integral parts of interlinking circuits rather than serially arranged stages in a one way process. In this account I shall attempt to identify some key aspects of our knowledge of the organisation of excitatory, inhibitory and neuromodulatory interactions in the central visual system that are likely to provide some insight into the way the elements of the system interact. During the course of this I shall pay particular attention to the role of layer VI cells in the visual cortex. The feedback from these cells to the dLGN provides an input to the geniculate circuitry greatly exceeding that deriving from retinal afferents. The same cells provide a feedforward projection to layer IV of the cortex and themselves receive direct geniculate input. It is clear that even the cortical and subcortical components of the visual system cannot be regarded as clearly distinct stages in a sequential process.

Basic synaptic circuit in the DLGN and visual cortex

The main elements of the circuitry in the dorsal lateral geniculate nucleus are summarised in figure 1A. The retinal afferents make synaptic contact with both the proximal dendrites of relay cells and the presynaptic dendrites of the intrinsic inhibitory interneurones of the dLGN. These interneurones are GABAergic (Sterling and Davis 1980; Sillito and Kemp 1983; Fitzpatrick et al. 1984; Montero 1986; Montero and Singer 1984, 1985; Montero and Zempel 1985) and their presynaptic dendrites, referred to as F2 terminals, form triadic synaptic arrangements with the retinal afferents and the relay cell dendrite. This synaptic structure, encapsulated by a glial sheet, is called a glomerulus. The essential logic of this arrangement seems to be that a retinal terminal would both directly excite the relay cell and initiate a short latency inhibitory input to it via the contact on the presynaptic dendrite. The axons of these same inhibitory interneurones make extraglomerular synaptic contact via "F1" terminals on the dendrites of relay cells (Montero 1987). A second level of inhibitory input derives from another group of GABAergic cells, the perigeniculate cells. These provide extraglomerular axonal synaptic input via "F1" terminals to the dendrites and cell body of relay cells and intrageniculate inhibitory interneurones. They also make contact via F1 terminals, with presynaptic dendrites in the synaptic glomeruli (Montero 1987). In addition the perigeniculate cells inhibit other perigeniculate cells and it seems that the presynaptic dendrites of the intrinsic inhibitory inter

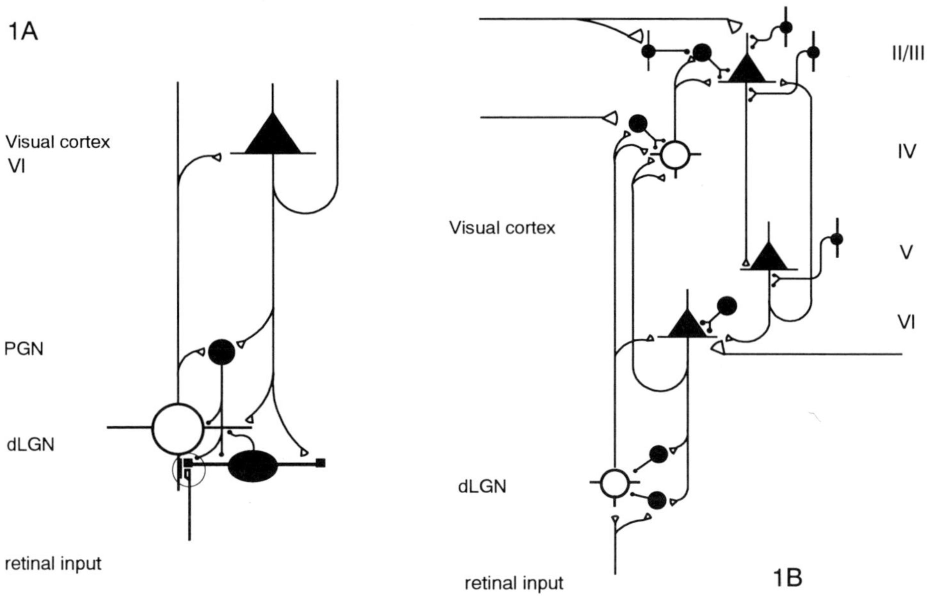

Fig. 1. Elements of the synaptic circuitry in the central visual system. **1A**: Connections in the dorsal lateral geniculate nucleus (*dLGN*) and its feedback from the visual cortex. Open terminals correspond to excitatory synapses and closed terminals to inhibitory synapses. The components linked to the triadic synapses in the synaptic glomeruli are highlighted by the faint circle. Here the dendrite of the relay cell is thickened to indicate a dendritic spine and the retinal afferent is presynaptic to both the relay cell and the presynaptic dendrite of the inhibitory interneurone. Conventional presynaptic contacts from axons are made by both the intrinsic inhibitory interneurone and the perigeniculate cells (*PGN*). Both these cell groups are GABAergic. **1B**: Pattern of connectivity seen in the visual cortex and its interactions with the dLGN. Pyramidal cells are shown as filled pyramids and other excitatory cells as open circles with three dendrites, all excitatory connections shown by open terminals. Inhibitory interneurones are shown as filled circles only or filled circles with two dendrites. All inhibitory contacts are shown by filled terminals. Long distance horizontal excitatory connections (e.g. between columns of similar orientation selectivity) are shown by large open terminals. Patterns of inhibitory contact include specific axo-axonic input from chandelier cells to pyramidal cells, basket cell type input to proximal dendrites and cell body and input from bitufted and neurogliaform cells to dendrites only. Note the presence of contacts between inhibitory interneurones and the circuit linking all layers of the cortex and the dLGN. Notional laminar locations are indicated to the right of the figure

neurones may also make contact with each other. The perigeniculate cells receive input from collaterals of the relay cells projecting to the visual cortex. Layer VI cells in the visual cortex provide a corticofugal projection which makes excitatory synaptic contacts (Dubin and Cleland 1977; Ahlsen et al. 1982; Lindstrom and Wrobel 1990b) on perigeniculate cells, the extraglomerular dendrites of relay cells and intrageniculate inhibitory interneurones and to a lesser extent, presynaptic dendrites (Weber et al. 1989). The corticofugal terminals appear to contact the dendrites of inhibitory interneurones three times as often as those of the relay cells (Weber et al. 1989).

The primary neuronal types in the visual cortex are summarised in figure 1B. The excitatory cells have spiny dendrites and are made up of pyramidal cells and spiny stellates, with the spiny stellates only occurring in layer IV. The inhibitory interneurones either lack dendritic spines or are sparsely spined, they can be broadly subdivided into basket cells, chandelier cells, neurogliaform cells and bitufted cells. The target distribution of inhibitory axon terminals varies with the type of inhibitory interneurone. For example, chandelier cells make synaptic contacts that appear to be restricted to the initial segment of pyramidal cells, whilst basket cells make contacts on the cell body and proximal dendrites. The neurogliaform and bitufted cells make contact only on dendritic shafts and spines with a bias to what appears to be small diameter distal dendritic processes (Somogyi 1989). This suggests a discrete functional role for the different groups of inhibitory interneurone. Although it once seemed that inhibitory synapses were concentrated in the region of the cell body, it is now clear (Somogyi 1989) that the majority are directed to dendritic shafts (58%) and spines (26%) with smaller numbers on the cell body (13%) and initial segment (2.5%). Despite the substantial advances in our knowledge of the morphology of the circuitry and the place of inhibitory interneurones in it, the functional significance of much of the detail still eludes us. There is no simple linear sequence in the pattern of connections relaying information through the visual cortex. This point is made in figure 8 for the excitatory connections between the cortical laminae and between visual cortex and dorsal lateral geniculate nucleus (DLGN). The representation here is highly simplified but it draws attention to the multiple connections between laminae and the mixture of feedforward and feedback interactions. Inputs reach the DLGN and visual cortex from the cholinergic, noradrenergic and serotinergic modulatory systems. These interact with the synaptic circuitry processing the visual input and seem to be concerned particularly with shifts in functional organisation linked with behavioural state.

Excitatory transmission in the central visual system

Our understanding of the events underlying excitatory transmission in the central nervous system has undergone major changes over the last decade. This follows from the growing realisation that excitatory amino acids mediate excitatory events in a wide range of locations and that their action is mediated by several types of receptor. In particular, three groups of receptor are commonly distinguished on the basis of the artificial agonist most selective for them. These are the n-methyl-d-aspartate (NMDA), kainate and AMPA (previously described as the quisqualate receptor) receptors. It is common practise to group the kainate and AMPA receptors and refer to them as non-NMDA receptors. In a functional sense the central significance of this is that whilst the non-NMDA receptors seem to mediate "classical" excitatory effects, evoking a rapid depolarization of the cell via a sodium conductance, the NMDA receptor ionophore exhibits a voltage dependent magnesium blockade such that its effectiveness varies with the degree of membrane depolarisation. As the cell becomes progressively more depolarized the level of blockade is diminished pari passu. Both sodium and calcium ions enter through the NMDA receptor ionophore. Events mediated via the NMDA receptor have been linked to LTP, plasticity and memory but it is becoming clear that NMDA receptors are also involved in the dynamics of excitatory processing in the central nervous system. Where they are so involved it makes the excitatory transfer particularly vulnerable to a range of other influences that affect membrane polarization.

Of particular interest is the fact that excitatory amino acids seem to be involved in the transfer of retinal information through the dLGN. Although it has been suggested that only non-NMDA receptors are involved (Crunelli et al. 1987), some of the original findings in a study by Kemp and Sillito (1982) seemed to be best explained by a contribution from NMDA receptors. If NMDA receptors are involved in the transfer of retinal information to dLGN cells, the voltage dependent Mg^{++} block of their channels would render this step in the visual pathway potentially susceptible to a wide range of other influences. This could be very important to the way we interpret the likely significance of the corticofugal projection and the neuromodulatory inputs to the dLGN. With these possibilities in mind we have used two new antagonists selective for NMDA receptors, APV and CPP and a non-

NMDA receptor antagonist acting at the AMPA (quisqualate) receptor, CNQX, to attempt to dissect out the contribution of the two categories of receptor to the visual responses of dLGN cells (Sillito et al. 1988; Sillito et al. 1990b, Sillito et al. 1990a).

The data obtained from this work were clear; selective blockade of either NMDA (Sillito et al. 1990b) or non-NMDA (Sillito et al. 1990a) receptors by local iontophoretic application of the appropriate antagonist could reduce or eliminate the visual response of dLGN cells. An example is given in figure 2A. The effects of blockade of NMDA receptors were most easily demonstrated because of the greater potency and selectivity of the antagonist CPP. In both X and Y cells the NMDA receptor blockade could entirely eliminate visual responses. The effects of CPP across the population of dLGN cells studied are summarised in figure 2C. Although CNQX was more complex to use, because of its action on the glycine site in the NMDA receptor, where

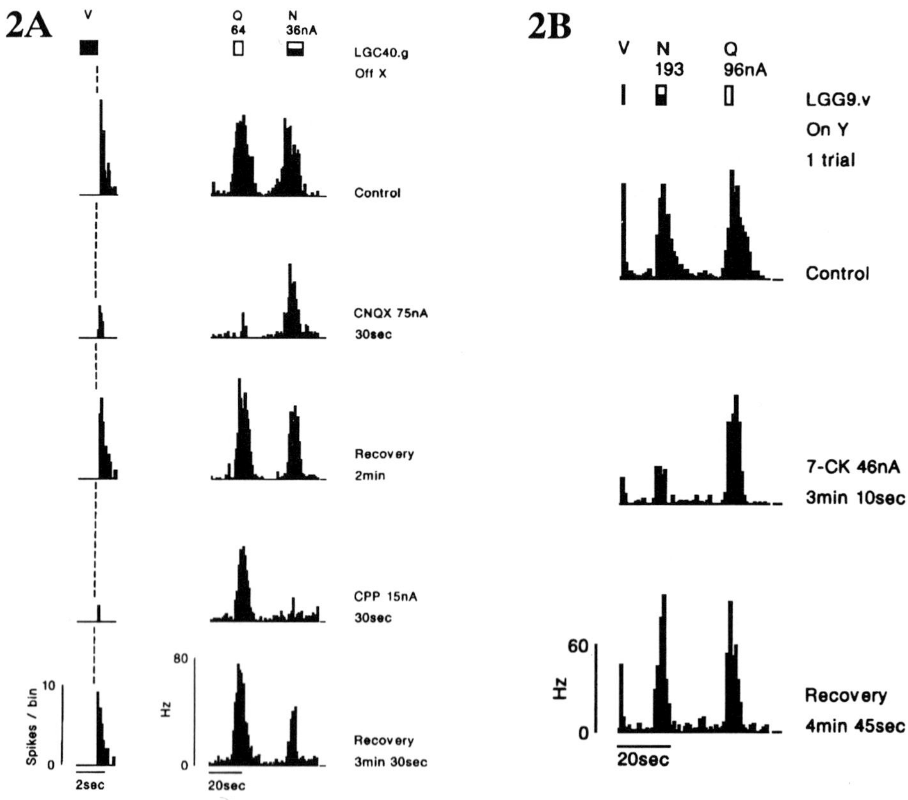

2C

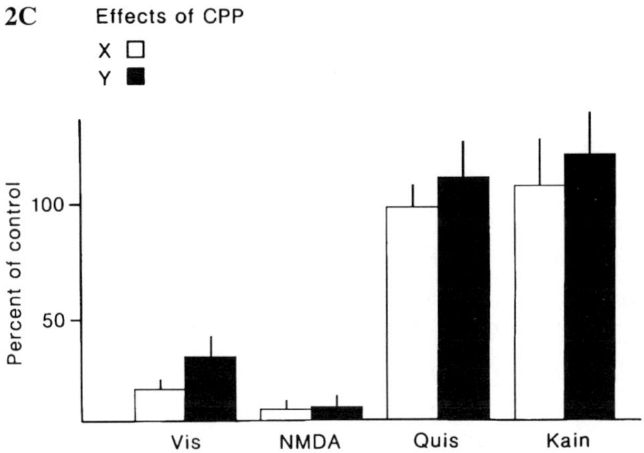

Fig. 2. 2A: Comparative action of CNQX and CPP on an off-centre X cell. PSTHs to the right show test sequences for drug applications plotted with 900 msec bins, those to the left document the visual response only, obtained in the same sequence but plotted with 100 msec bins. The dotted line indicates time of offset of the visual stimulus. The sequence and duration of the drugs and visual stimulus are given above the records. Records show 1 trial and in sequence the response to the visual stimulus and iontophoretic pulses of quisqualate (*Q*) and NMDA (*N*). The drug ejection currents are indicated above the records. Both CNQX (75nA onset 30 secs before record taken) and CPP (30nA onset 30 secs before record) reduce the visual response, but the largest effect is seen with CPP. **2B**: The effect of the 7-CK, an antagonist for the glycine site on the NMDA receptor, on the responses of an "on" centre Y cell in the cat dorsal lateral geniculate nucleus. The peristimulus histograms show the response of the cell to a spot of light flashed on and off within the receptive field centre and iontophoretic pulses of NMDA and the non-NMDA receptor agonist, quisqualate. The cell gives a powerful excitatory response to all three events. Iontophoretic application of 7-CK produces a strong and selective reduction of the responses to the visual stimulus and NMDA. Cessation of antagonist application is followed by recovery of the responses. Symbols above record show duration of the flash and drug pulses and the figures give the iontophoretic ejection current for NMDA (*N*) and quisqualate (*Q*). For the antagonist and recovery, the times refer to the period since onset and cessation of antagonist application respectively. Each record represents 1 trial plotted with 1000 msec bins. The calibration bars indicate response frequency and time. **2C**: Histogram summarising the action of CPP on the population of X and Y cells. Each column shows the mean response during APV application expressed as percentage of control. Error bars show standard error of the mean. Open columns refer to X cells and closed columns to Y cells

we were able to obtain pharmacologically selective blockade of responses to non-NMDA receptor agonists, potent effects on visual responses were also observed (see figure 2A). One possibility here, particularly in the light of the in vitro work in this field, was that the effects of the NMDA receptor antagonists reflected a modulation of a corticofugal influence itself mediated via NMDA receptors. Thus the visual response would be conditional on this background influence. Several factors would militate against this interpretation at its simplest level. Firstly the background discharge levels of layer VI cells are very low and, secondly, the small stationary flashing spots we used to generate the visual response in the dLGN cells are singularly ineffective in driving layer VI cells (Gilbert 1977; Harvey 1980; Tsumoto and Suda 1980). However, we checked our protocol in a series of experiments carried out on cats with areas 17 and 18 removed (Salt and Sillito 1989). Under these conditions dLGN cells responded briskly to visual stimuli and their responses could be selectively antagonised by iontophoretic application of CPP as in the normal preparation. This observation should not be taken to imply that the corticofugal system has no effect, merely that in this particular experimental protocol, designed to address the pharmacology of the retinal input, it is not contributing to the observations. The point of note here is that the stimulus we were using for the visual activation of the dLGN cells was a small flashing spot of light, this is not an effective stimulus for layer VI cortical cells providing the feedback (e.g. Gilbert 1977).

In vitro work recently demonstrated that activation of the NMDA receptor is subject to an allosteric facilitation by glycine acting at a strychnine insensitive site within the NMDA receptor complex (Johnson and Ascher 1987). We thus examined the extent to which retinogeniculate transmission is influenced by modulation from the strychnine insensitive glycine receptor in vivo. We utilised the same protocol as for our work with CPP and CNQX. Iontophoretic application of either HA-966 or 7-CK, antagonists of glycine at the site in the NMDA receptor complex, greatly reduced and in some cases blocked the transfer of visual information as is shown for 7-CK in figure 2B (Levy et al. 1990). This would indicate that it might be possible to demonstrate visual response enhancement by activation of the glycine receptor. We attempted to obtain facilitation of the responses to NMDA and visual stimulation by iontophoretically applying a glycine analogue, D-serine, either with the experimental paradigm used for studying antagonist effects or by separate synchronised pulses timed to coincide with the visual stimulus and NMDA pulse. We were unable to obtain any significant enhancement of visual or NMDA responses. Given the effectiveness of the two antagonists, this observation would support the view that for the retino-geniculate synapses in vivo, the levels of endogenous glycine, or other substance acting on the glycine site in the NMDA receptor complex, are high.

Despite certain complexities in interpretation, the present findings lead to a fairly clear, albeit preliminary, overview of factors that seem to influence excitatory transmission from retinal afferents to dLGN cells. A diagrammatic summary of this is given in figure 3. The retinal ganglion cell neurotransmitter acts on both non-NMDA and NMDA receptors. The influence of the non-NMDA receptors will generate membrane depolarization from levels of hyperpolarization where the Mg^{++} blockade negates the influence of the NMDA receptor. As the level of membrane depolarization increases the contribution from the NMDA receptors comes into play. This in turn is dependent on activation of the glycine site in the NMDA receptor complex. There may be two components to the glycinergic modulation, one relating to the initiation of NMDA receptor activation and the other preventing its desensitization in the face of repeated and prolonged activation (Johnson and Ascher 1987; Mayer et al. 1989; Thompson et al. 1989). The high background discharge of retinal ganglion cells and the rapid and repeated changes in frequency elicited by the ever shifting retinal image underline the potential significance of the latter facet of the glycinergic effects. The influence exerted by glycine might be varied either by processes that alter the extracellular concentrations of glycine or by an endogenous glycine antagonist, such as kynurenate (Birch et al. 1988). The large part of the visual response thus appears to be mediated at the level where both NMDA and non-NMDA receptors are contributing to the depolarization. The background discharge levels of retinal ganglion cells together with the facilitatory and disinhibitory influence of the cholinergic input are contributing factors to the kinetics of the transmission in vivo (Sillito et al. 1988). The voltage dependent blockade of the NMDA receptor must ensure that hyperpolarizing or depolarizing inputs serving to move the cell in or out of the domain of the blockade will not have a simply additive interaction with those establishing the initial situation. This may be important both when analyzing the contribution from neuromodulatory inputs such as the cholinergic input and the stimulus dependent inhibitory effects which can be complex and involve corticofugal feedback (Murphy and Sillito 1987, 1989). Even the response to a flashed stimulus is likely to involve the simultaneous suppression of an

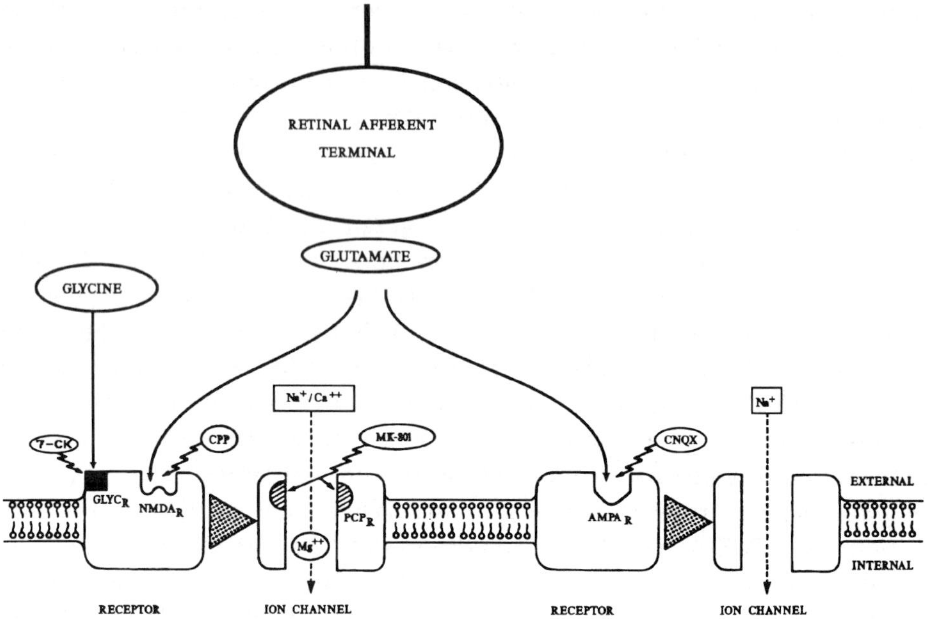

Fig. 3. Schematic summary of the findings regarding excitatory amino acid receptors and the transfer of retinal information. Retinal afferents in the dLGN, release a transmitter, possibly glutamate, that acts at both NMDA and non-NMDA (AMPA) receptors. The mean background discharge levels of retinal ganglion cells are high (41Hz) and this produces a constant background release of the retinal neurotransmitter which opens Na^+ channels in the dLGN relay cell via the AMPA receptor. As the cell membrane depolarizes and the Mg^{++} block of the NMDA receptor ion channel is lifted, further depolarization follows from the retinal neurotransmitter acting at the NMDA receptor. The visual input in vivo causes constantly shifting increases or decreases in the background activity of the retinal ganglion cells. Blockade of either the NMDA receptors with CPP or the AMPA (non-NMDA) receptor with CNQX can block the transfer of visual information. Both the initial activation of the NMDA receptor and its desensitization in the face of repeated activation seem to be influenced by the action of glycine at a site within the NMDA receptor complex. Blockade of the glycine site with either 7-CK or HA-966 will reduce or block visual responses in vivo, suggesting that normal visual driving is dependent not only on activation of the NMDA receptor, but also on the presence of glycine (or another substance acting at the glycine receptor) and its interaction with the glycine site. In addition, substances acting at the phencyclidine (PCP) receptor in the ion channel of the NMDA receptor could also, via their blockade of the ion channel, reduce the effectiveness of the transfer of visual information. Thus the translation of the output from a retinal afferent into an excitatory response in the postsynaptic relay cell is conditional upon a range of interacting processes, which imply a level of functional complexity that has not been generally associated with this level of the visual system

inhibitory drive as well as the initiation of an excitatory barrage (Sillito and Kemp 1983). Further to the latter point, the triadic synapses on relay cell dendrites with their potential for local circuit action via the presynaptic dendrite of the inhibitory interneurone (Famiglietti and Peters 1972; Rapisardi and Miles 1984), raise the possibility of a local gating that modulates the contribution from the NMDA receptor. This would influence transmission at a specific location in the dendritic field of the relay cell. Detailed comprehension of the significance of the various components of retinogeniculate excitatory transmission will require a synthesis encompassing all these issues.

In the visual cortex the balance of the evidence favours the view that NMDA and non-NMDA receptors contribute to excitatory transmission, with the proviso that in layer IV, NMDA receptors seem to play a role in early life, but not in the adult. From one viewpoint this can and has been linked to the plasticity exhibited by the visual cortex in early life. On the other hand it is particularly interesting that the adult visual system apparently utilises NMDA receptors for the transfer of visual information at the retinogeniculate synapse, but not the geniculocortical synapse in layer IV. Where NMDA receptors are involved in the visual cortex, the points outlined above in relation to the retinogeniculate transfer apply.

Corticofugal influences on inhibitory mechanisms shaping the transfer of information from dLGN to striate cortex

Cells in the dLGN have concentrically organised "on" or "off" centre receptive fields, with centre-surround antagonism, and are superficially very similar to those of retinal ganglion cells (Hubel and Wiesel 1961). However, the degree of surround antagonism of centre responses is significantly higher in dLGN cells than retinal ganglion cells. This can be linked to IPSPs generated by GABAergic inhibitory interneurones with receptive fields overlying the surround and centre surround border (Singer et al. 1972; Singer and Creutzfeldt 1970; Sillito and Kemp 1983). This point is most simply illustrated by examining the effect of a local GABA blockade on the responses of a dLGN cell to a stationary flashing stimulus of varying diameter. A example is given in figure 4C. Under control conditions, increasing stimulus dia

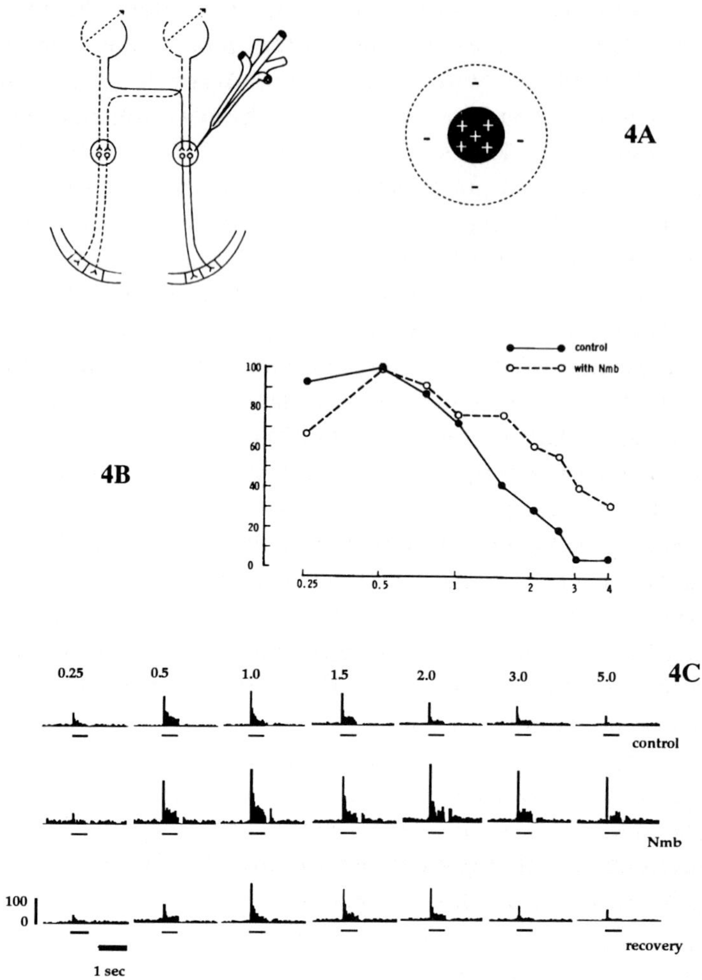

Fig. 4. The effect of inhibitory blockade induced by iontophoretic application of the GABA antagonist N-methylbicuculline (*Nmb*) on centre surround antagonism in the dLGN. **4A**: Summary diagram showing iontophoretic pipette in the dLGN of a schematic visual pathway and the concentric receptive field organisation of a dLGN cells. **4B**: Curves showing the effect of varying the diameter of a stationary flashing spot on the responses of an on-centre X cell. The response magnitude on these curves is expressed as a percentage of the maximum control response and the range of stimulus diameters used extended from 0.25-4.0°. In the presence of the GABA antagonist (*Nmb*) the attenuation of the response at larger stimulus diameters is diminished, reflecting a blockade of the input from GABA cells enhancing the inhibitory surround. **4C**: PSTHs showing effect of varying stimulus diameter for an on centre Y cell. The diameter of the flashing spot of light (0.5 sec duration), centred over the receptive field, is increased from 0.25° to 5.0°. Under control conditions there is marked

meter so that it expands within the centre and then crosses into the surround, results in a rise then a sharp fall in response magnitude. A component of this fall reflects centre-surround interaction at retinal levels, but there is also a significant contribution from intrageniculate mechanisms as indicated by the responses during Nmb application. In the presence of the GABA blockade induced by iontophoretic application of N-methylbicuculline (Nmb) responses to the larger diameter stimuli are increased in magnitude relative to those elicited from the centre. This point is further emphasised by the curves plotted in figure 4B. During Nmb application the cell's responses reflect the level of surround antagonism associated with retinal ganglion cells. Comparing the responses of X and Y cells it is clear that although the absolute degree of surround antagonism of centre responses is lower in Y cells than X cells, it is still enhanced by GABAergic inhibitory mechanisms (Sillito and Kemp 1983).

Responses of visual cortical cells are routinely documented in terms of the selectivity they exhibit to the orientation, length and direction of motion of moving bar stimuli. These types of stimuli evoke good responses from visual cortical cells whilst stationary flashing spots are relatively ineffective. In terms of unravelling the corticofugal system's contribution to visual processing in the dLGN it is thus essential to examine dLGN cell responses with the type of visual stimuli that will effectively drive layer VI cells in the visual cortex. A moving bar of varying length provides a stimulus that can be compared with the responses to a flashing spot of varying diameter, insofar as the variation in length can be adjusted so that it increases within the receptive field centre and then progressively encroaches on the surround mechanism. It is clear that the response of a dLGN cell to a bar of increasing length should invoke the surround inhibitory mechanisms. This does occur, the response to a bar declines dramatically with increasing length (Schiller et al. 1976; Cleland et al. 1983; Jones and Sillito 1987, 1991). Thus dLGN cells are "length tuned" because they give the largest response to a bar of a certain optimal length . This is illustrated in figure 5A. This response property was first reported by Hubel and Wiesel (1965, 1968) for the so-called hypercomplex cells in the visual

---

response attenuation beyond 1.5°, but this is greatly reduced during Nmb application (80nA). For the PSTHs the bin size is 50 msecs and vertical calibration indicates range corresponding to 0-100 counts/bin.

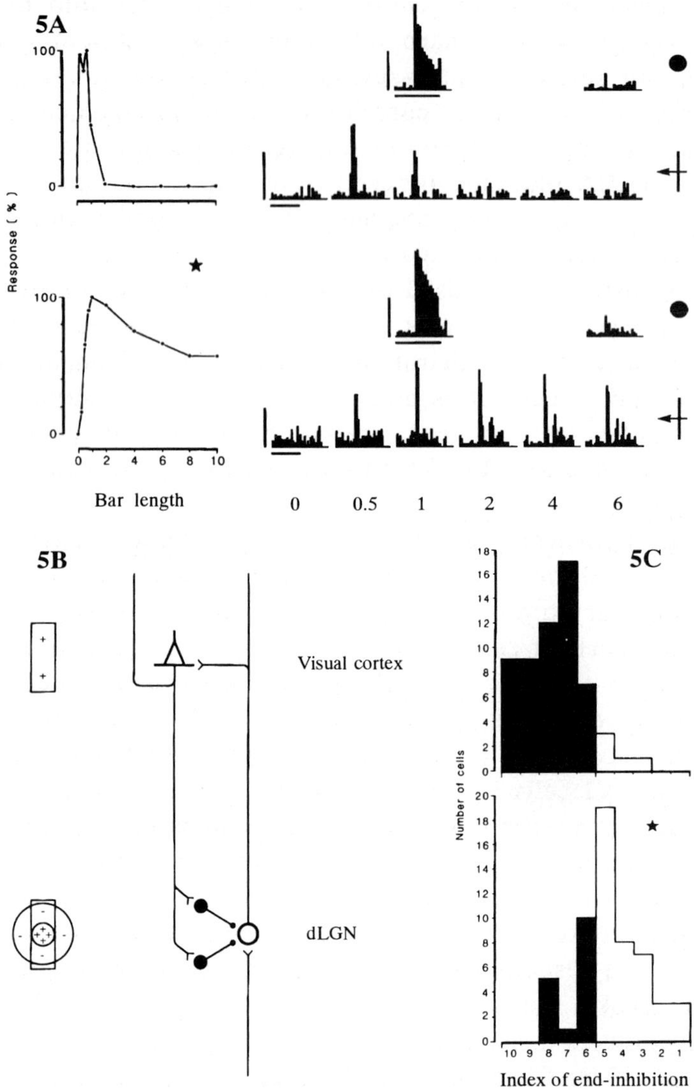

Fig. 5. The influence of corticofugal feedback on the length tuning of dLGN cells to a moving bar of light. As bar length increases and crosses the surround it only activates part of the surround, but corticofugal feedback increases the drive to the inhibitory neurones at this stage (**5B**). **5A**: The records document the responses of two on-centre Y cells, with fields at the same eccentricity in the same preparation, one recorded in the left dLGN with corticofugal feedback and the other in the right dLGN without corticofugal feedback (Areas 17 and 18 of the visual cortex removed by aspiration). The length tuning curves showing responses expressed as a percentage of the maximum are illustrated to the left and samples of the peristimulus histograms for the actual response shown to the

cortex, a group of cells at that time considered to follow from complex cells in a hierarchical processing sequence. In the cortex the response reduction has been attributed to inhibitory zones, lying to either end of the receptive field centre, the so-called "inhibitory end-zones". A response attenuation of 50% with increasing stimulus length has been considered to be a criterion for placing cortical cells in the hypercomplex category (Yamane et al. 1985). In the cat dLGN, for X and Y cells with clear centre-surround antagonism, the mean response reduction with increasing stimulus length is 71% (n=186; Jones and Sillito 1987, 1991).

The presence of this putative cortical response property at the level of the dLGN raises a number of issues which question some of the background assumptions regarding the mechanisms underlying receptive field organisation at both cortical and geniculate levels. Firstly, there is the immediate suggestion that because layer VI cells are well activated by moving bars (Gilbert 1977; Grieve and Sillito 1991) a component of the dLGN cell length tuning may reflect their influence. The corticofugal system provides the major synaptic input to the dLGN and its connections seem to be strongly biased towards inhibitory interneurones (Weber et al. 1989). If the feedback from layer VI cells enhanced the activity of inhibitory interneurones in the dLGN it could well reinforce the surround antagonism of dLGN cells and contribute to their strong length tuning. A brief consideration of the comparative geometry of the stimulus configuration for moving bars,

---

right. Immediately above these there are two PSTHs documenting the cells response to a 1° and 6° diameter flashing spot. The cell with corticofugal feedback shows a high level of length tuning to the drifting bar stimuli, and strong centre-surround antagonism as revealed by the flashing spots. The cell without corticofugal feedback (* shows equally strong centre-surround antagonism to the flashing spots, but poor length tuning to the moving bars. **5C**: Histograms summarize the distribution of length tuning in the population of cells (59) studied with corticofugal feedback and those (56) without (*). This is expressed as an index of end-inhibition, where cells with the strongest end-inhibition (total suppression of resting discharge at longer lengths) are in group 10 (left side of histogram) and those with none in group 1 (right side). The shaded portion of the PSTHs identifies those cells that if studied in the cortex, would have been classified as hypercomplex. There is a strong shift to the right in the population without feedback. Scale bars under PSTHs show 2 second period and those to the left range for 0-50 impulses per second. All PSTHs averaged for 20 trials. Figures modified from Murphy and Sillito 1987

as opposed to a flashing circle of light, makes it clear that a bar of similar width to the receptive field centre but long enough to cover the surround will stimulate a smaller component of the surround than a circle of the same diameter, and hence evoke a lower degree of centre-surround antagonism. However, feedback from cortical cells well activated by moving bars, to inhibitory interneurones contributing to centre-surround antagonism at the level of the dLGN, could reinforce the surround inhibition elicited by bars. These ideas are summarised by the diagram in figure 5B.

The key issue here is whether removing the corticofugal feedback influences the length tuning of dLGN cells. It turns out it does, in the absence of the feedback there is a substantial reduction in the length tuning of both X and Y cells in the dLGN under circumstances where centre-surround antagonism as tested by flashing spots of varying diameter was unaffected. This is illustrated in figure 5A which compares the length tuning curves of two on centre Y cells recorded in left and right dLGNs of a preparation with areas 17 and 18 of the visual cortex removed on one side. Although the cell lacking corticofugal feedback showed a much reduced response attenuation with increasing stimulus length the response attenuation caused by increasing the diameter of a stationary flashing spot from 1° to 6° was similar in both cases. Taking the population of dLGN cells, subdivided into categories on the basis of an index of end-inhibition, there is a very significant difference in the distribution of length tuning in groups with and without feedback (Figure 5C Index of end-inhibition histograms). The mean response reduction shifts from 71% to 43%. This suggests the feedback facilitates the drive from GABAergic inhibitory interneurones as bar lengths increase beyond the dimensions of the dLGN cell receptive field centre. The effect of surround inhibition can be argued to effectively enhance the resolution of the receptive field to a discontinuity in contrast between field centre and surround. The corticofugal feedback driving the intrageniculate inhibitory mechanisms, would seem to optimise this effect for thin contrast contours, so that the resolution of the field for a discontinuity over the field centre is retained despite the reduced area of surround activated by the stimulus.

The presence of a corticofugal influence on inhibitory mechanisms in the dLGN raises the question of orientation bias in their operation. The projection which derives primarily from areas 17 and 18 is broadly retinotopically organised so that there are reciprocal projections between dLGN and cortical locations subserving the same region of visual space (Hollander 1970; Kawamura et al. 1974; Updyke 1975). Layer VI cells are orientation tuned and hence either each location in the dLGN effectively receives feedback from a complete subset of cortical orientation columns or there must be a degree of orientation bias to the feedback affecting any given cell (Figure 6B). The problem has been examined recently (Sillito et al. 1991) by a series of experiments utilising a visual stimulus subdivided into an inner window located over the receptive field centre, and an outer window. (see figure 6A) The diameter of the inner window was chosen to match the value for the optimal length assessed from a length tuning curve constructed for the cell. The motion of the inner and outer stimuli were phase locked so that when both were at the same alignment they appeared as a single bar or grating moving over the receptive field. The effect of varying the orientation alignment of the two components of the stimulus was then documented. For dLGN cells the overall circular symmetry of the receptive field might be expected to result in similar magnitude inhibitory effects from the surround, irrespective of the orientation alignment of the two components of the stimulus. On the other hand, layer VI cortical cells with non-endstopped orientation tuned fields respond best to the aligned condition (Figure 6C). Thus the corticofugal influence driving the inhibitory processes enhancing length tuning in dLGN cells should be most effective for the aligned condition of this stimulus. Furthermore, if such an influence derives from a complete subset of orientation columns, this should apply for the alignment condition at any absolute orientation of the overall stimulus. The data from dLGN cells show that maximal suppression of the response to the inner stimulus is seen for the stimulus alignment condition (Figure 6C) and that for a given cell this alignment effect obtains at a range of different overall orientations for the alignment condition. The plots in figure 6C for a dLGN cell show the response elicited at varying orientations of the inner stimulus for three different orientations of the outer stimulus. The essential point is that there is a clear shift in the focus of the smallest response to follow the orientation of the outer stimulus.

The orientation alignment effects demonstrated by these procedures might be argued to follow from receptive field elongation of the type described by several laboratories for retinal ganglion cells and considered to underlie the orientation bias seen in some cells at retinal and geniculate levels (Hammond 1974; Levick and Thibos 1980, 1982; Vidyasagar 1984; Shou and Zhou 1986 but note Soodak et al. 1987).

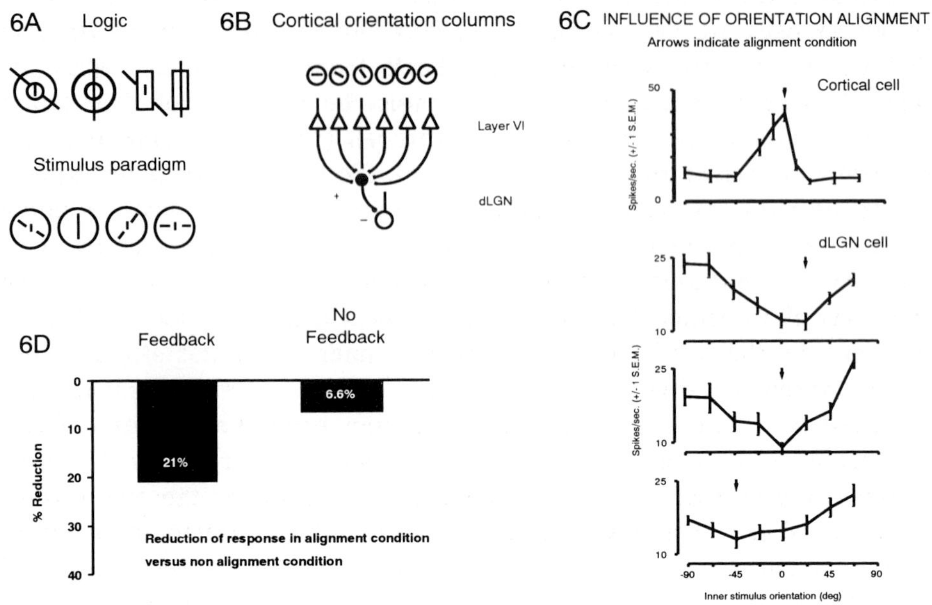

Fig. 6. Orientation sensitive feedback from cortex to dLGN. Layer VI cells in the cortex have orientation selective fields. Thus the cortically induced enhancement of centre-surround interaction should reflect some of the characteristics associated with cortical fields. The logic of an experiment to investigate this is shown in figure **6A**. A bipartite stimulus was used to examine dLGN cell fields as shown in the stimulus paradigm. The inner component of the stimulus was located over the receptive field centre, and the orientation of the inner and outer components could be varied. The motion of the inner and outer components was phase locked so that when in alignment they appeared as a single stimulus moving over the receptive field. Inner and outer stimulus orientation were varied on a randomised interleaved sequence. The primary assumption of the experiment is that the inhibitory effect elicited from the surround of the dLGN cell receptive field should not be sensitive to the relative alignment of the two components of the stimulus, because of the circular concentric arrangement. Conversely the fields of the visual cortical cells driving the corticofugal feedback should be optimally activated by the orientation aligned condition of the stimulus. This is shown by the tuning curve for a cortical cell at the top of **6C**. The arrow above the curve indicates the alignment condition. As the orientation alignment of the stimulus is varied it is clear that maximal responses are obtained as the inner and outer stimuli approach and reach alignment. Thus the corticofugal contribution to length tuning should be maximal when the inner and outer components of the stimulus are in alignment. The second curve in **6C** shows the effect of the alignment condition on a dLGN cell. This clearly shows a maximal effect as the two components of the stimulus approach and reach orientation alignment. In figure **5B** we show the inhibitory interneurones in the dLGN influencing a given relay cell, receiving feedback from the cortex at a single orientation. Does this occur or is the arrangement

There are several arguments against this, the main being that elongation in a particular plane cannot account for an alignment effect that follows the overall orientation of the alignment condition around the "clock", as suggested by the data in figure 6B. It is also not clear that a simple elongation of the field could account for the alignment effect even at a single orientation. In essence the data requires an inhibitory influence sensitive to the orientation alignment of a contour crossing centre and surround at any given orientation. However, the main argument is that the orientation alignment effect is radically reduced when the cortical feedback is removed by chemical inactivation or lesions, as is shown in figure 6D. There is still apparently a very small effect left in the absence of feedback, but this is not statistically significant and we cannot be sure that it does not represent some element of residual feedback left by our inactivation procedure. Thus whilst a subcortical contribution to such an effect cannot be excluded, the simplest explanation is that the effect follows from the cortex, and that an entire subset of orientation columns from the visual cortex generate the feedback effects influencing any given dLGN cell. This feedback ensures that cells are sensitive to the orientation alignment of contours crossing their receptive field centre and surround mechanisms. The outcome of this would seem to be that the output from the dLGN would be sensitive to discontinuities in the orientation domain for contours moving through visual space. A perfectly straight contour would produce a relatively uniform output from the rows of dLGN cell fields it engaged, with peaks at either end. Discontinuities in the orientation along the length of the contour would result in peaks in the output

---

shown in figure **6A** more accurate? Here there is feedback from cortical cells in an entire subset of orientation columns. If this model applies, the alignment effect should be seen at any given overall orientation. The curves for the dLGN cell in the lower three records of **6C** show the effect of varying the inner stimulus orientation for three different orientations of the outer stimulus as indicated by the arrows above the records. Maximum suppression is clearly seen as the stimuli approach and reach the alignment condition for each of three different alignment conditions illustrated. Thus it seems that feedback for any given locus in the dLGN derives from an entire subset of orientation columns. **6D**: Effect of removing feedback on the sensitivity of the dLGN cell field to the alignment condition. Histograms show for the population of cells, the increased surround reduction of centre response associated with the aligned condition over the non aligned effects. With feedback the aligned position produces a highly significant 21% increase in the surround effect, this falls to a non-significant 6.6% in the absence of feedback. See text for further details

from those cells with fields crossed by the discontinuity, because the corticofugal feedback driving the inhibition would be reduced at these points.

The cortical step in the mechanisms underlying length tuning

The length tuned receptive field was the first attribute of visual cortical cell response properties to be clearly linked to a model involving inhibitory interneurones in the original work of Hubel and Wiesel (1965, 1968). In their hierarchical scheme these cells, described as hypercomplex, were seen as a processing step beyond the level of complex cells. Two possible synaptic mechanisms as summarised in figure 7A, were suggested. The main point is that a cell with a short excitatory receptive field receives inhibitory input from either a single cell with an overlapping but longer receptive field, or two cells with receptive fields displaced to either side of the excitatory field. In both cases elongation of a stimulus beyond the excitatory field would increase the magnitude of the inhibitory input converging on the hypercomplex cell. The field was seen as possessing inhibitory end-zones and it is a common practise to describe cells with length tuned receptive fields as being end-stopped. The first direct test of this hypothesis came from iontophoretic experiments examining the effect of bicuculline on the responses of hypercomplex cells in layers II and III of area 17 (Sillito and Versiani 1977). The data from these experiments was interesting because hypercomplex cell length tuning was reduced by inhibitory blockade, but was not eliminated, suggesting the presence of a length tuned excitatory input. An example of the effects of inhibitory blockade on one of the cells examined in this work is given in figure 7C. The presence of a length tuned excitatory input to superficial layer hypercomplex cells is in accord with the demonstration that many layer IV simple family cells also have "hypercomplex" or "length tuned" fields. In layer IV, which receives the major component of the input from the dLGN, the length tuning of simple cells is most easily explained by an excitatory input from length tuned dLGN cells. As the layer VI cells providing the corticofugal feedback to the dLGN also provide an extensive collateral projection to layer IV it is of interest to question the nature of their influence on responses in the length domain at this level. It is clear from electrophysiological and anatomical studies that layer VI cells can exert both excitatory and inhibitory effects in layer IV cells (Ferster and Lindstrom 1984 a,b; Somogyi 1989). The anatomical data suggest that only 14% of layer VI cell terminals contact GABAergic cells suggesting a strong bias towards connections on excitatory interneurones. However, in terms of a contribution to visual processing, considerable emphasis has been given to the capacity for layer VI cells to drive inhibitory interneurones in layer IV. In particular Bolz and Gilbert (1986) have asserted that layer VI cells establish the end-inhibition generating the length tuning layer IV hypercomplex cells. The logic for this view lay in the original surmise of McGuire et al. (1984) that layer VI cell collaterals arborising in layer IV terminated primarily on the smooth dendritic processes of what seemed likely to be inhibitory interneurones. This, linked to Gilbert's (1977) finding that layer VI cells have the longest receptive fields found in the striate cortex, led to the conclusion that cells with long receptive fields provided a predominantly inhibitory influence on layer IV. This connection from VI to IV seemed to be the realisation of the circuit illustrated in figure 7A and Bolz and Gilbert reported that localised blockade of activity in layer VI eliminated the length tuning of layer IV simple cells. This appeared to reflect the loss of an inhibitory input generating the hypercomplex cell end-zone inhibition because the excitatory responses to short bars were unchanged.

This observation could however, be explained by the loss of the reflected feedback to the dLGN. Against this view, is the fact that the changes in the length tuning of dLGN cells seemed to require loss of the feedback from both areas 17 and 18 (Murphy and Sillito 1987). Localised inactivation of a small patch of layer VI in the same orientation column as the overlying layer IV cells studied (Bolz and Gilbert 1986) would thus seem unlikely to precipitate a major change in the length tuning of the input dLGN cells. As the major component of the input from VI to IV seems to be excitatory to spiny cells, local inactivation of VI might be expected to reveal the withdrawal of a facilitatory influence in IV. Indeed, very recent work indicates that localised blockade of layer VI cells does reveal changes commensurate with the loss of an excitatory drive to cells in the overlying layer IV (Grieve and Sillito 1990b, 1991). In these experiments, blockade of layer VI was produced by localised iontophoretic application of either GABA or the potent $GABA_A$ receptor agonist, muscimol. A multibarreled iontophoretic electrode and a tungsten in glass recording electrode were

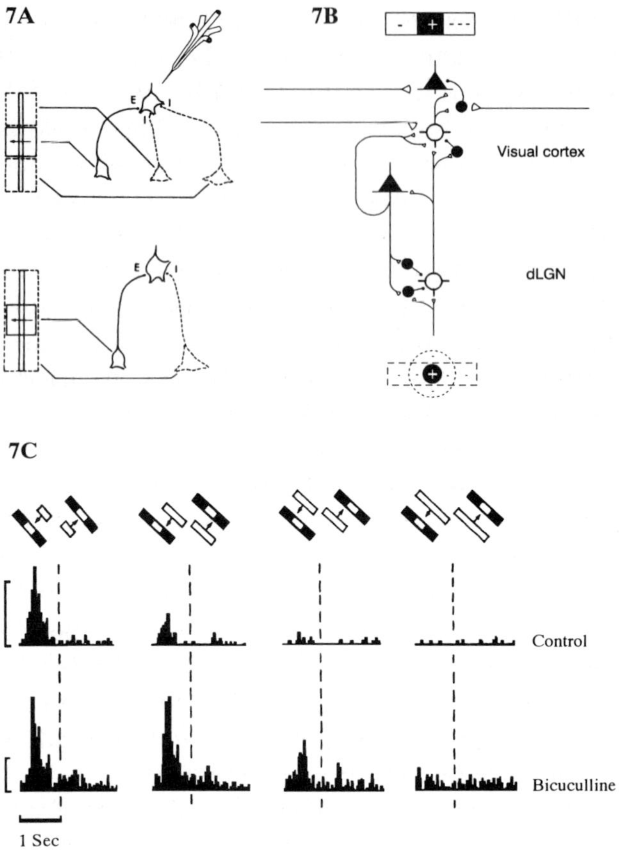

Fig. 7. Intracortical inhibitory influences on the hypercomplex cell field. **7A**: Concept diagram summarising Hubel and Wiesel's original suggestions regarding the synaptic connections generating hypercomplex cell orientation tuning. **7B**: Schematic diagram summarising some of the factors now thought to contribute to length tuning. Centre-surround antagonism in the dLGN cell receptive field following from both the retinal input characteristics and intrageniculate GABAergic inhibitory mechanisms establishes the first stage of length tuning. Feedback from layer VI cells in the visual cortex to the GABAergic inhibitory interneurones enhances the inhibitory drive attenuating the response to longer bars. This is summarised by the circular (subcortical) and rectangular (cortically derived) inhibitory fields in the receptive field schematic at the bottom of the figure. The input from dLGN to cortex carries these influences forward and provides direct excitatory input to layer IV simple cells and a disynaptic inhibitory drive via GABAergic cells. The collateral excitatory input from layer VI to IV reinforces excitatory responses to short bar lengths (see figure 8). Thus length tuning is established at the level of the dLGN and modulated by an intracortical thresholding inhibition and selective facilitation at short bar lengths. Longer distance excitatory connections from

carefully aligned so that they sampled cells in layers VI and IV with receptive fields of the same orientation selectivity and location in visual space. During blockade of layer VI two patterns of effect were observed on length tuned cells in the overlying layers III and IV. Either the visual responses to all stimuli were reduced in a non-specific manner, or the responses to the short optimal length stimuli were selectively reduced with respect to those to the longer non-optimal stimuli. None of the cells studied revealed a selective increase in the responses to longer length non-optimal stimuli commensurate with a loss of end-zone inhibition. This applied even in cases where the blockade of layer VI was continued until there were direct effects on layer IV cell excitability. Where the responses to the shorter stimuli were selectively reduced, the length tuning was in turn reduced, but this followed from the relative reduction of short as opposed to long bar responses (Figure 8A). This suggests the loss of an excitatory influence from layer VI cells with short receptive fields and the ideas are summarised in the diagram of figure 8B. The data would thus seem to be explained by a facilitatory input from layer VI cells to hypercomplex cells in the immediately overlying layer IV with overlapping receptive fields. The relative "resistance" of the responses to longer length stimuli may well reflect the presence of horizontally directed facilitatory inputs from more remote regions of layer VI or IV. These could be activated by the ends of the elongated stimulus driving cells in laterally displaced columns of similar orientation selectivity. It is already known that there are horizontal facilitatory connections between columns of similar orientation selectivity (Tso et al. 1986; Gilbert and Wiesel 1989; Engel et al. 1990). The cases where the responses to both the optimal short stimuli and the long stimuli

---

columns of similar orientation selectivity may provide either facilitatory or inhibitory drive strengthening or weakening the end-zone influences to one or the other side of the field. 7C: The PSTHs here show a test of the original model in 7A, by utilising iontophoretic application of bicuculline to block the inhibitory inputs to the cell. The hypercomplex cell receptive field is shown schematically above these records, with central excitatory region (open rectangle) and inhibitory end-zones (closed rectangles). The visual stimulus used to test this field is shown by the open bar and arrow. Bicuculline application (50nA) reduces the strength of the end-inhibition, particularly to one side of the field, but does not block the length tuning. The cell still fails to respond to the bar extended to either side of the field, suggesting a length tuned excitatory input. Records averaged for 25 trials. Bin size is 50 msecs and vertical calibrations indicate range corresponding to 0-25 counts per bin

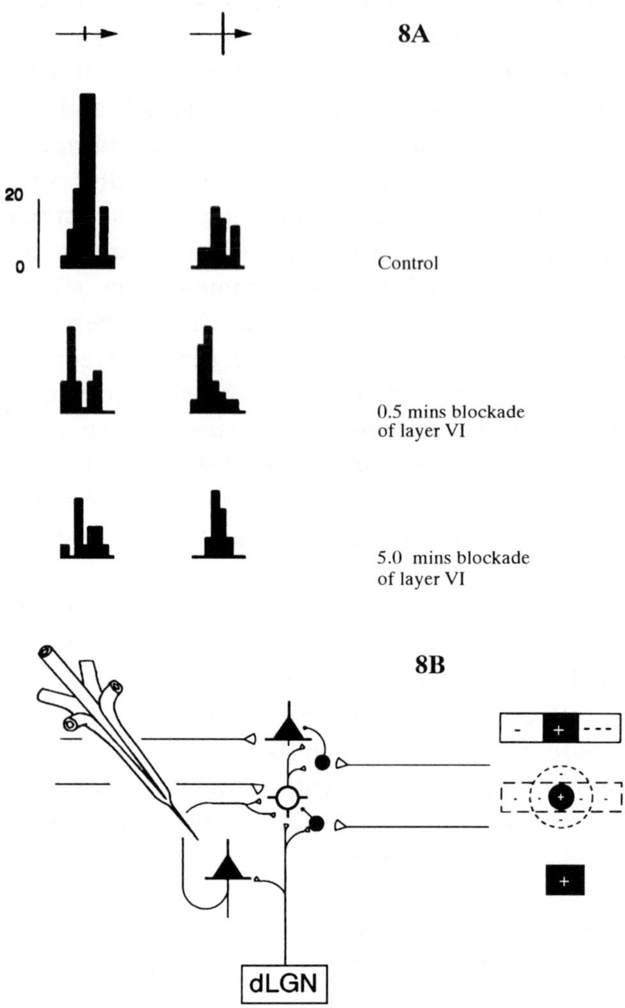

Fig. 8. Facilitatory effect of layer VI cells on response of layer IV hypercomplex cells to short bar lengths. **8A**: PSTHs document the responses to a short optimal length bar and a long bar crossing the receptive field of layer IV simple cell. Blockade of layer VI by iontophoretic application of the $GABA_A$ agonist muscimol (25nA) for 0.5 minutes reduces the response to the short bar but has no significant effect on the response to the long bar. Continued application of muscimol to 5.0 minutes causes a further reduction in the short bar response and a slight reduction of the long bar response. **8B**: Circuit being tested by the GABA application in layer VI. Schematic receptive fields to the right of the circuit diagram summarise some of the influences that may underlie these effects. The primary suggestion is that an excitatory drive from layer VI cells with receptive fields showing rapid spatial summation provide the critical stimulus locked facilitation to enable the layer IV cell to overcome

declined together could reflect cells that lack longer distance facilitatory inputs.

An interpretation of the likely contribution that layer VI cells could have to cortical mechanisms underlying length tuning has been confused by a widespread acceptance of the view that they typically have very long fields of 8° or more long (Gilbert 1977; Bolz and Gilbert 1986). These might seem to be ideally suited to generating the inhibitory end-zones for the model in fig 9 but in reality are not compatible with the data from quantitative studies of the inhibitory mechanisms underlying length tuning. Careful quantitative study of simple type hypercomplex cells (Kato et al. 1978; Yamane et al. 1985) suggests that the spatial extent of the inhibitory end zone region is much more restricted than that which would derive from an input summing to 8° or more. Specifically, the central excitatory region is on average 1.5° in length (Kato et al. 1978) and the maximum response reduction occurs when the stimulus is increased in length by a further 1.3° (Yamane et al. 1985). This implies a very steep slope in the curve for the decrement in response with length. Thus the inhibitory input would appear to be driven by a mechanism exhibiting its primary rise in response magnitude for stimulus lengths in the range 1.5-2.8°. Alternatively, if the end inhibition were derived from the summed action of separate inhibitory fields, offset to either end of a central excitatory zone (figure 9), the mechanisms driving these two inhibitory fields would need to show an even more rapid rise in response magnitude. In this latter case, the major change in response magnitude should occur for lengths up to 0.7°, or slightly more according to the degree of overlap of the two zones with the central excitatory field. Thus the link between hypercomplex cell inhibitory fields and layer VI cells with long receptive fields is not compelling. Similar arguments apply if one considers the underlying mechanisms necessary to generate the corticofugal enhancement of dLGN cell tuning. The facilitatory effects discussed above in relation to the layer VI cell influence on IV also need a mechanism showing rapid spatial summation. There is in fact not a problem, many layer VI cells do have short fields (Grieve and Sillito 1990a, 1991) with 61% of the population showing summation to 4° or less. Careful reading of the literature shows several other

---

feedforward inhibitory influences. See the text and discussion of figure 11 for further explanation. PSTHs averaged for 5 trials and bin size is 150 msecs.

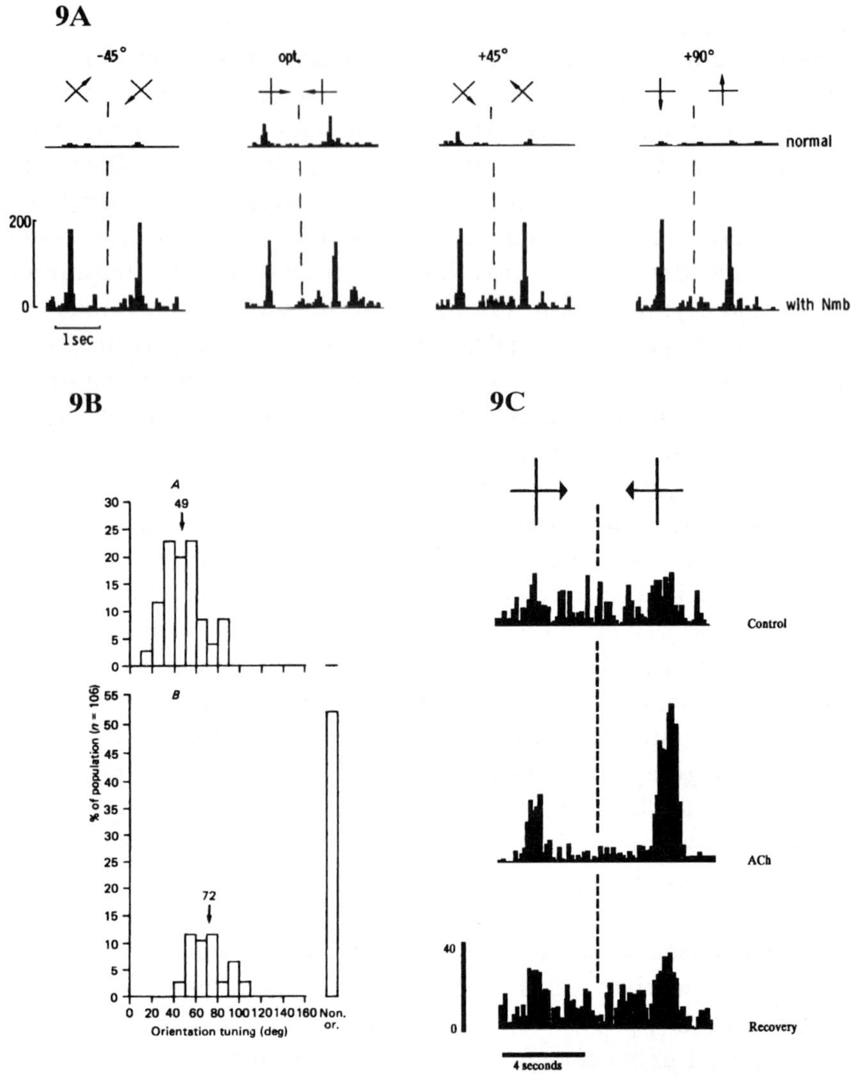

Fig. 9. Drug induced changes in orientation and direction tuning. **9A**: PSTHs show responses of a simple cell to a moving bar of varying orientation before and during inhibitory blockade. Iontophoretic application of the GABA antagonist bicuculline (*Nmb*) causes a large increase in response magnitude and the appearance of responses at non-optimal orientations which exceed those to the optimal. Vertical calibration indicates range for 0-200 counts/50msec bin. See text for discussion of the effect. **9B**: Histogram to the left of the figure shows the distribution of orientation tuning in a population of 106 complex cells before (*A*) and during inhibitory blockade (*B*). The orientation tuning of the cells is derived from the width of the tuning curve at half height. Cells losing orientation

authors have identified this fact but it seems to have lost its way in the face of the view that layer VI cells have very long fields. Indeed, some do have long fields, but they are in the minority (Grieve and Sillito 1991).

Although the available findings seem to present contradictory views of the inhibitory processes underlying the generation of length tuned receptive fields, there are many common themes which begin to generate a coherent overview. A major component of the excitatory input from the dLGN to the cortex seems to be length tuned (Schiller et al. 1976; Rose 1979; Cleland et al. 1983; Jones and Sillito 1987, 1991), thus there is no need to identify a special mechanism to establish length tuning in cortical cells. Indeed, the converse really applies, the problem is how it may be eliminated. Hypercomplex cells outside layer IV seem to receive a length tuned excitatory input (Sillito and Versiani 1977) and this could derive either from layer IV hypercomplex cells or a direct input from length tuned dLGN cells. There is strong evidence for the view that intracortical inhibitory mechanisms contribute to the inhibitory influences in cortical hypercomplex cell receptive fields (Sillito and Versiani 1977; Sillito 1977a; Kato et al. 1978; Orban et al. 1979a,b). The length selectivity of layer IV cells could be enhanced in the cortex by any inhibitory mechanism that decreased the excitability of layer IV hypercomplex cells, so that only the maximal response point in the length tuning curve of the geniculate input drove them to threshold. The available data suggest that intracortical excitatory interactions are important here (Ferster and Lindstrom 1984 a,b; Grieve and Sillito 1991). The geniculate input

---

tuning during bicuculline application are shown in the "Non or" column to the right of the figure (B). Arrows show median orientation tuning for those cells showing selectivity. **9D**: Influence of acetylcholine (*ACh*) on response magnitude, direction selectivity and resting discharge. The records show the effect of iontophoretically applied ACh on the visual response of a layer IV simple cell to an optimally oriented bar passing forwards and backwards over the receptive field. Under control conditions this cell gave weak bidirectional responses to the stimulus. Iontophoretic application of ACh (20nA) reduced the background activity and greatly increased the visual responses, but in particular enhanced the directional selectivity. This is likely to reflect two different components of action of ACh. Firstly, a direct excitation of adjacent inhibitory interneurones influencing background discharge and directional selectivity, and secondly, an action on the voltage dependent and calcium dependent potassium channels underlying the after hyperpolarization of the cell recorded from (see text for further discussion). The records are averaged for 10 trials and plotted with 150 msec bins

would drive both layer IV cells and layer VI cells. The stimulus locked nature of the facilitatory input from layer VI to layer IV seems to be a critical factor in establishing the level of summation necessary for the expression of the full excitatory response in layer IV hypercomplex type simple cells. It is important to note that the corticofugal projection from layer VI to the dLGN seems to enhance the length tuning of the input dLGN cells by increasing the gain of inhibitory mechanisms acting on them (Murphy and Sillito 1987). These same layer VI cells provide the recurrent projection to layer IV, and their apical dendrites pass up to layer IV where they can collect input from both geniculate afferents and the terminals of intracortical cells. They also receive input from geniculate afferents to layer VI. From this viewpoint it is apparent that we are looking at the function of a circuit with interlinked elements. In this circuit, the layer VI cells seem to play a crucial role in regulating the access of visual information to the cortex by their subcortical influence on the responses of dLGN cells and their cortical influence at the primary site of termination of dLGN cell axons in layer IV. The stress here on a facilitatory influence in layer IV and an inhibitory influence in the dLGN is consistent with biases suggested by the anatomical evidence and much of the recent physiological data. The overall balance of the two patterns of effect would seem to be complementary and clearly has interesting functional consequences. The suggestions discussed here are summarised in figure 7B.

Receptive field length and mechanisms underlying orientation tuning

In the cortex, cells with hypercomplex fields are not in reality a sharply defined subgroup, but one end of a spectrum of cells extending from those with very powerful end stopped fields to those with none (e.g. Rose 1979; Yamane et al. 1985). Consideration of the mechanisms underlying the generation of their response properties is possibly better placed in the perspective of those processes that may contribute to the fields of cells showing little or no end stopping in their fields. The end stopping of dLGN cells poses an interesting problem for models of the synaptic convergence underlying non length tuned fields. The arguments here are in turn crucial to our understanding of the way orientation tuned fields might be established by the convergence of geniculate afferents. Were the input to a simple cell to derive from a single geniculate cell or a group of geniculate cells with strongly overlapping fields, it is immediately apparent that it would have an endstopped receptive field. However, the geniculate input to layer IV spiny cells forms only a small part of their excitatory input, the rest derives from intracortical sources. In the orientation domain, the primary long distance excitatory connections occur between columns of similar orientation selectivity (Tso et al. 1986; Gilbert and Wiesel 1989; Engel et al. 1990). Thus extending the length of a bar along the axis of the optimal orientation of a cell will elicit facilitatory effects from columns of similar orientation. Clearly this type of connection would serve to offset the decrement in response from the primary geniculate input. Thus varying the strength of these laterally directed excitatory influences gives the capability of varying degrees of reduction in the length tuning of cortical cells. An alternative view is that the input to a layer IV spiny cell derives from a group of dLGN cells with receptive fields forming a row through visual space along the axis of the optimal orientation. This type of arrangement is frequently considered to account for the mechanisms establishing orientation tuned fields in layer IV (Hubel and Wiesel 1962). A short bar moving over the centre of the receptive field of the input dLGN cell contributing to the centre of the simple cell field, would evoke a maximal response from the input cell. Increasing stimulus length would cause a decline in the response from the central input cell but start to recruit input from adjacent input cells, however their input in turn would decline as bar length further increased. To avoid response decline at longer bar lengths it is necessary to increase the number of input cells or synaptic weighting for locations displaced from the simple cell receptive field centre. This has the corollary that two short bars spatially displaced from the centre and moved over the ends of the field would evoke strong responses; this does not appear to happen. Mapping the field of a simple cell with small stationary flashing stimuli shows that the primary excitatory effects are elicited from the central region of the field and are not balanced by strong inputs from the ends (e.g. Creutzfeldt et al. 1974b; Jones and Palmer 1987). Thus from the geniculate data one would predict length tuning in these cells because the drive from their input will fall as stimulus length increases. Many of such cells do not show length tuned fields.

The conclusion here must be that a long stimulus provokes effects in the circuitry that are not revealed by short stimuli.

How do these issues link with the evidence regarding the mechanisms underlying orientation selectivity? The relation between the pattern of convergence of geniculate inputs and the generation of orientation selectivity has been the centre of an extensive controversy in the field since Hubel and Wiesel first formulated their ideas in the early sixties. In their model, the mechanisms underlying the orientation selectivity of essentially all cells in the visual cortex involve precisely organised excitatory connections, firstly in terms of the geniculate input to simple cells, but subsequently between cortical cells to conserve the selectivity established in simple cells. The view was first questioned by the intracellular and electrophysiological analysis carried out by Creutzfeldt's laboratory (Creutzfeldt and Ito 1968; Creutzfeldt et al. 1974 a,b). These experiments emphasised the importance of inhibitory mechanisms to the responses of visual cortical cells and provided evidence indicating that the receptive fields of some cortical cells were virtually circular despite their orientation tuning. The latter led to the suggestion that intracortical inhibition was structuring the response of these cells in the orientation domain with the logical consequence that the inhibition would be maximal at 90° to the cells optimal orientation. However, this interpretation, based largely on an appraisal of receptive field shape, had to be balanced by their intracellular observations which showed that in most cells, inhibition as well as excitation appeared to be less marked during stimulation in the non-optimal orientation. Very similar findings in recent times by Ferster (1986, 1987) have essentially confirmed this latter point, stimuli crossing the receptive field at orientations orthogonal to the optimal elicited few EPSPs and IPSPs. If intracortical inhibition were shaping orientation tuning in the simple manner envisaged, it is logical to anticipate both EPSPs and IPSPs in response to this stimulus.

There are essentially two problems here, the first is that many orientation tuned cortical cells seem to lack the elongated excitatory field necessary to enable excitatory convergence to establish orientation tuning. The second is that when tested by intracellular techniques, they appear to lack either the excitatory or inhibitory inputs that models involving inhibitory mechanisms would predict. These problems are put into a sharper perspective by the data obtained using iontophoretic application of the GABA antagonist bicuculline to produce a localised block of GABA mediated inhibitory processes acting on visual cortical cells (Sillito 1974, 1975a,b, 1977a,b, 1979, 1984; Sillito et al. 1980; Tsumoto et al. 1979). During this blockade, when it may be presumed that local GABA synapses are also blocked, the data showed that orientation selectivity in virtually all cortical cells could be reduced and in some even eliminated. For complex cells about half the population showed a broadening of the orientation tuning and half changes that essentially eliminated the original bias (Sillito 1979). This is summarised by the histograms in figure 9B. In the case of simple cells orientation tuning seemed to be more resistant to inhibitory blockade and early experiments showed only a broadening of the orientation tuning curve (Sillito 1974, 1975b) but more potent blockade of their inhibitory inputs (Tsumoto et al. 1979; Sillito et al. 1980) eliminated orientation tuning. The effects of inhibitory blockade on a simple cell are illustrated in figure 9A. It is absolutely clear that the blockade enables previously ineffective excitatory inputs to drive the cell. Support for the presence of suppressed excitatory influences comes from Eysel's recent work (see this volume). Essentially his observations demonstrate that local inactivation of groups of cortical cells adjacent to a cell under study, reveal excitatory responses in that cell to previously ineffective orientations. It seems the inactivation is switching off a neural influence that normally suppresses responses to some orientations. These data seem to be most easily explained by the presence of a cross orientation inhibitory influence and several other studies (Sillito 1979; Ramoa et al. 1986; Morrone et al. 1982; Morrone and Burr 1986) have demonstrated a cross orientation suppression of elevated background discharge levels produced either by a conditioning visual stimulus or iontophoretic application of an excitatory amino acid.

The particularly interesting thing here is the consistency of the inconsistent observations derived from the different experimental approaches. There is apparently good evidence to support each of the virtually orthogonal interpretations of the mechanisms underlying orientation tuning. Certainly one of the difficulties in resolving these issues lies in the tendency to assume there is one mechanism establishing orientation tuning for all cells. This is clearly unlikely, the data obtained with pharmacological blockade of inhibitory synapses underline the fact that from this yardstick, the contribution of inhibitory mechanisms to orientation tuning varies across the population of cells (Sillito 1975b, 1979, 1984). Indeed it seems most likely that in many cases the orientation tuning of given cells will depend on several mechanisms. The cortex seems to be able to express orientation selectivity in the absence of a functioning layer IV (Malpeli et al. 1981; Malpeli 1983; Malpeli et al. 1986). Thus the mechanism for generating orientation selectivity would seem to be expressed independently in several laminar locations, a view which matches conclusions drawn from the earlier data obtained with GABA blockade (Sillito 1979; Sillito et al. 1980; Sillito 1984).

Is it possible to relate the various threads of these arguments together in a way that matches the available experimental data? Any attempt to proceed with this has to consider the profile of the geniculate input to the cortex elicited by a moving bar of light. It is apparent that the length tuning of dLGN cells will result in a minimal output to cortex from those dLGN cells covered by the centre of the bar, with the strongest output from fields at the ends of the bar where only part of the surround mechanism is covered by the stimulus. These inputs elicited by the ends of the bar should drive the central regions of the fields of cortical cells with similar orientation, but a location spatially shifted along the axis of the optimal orientation. It is at this point that the intracortical connections from columns of like orientation selectivity may be critical. The suggestion I make here is that time locked facilitation from the intracortical connections interacts with and reinforces the reduced drive from the dLGN cells so that the cell response is enabled. A stimulus rotated away from the optimal orientation loses this facilitation and the cell responds little if at all. However, one would predict that an orthogonally oriented bar, reduced in length until it is of the same dimensions as the dLGN input field centre could provoke a response if moved over the field because the direct geniculate input should be maximal. Interestingly this does seem to occur (e.g. Wörgötter and Eysel 1989). On the other hand, increasing the length of the orthogonally oriented stimulus will radically reduce the magnitude of the dLGN input cell responses because of their length tuning but will not bring in any compensatory intracortical facilitation because the ends of the bar are not activating the correct columns. At this point it is clear that the excitatory input from an incorrectly oriented elongated bar would be low, much as the intracellular studies show. The critical issue is the intracortical facilitation and the threshold for the effectiveness of this may be modulated by feedforward inhibitory effects driven by dLGN terminals which also contact non spiny GABAergic cells. The input from these, for the same reasons, could be greater for optimal orientations. In this argument the central assumptions are the length tuning of dLGN cells and the intracortical facilitatory connections between columns of like orientation. Although this may seem to require orientation selectivity to be set up in other columns to achieve the facilitation, in the first instance one need not regard the columns as orientation tuned, but simply strongly connected points on a map of visual space in the cortex which are simultaneously activated by a bar of particular orientation. The orientation follows from this pattern of excitatory connection across the cortex, the length tuning of the dLGN input and local thresholding feedforward inhibition. These interactions involve the corticofugal feedback to the geniculate inhibitory circuitry enhancing length tuning as well as the intracortical connections. It is also at this stage worth reconsidering the possibility that the inhibitory interneurones mediating the local thresholding, feedforward inhibition may in some cases receive an excitatory drive from adjacent columns of differing orientation selectivity (but in the same hypercolumn). This might normally simply increase the excitability level of the inhibitory cells without driving them to threshold, but coupled with the direct geniculate input in their own column serve to modulate the thresholding effect. Any process that increased the excitability of the cells controlled by these local inhibitory interneurones, for example local iontophoretic application of an excitatory amino acid or a small visual conditioning stimulus might also facilitate the interneurones themselves and enable them to be driven by the cross orientation inputs converging on them. In this way the presence of cross orientation inhibitory effects could be brought out (Sillito 1979; Ramoa et al. 1986; Morrone et al. 1982; Morrone and Burr 1986).

Considering the issue of pharmacological blockade of inhibition in this model it is important to ask how the excitatory and inhibitory events may interplay in the circuitry. Where NMDA receptors have a role in visual responses the duration of the EPSP provides a broader window of excitation for the correlation of effects from several inputs to a cell. Their voltage dependency introduces a further facet to our understanding of the potential impact of inhibitory inputs in terms of the capacity of the inhibition to suppress the regenerative development of an excitatory response that can follow the initiation of effects via NMDA receptors. Inhibitory blockade will release a cell from local feedforward inhibition and other inhibitory inputs converging on all but the far distal dendrites of pyramidal cells. Where NMDA receptors are involved the loss of the hyperpolarizing influence may enable their effect at lower levels of excitatory drive to the cell and because of the duration of the EPSPs so generated open a wider temporal window for the summation of visually driven excitatory inputs. This alone may generate enough facilitation to enable cells to respond to direct geniculate input without the permissive influence of the iso-orientation intracortical facilitation. This effect does not require cross orientation inhibition. It is becoming clear that some cortical cells, those in layer III for example, can utilise excitatory inputs from a range of different inputs to express the same overt receptive field properties. Thus layer III complex cells seem to respond similarly whether driven by inputs originating in the A laminae of the dLGN via layer IV, the C laminae of the dLGN, area 18 or all of these (Malpeli 1983; Malpeli et al. 1986; Schwark et al. 1986). This multiple sourcing of inputs poses problems for gain control, and it may be that particular inputs are regulated by the bitufted and neurogliaform GABAergic cells synapsing at specific locations on dendrites. Lifting this type of inhibitory control may bring a massive barrage of facilitatory influence to bear on cells and generate significant non-linearities in the way the effects of the inputs sum.

Final comment

Much of the present debate about the circuitry in the central visual system, the way it is organised and its functional import is based on data derived from the use of restricted and very simple stimulation paradigms. The choice of these reflect the underlying dogma concerning what happens at each level in the system. It is going to be necessary to produce stimulus configurations and tests that explore the impact of context across the map of the neural representation of visual space on the tuning and response properties of a cell at any given location in that map. Using drifting, bipartite oriented stimuli, the dLGN cell begins to reveal the presence of the massive feedback from the orientation sensitive system in the cortex. In the visual cortex different layers of influence are superimposed in ways that vary with the nature of the stimulus. The system seems to utilise several inputs to achieve the same end as far as simple response properties go and we have yet to dissect out the full significance of this in terms of our experimental approaches. It is also essential to take note of the fact that the organisation of the central circuitry is very dependent on the pattern of neurmodulatory input. At geniculate levels the cholinergic system for example depolarizes relay cells via a nicotinic mechanism (Sillito et al. 1983; McCormick and Prince 1987, 1990; McCormick and Pape 1988, 1990) and hyperpolarizes perigeniculate cells (Sillito et al. 1983; McCormick and Prince 1987, 1990) and intrinsic inhibitory interneurones via a muscarinic mechanism (McCormick and Pape 1988). The increased activity of the cholinergic input in the waking state will thus result in a degree of disinhibition and direct excitation of relay cells, consequently helping to enable NMDA receptor mediated effects. There are some qualifications applying here. Although the cholinergic input may hyperpolarize inhibitory interneurones it does not eliminate their influence. In particular, short range inhibitory interactions appear to be very effective in the presence of ACh although long range processes are diminished (Sillito et al. 1983; Eysel et al. 1986; Murphy and Sillito 1989). In the visual cortex the pattern of influence of the cholinergic system on the cortical circuitry is somewhat different to that seen in the dLGN. There is a direct depolarising influence on inhibitory interneurones which can drive a discharge and will contribute to their normal background activity (McCormick and Prince 1985). In addition, pyramidal cell responses are modulated via an action on the voltage dependent potassium channel underlying the M current, and the calcium dependent potassium channel (Halliwell and Adams 1982; Bernardo and Prince 1982; McCormick and Prince 1985, 1990; McCormick et al. 1985). In both cases the effectiveness of these currents is diminished by ACh. The impact on pyramidal cells will be to facilitate their responses to an existing excitatory input, allowing higher frequency discharge because of the reduction of the after hyperpolarization linked to the two potassium channels. This contrasts with the strong excitatory and at least partial disinhibitory effects on the geniculate circuitry. The gain of the intracortical inhibitory mechanisms will be enhanced by activity in the cholinergic system. This is exemplified by the action of ACh on the stimulus specific responses of visual cortical cells. Responses to optimal stimuli are enhanced, and selectivity in a significant number of cases is increased commensurate with facilitatory effects on the inhibitory circuitry generating response selectivity (Sillito and Kemp 1983; Sillito and Murphy 1988; Murphy and Sillito 1990). An example of the action of ACh on the responses of a visual cortical cell is given in figure 9C. In the absence of significant cholinergic input the extracellular response of this cell could give a very misleading impression of the way it would participate in vision in the waking state. Even intracellular analysis could fail to detect the mechanisms underlying its direction selectivity, they seem to be revealed by the cholinergic drive implementing the facilitation necessary for the inhibitory interneurones to provide effective drive. It is as yet, far from clear how the various modulatory inputs interact in the circuitry, but the specific patterns of termination of the different inputs and the range of ion channels influenced indicates a substantive capacity to evoke change.

References

Ahlsen G, Grant K, Lindstrom S (1982) Monosynaptic excitation of principal cells in the lateral geniculate nucleus by corticofugal fibres. Brain Res 234:454-458

Bernardo LS, Prince DA (1982) Cholinergic excitation of mammalian hippocampal pyramidal cells. Brain Res 249:315-331

Birch PJ, Grossman, CJ, Hayes AG (1988) Kynurenic acid antagonises responses to NMDA via an action at the strychnine-insensitive glycine receptor. Eur J Pharmacol 154:85-88

Bolz J, Gilbert CD (1986) Generation of end-inhibition in the visual cortex via interlaminar connections. Nature 320:362-365

Cleland BG, Lee BB, Vidyasagar TR (1983) Response of Neurons in the Cat's Lateral Geniculate Nucleus to Moving Bars of Different Length. J Neurosci 3:108-116

Creutzfeldt OD, Ito M (1968) Functional Synaptic Organisation of Primary Visual Cortex Neurones in the Cat. Exp Brain Res 6:324-352

Creutzfeldt OD, Innocenti GM, Brooks D (1974a) Vertical Organisation in the Visual Cortex (Area 17) in the Cat. Exp Brain Res 21:315-336

Creutzfeldt OD, Kuhnt U, Benevento LA (1974b) An Intracellular analysis of visual cortical neurones to moving stimuli: Responses in a co-operative neuronal network. Exp Brain Res 21:251-274

Crunelli V, Kelly JS, Leresche N, Pirchio M (1987) On the excitatory post-synaptic potential evoked by stimulation of the optic tract in the rat lateral geniculate nucleus. J Physiol 384:603-618

Dubin MW, Cleland BG (1977) Organization of Visual Inputs to Interneurons of Lateral Geniculate Nucleus of the Cat. J Neurophysiol 40:410-427

Engel AK, König P, Gray CM, Singer W (1990) Stimulus-dependent neuronal oscillations in cat visual cortex: Inter-columnar interaction as determined by cross-correlation analysis. Eur J Neurosci 2:588-606

Eysel UT, Pape HC, Van Schayck R (1986) Excitatory and differential disinhibitory actions of acetylcholine in the lateral geniculate nucleus of the cat. J Physiol 370:233-254

Famiglietti EW, Peters A (1972) The synaptic glomerulus and the intrinsic neurons in the dorsal lateral geniculate nucleus of the cat. J Comp Neurol 144:285-334

Ferster D, Lindstrom S (1984a) Synaptic Excitation of Neurones in Area 17 of the Cat by Intracortical Axon Collaterals of Cortico- geniculate cells. J Physiol 367:233-252

Ferster D, Lindstrom S (1984b) Augmenting Responses Evoked in Area 17 of the Cat by Intracortical Axon Collaterals of Cortico-geniculate cells. J Physiol 367:217-232

Ferster D (1986) Orientation Selectivity of Synaptic Potentials in Neurons of Cat Primary Visual Cortex. J Neurosci 6:1264-1301

Ferster D (1987) Origin of Orientation-Selective EPSPs in Simple Cells of Cat Visual Cortex. J Neurosci 7:1780-1791

Fitzpatrick D, Penny GR, Schmechel DE (1984) Glutamic acid decarboxylase-immunoreactive neurons and terminals in the lateral geniculate nucleus of the cat. J Neurosci 4:1809-1829

Gilbert CD (1977) Laminar differences in receptive field properties of cells in cat primary visual cortex. J Physiol (Lond) 268:391-421

Gilbert CD, Wiesel TN (1989) Columnar Specificity of Intrinsic Horizonal and Corticocortical Connections in Cat Visual Cortex. J Neurosci 9/7:2432-2442

Grieve KL, Sillito AM (1990a) The role of feedback from layer VI to IV in the generation of length tuning in the visual cortex of the anaesthetized cat. J Physiol 429:48P

Grieve KL, Sillito AM (1990b) The length summation properties of layer VI cells in the visual cortex and hypercomplex cell end zone inhibition. Exp Brain Res:In press

Grieve KL, Sillito AM (1991) A re-appraisal of the role of layer VI of the visual cortex in the generation of cortical end-inhibition. Exp Brain Res:In press

Halliwell JV, Adams PR (1982) Voltage-clamp analysis of muscarinic excitation in hippocampal neurons. Brain Res 250:71-92

Hammond P (1974) Cat retinal ganglion cells: size and shape of receptive field centres. J Physiol 242:99-118

Harvey AR (1980) A physiological analysis of subcortical and commissural projections of areas 17 and 18 of the cat. J Physiol 302:507-534

Hollander H (1970) The projection from the visual cortex to the lateral geniculate body (LGB). An experimental study with silver impregnation methods in the cat. Exp Brain Res 21:430-440

Hubel DH, Wiesel TN (1961) Integrative activity in the cat's lateral geniculate body. J Physiol 155:385-398

Hubel DH, Wiesel TN (1962) Receptive fields binocular interaction and functional architecture in the cat's visual cortex. J Physiol 160:106-154

Hubel D, Wiesel TN (1965) Receptive fields and functional architecture in two nonstriate visual areas (18 and 19) of the cat. J Neurophysiol 28: 229-289 Hubel D, Wiesel TN (1968) Receptive fields and functional architecture of monkey striate cortex. J Physiol 195:215-243

Johnson JW, Ascher P (1987) Glycine potentiates the NMDA response in cultured mouse brain neurons. Nature 325:529-531

Jones HE, Sillito AM (1987) The length tuning of cells in the feline dorsal lateral geniculate nucleus (dLGN). J Physiol (Lond) 390: 32P

Jones HE, Sillito AM (1991) The length response properties of cells in the feline dorsal lateral geniculate nucleus (dLGN). J Physiol: In press

Jones J, Palmer LA (1987) The two-dimensional spatial structure of simple receptive fields in cat striate cortex. J Neurophysiol 5:86-1187-1211

Kato H, Bishop PO, Orban GA (1978) Hypercomplex and Simple/Complex Cell Classifications in Cat Striate Cortex. J Neurophysiol 14:1071-1095

Kawamura S, Sprague J, Nimi K (1974) Corticofugal projections from the visual cortices to the thalamus, pretectum and superior colliculus in the cat. J Comp Neurol 158:339-362

Kemp JA, Sillito AM (1982) The nature of the excitatory transmitter mediating X and Y cell inputs to the cat dorsal lateral geniculate nucleus. J Physiol 323:377-391

Levick WR, Thibos LN (1980) Orientation Bias of Cat Retinal Ganglion Cells. Nature 286: 389-390

Levick WR, Thibos LN (1982) Analysis of Orientation Bias in Cat Retina. J Physiol 329:243-261

Levy, R.H., Jones, H.E. and Sillito, A.M. (1990) The actions of ionophoretically applied 7-chlorokynurenate and HA-966 on sensory transmission in the dorsal lateral geniculate nucleus (dLGN) of the anaesthetized cat. J Physiol 426:108P

Lindström S, Wróbel A (1990a) Frequency dependent corticofugal excitation of principal cells in the cat's dorsal lateral geniculate nucleus. Exp Brain Res 79:313-318

Lindström S, Wróbel A (1990b) Private inhibitory systems for the X and Y pathways in the dorsal lateral geniculate nucleus of the cat. J Physiol (Lond) 429:259-280

Malpeli JG, Schiller H, Colby C (1981) Response Properties of Single Cells in Monkey Striate Cortex During Reversible Inactivation of Individual Lateral Geniculate Laminae. J Neurophysiol 46:1102-1119

Malpeli JG (1983) Activity of Cells in Area 17 of the Cat in Absence of Input From Layer A of Lateral Geniculate Nucleus. J Neurophysiol 49:595-610

Malpeli JG, Lee C, Schwark HD, Weyand TG (1986) Cat Area 17 I Pattern of Thalamic Control of Cortical Layers. J Neurophysiol 56:1062-1073

Mayer ML, Vyclicky L, Clements J (1989) Regulation of NMDA receptor desensitization in mouse hippocampal neurons by glycine. Nature 338:425-427

McCormick DA, Connors BW, Lighthall JW, Prince DA (1985) Comparative electrophysiology of pyramidal and sparsely spiny stellate neurons of the neocortex. J Neurophysiol 54:782-806

McCormick DA, Prince DA (1985) Two types of muscarinic response to acetylcholine in mammalian cortical neurons. Proc Nat Acad Sci 82:6344-6348

McCormick DA, Prince DA (1987) Actions of acetylcholine in the guinea pig and cat medial and dorsal lateral geniculate nucleus, in vitro. J Physiol 3920:147-165

McCormick DA, Pape HC (1988) Acetylcholine inhibits identified interneurons in the cat lateral geniculate nucleus. Nature 334:246-248

McCormick DA, Prince DA (1990) Pirenzepine discriminates among ionic responses to acetylcholine in guinea-pig cerebral cortex and reticular nucleus of thalamus. TIPS 1986-1986

McGuire BA, Hornung J P, Gilbert CD, Wiesel TN (1984) Patterns of synaptic input to layer 4 of cat striate cortex. J Neurosci 4:3021-3033

Montero VM, (1986) Localization of Y-Aminobutyric Acid (GABA) in Type 3 Cells and Demonstration of Their Source to F2 Terminals in the Cat Lateral Geniculate Nucleus: A Golgi-Electron-Microscopic GABA-Immunocytochemical Study. J Comp Neurol 254:228-245

Montero VM, Singer W (1984) Ultrastructure and Synaptic Relations of Neural Elements Containing Glutamic Acid Decarboxylase (GAD) in the Perigeniculate Nucleus of the Cat. Exp Brain Res 56:115-125

Montero VM, Singer W (1985) Ultrastructural Identification of Somata and Neural Processes Immunoreactive to Antibodies Against Glutamic Acid Decarboxylase (GAD) in the Dorsal Lateral Geniculate Nucleus of the Cat. Exp Brain Res 59:151-165

Montero VM, Zempel J (1985) Evidence for Two Types of GABA-Containing Interneurons in the A-Laminae of the CAt Lateral Geniculate Nucleus: a Double-Label HRP and GABA- Immunocytochemical Study. Exp Brain Res 60:603-609

Montero VM (1987) Ultrastructural Identification of Synaptic Terminals From the Axon of Type 3 Interneurones in the Cat Lateral Geniculate Nucleus. J Comp Neurol 264:268-283

Morrone MC, Burr DC, Maffei L (1982) Functional implications of cross-orientation inhibition of cortical visual cells. I. Neurophysiological evidence. Proc R Soc Lond B216:335-354

Morrone MC, Burr DC (1986) Evidence for the existence and development of visual inhibition in humans. Nature 321:235-237

Murphy PC, Sillito AM (1987) Corticofugal feedback influences the generation of length tuning in the visual pathway. Nature 329(6141):727-729

Murphy PC, Sillito AM (1989) The binocular input to cells in the feline dorsal lateral geniculate nucleus. J Physiol (Lond) 415:393-409

Murphy PC, Sillito AM (1990) Cholinergic enhancement of direction selectivity in the visual cortex of the Cat. Neuroscience. 40:13-20.

Orban GA, Kato H, Bishop PO (1979a) End-Zone Region in Receptive Fields of Hypercomplex and Other Striate Neurons in the Cat. J Neurophysiol 42:818-832

Orban GA, Kato H, Bishop PO (1979b) Dimensions and Properties of End-Zone Inhibitory Areas in Receptive Fields of Hypercomplex Cells in Cat Striate Cortex. J Neurophysiol 42:833-849

Ramoa AS, Shadlen M, Skottun BC, Freeman RD (1986) A comparison of inhibition in orientation and spatial frequency selectivity of cat visual cortex. Nature 321:237-239

Rapisardi SC, Miles TP (1984) Synaptology of retinal terminals in the dorsal lateral geniculate nucleus of the cat. J Comp Neurol 223:515-534.

Rose D (1979) Mechanisms Underlying the Receptive Field Properties of Neurons in Cat Visual Cortex. Vision Res 19:533-544

Salt TE, Sillito AM (1989) The NMDA-receptor mediated component of the visual response of cells in the feline dorsal lateral geniculate nucleus (dLGN) in the absence of corticofugal feedback. J Physiol 418:108P

Schiller PH, Finlay BL, Volman S (1976) Quantitative studies of single-cell properties in monkey striate cortex I Spatiotemporal organization of receptive fields. J Neurophysiol 39:1288-1319

Schwark HD, Malpeli JG, Weyand TG, Lee C (1986) Cat Area 17 II Response Properties of Infragranular Layer Neurons in the Absence of Supragranular Layer Activity. J Neurophysiol 56:1074-1087

Shou T, Zhou Y (1986) The orientation bias of LGN neurons shows topographic relation to area centralis in the cat retina. Exp Brain Res 64:233-236

Sillito AM (1974) The effectiveness of bicuculline as an antagonist of GABA and visually evoked inhibition in the cat's striate cortex. J Physiol 250:287-304

Sillito AM (1975a). The effectiveness of bicuculline as an antagonist of GABA and visually evoked inhibition in the cat's striate cortex. J Physiol (Lond) 250:287-304

Sillito AM (1975b) The contribution of inhibitory mechanisms to the receptive field properties of neurones in the striate cortex of the cat. J Physiol (Lond) 250:305-329

Sillito AM (1977a) The spatial extent of excitatory and inhibitory zones in the receptive field of superficial layer hypercomplex cells. J Physiol (Lond) 273:791-803

Sillito AM (1977b) Inhibitory processes underlying the directional specificity of simple complex and hypercomplex cells in the cat's visual cortex. J Physiol 271:699-720

Sillito AM, Versiani V (1977) The contribution of excitatory and inhibitory inputs to the length preference of hypercomplex cells in layers II and III of the cat's striate cortex. J Physiol (Lond) 273:775-790

Sillito AM (1979) Inhibitory Mechanisms Influencing Complex Cell Orientation Selectivity and Their Modification At High Resting Discharge Levels. J Physiol 289:33-53

Sillito AM, Kemp JA, Milson JA, Berardi N (1980) A re-evaluation of the mechanisms underlying simple cell orientation selectivity. Brain Res 194:517-520

Sillito AM, Kemp JA, Berardi N (1983) The cholinergic influence on the function of the cat dorsal lateral geniculate nucleus (dLGN). Brain Res 280:299-307

Sillito AM, Kemp JA (1983) The influence of GABAergic inhibitory processes on the receptive field structure of X and Y cells in the cat dorsal lateral geniculate nucleus (dLGN). Brain Res 277:63-77

Sillito AM (1984) Functional considerations of the operation of GABAergic inhibitory processes in the visual cortex. Cerebral Cortex 2A:91-172

Sillito AM, Murphy PC (1988). GABAergic processes in the central visual system. In: Avioli M, Reader TA, Dykes RW, Gloor P (eds) Neurotransmitters and cortical function. Plenum Publishing Corporation, pp 167-185

Sillito AM, Murphy PC, Moody I (1988). The Modulation of the Retinal Relay to the Cortex in the Dorsal Lateral Geniculate Nucleus. Eye Suppl. 2:221-232

Sillito AM, Murphy PC, Salt TE (1990a) The contribution of the non-N-methyl-D-aspartate group of excitatory amino acid receptors to retinogeniculate transmission in the cat. Neuroscience 34:273-280

Sillito AM, Murphy PC, Salt TE, Moody CI (1990b) Dependence of retinogeniculate transmission in cat on NMDA receptors. J Neurophysiol 63:347-355

Sillito AM, Murphy PC, Cudeiro J (1991) Orientation domain substructure to centre surround interactions in the dorsal lateral geniculate nucleus (dLGN) of the anaesthetized cat. J Physiol

Singer W, Creutzfeldt OD (1970) Reciprocal Lateral Inhibition of On- and Off-Center Neurones in the Lateral Geniculate Body of the Cat. Exp Brain Res 10:311-330

Singer W, Poppel E, Creutzfeldt OD (1972) Inhibitory interaction in the cat's lateral geniculate nucleus. Exp Brain Res 14:210-226

Somogyi P (1989) Synaptic organisation of GABAergic neurons and $GABA_A$ receptors in the lateral geniculate nucleus and visual cortex. In: Lam DKT, Gilbert CD (eds) Neural Mechanisms of Visual Perception. Neural mech Portfolio Pub Co: pp 35-62

Soodak RE, Shapley R, Kaplan E (1987) Linear Mechanism of Orientation Tuning in the Retina and Lateral Geniculate Nucleus of the Cat. J Neurophysiol 58:267-275

Sterling P, Davis TL (1980) Neurons in cat lateral geniculate nucleus that concentrate exogenous[3H]-y-aminobutyric acid(Gaba). J Comp Neurol 192:737-749

Thompson AM, Walker VE, Flyn DM (1989) Glycine enhances NMDA receptor mediated synaptic potentials in neocortical slices. Nature 338:422-424.

Ts'o DY, Gilbert CD, Wiesel TN (1986) Relations Between Horizontal Interactions and Functional Architecture in Cat Striate Cortex as Revealed by Cross-Correlation Analysis. J Neurosci 6:1160-1170

Tsumoto T, Eckart W, Creutzfeldt OD (1979) Modification of Orientation Sensitivity of Cat Visual Cortex Neurons by Removal of GABA-Mediated Inhibition. Exp Brain Res 34:351-363

Tsumoto T, Suda K (1980) Three Groups of Cortico-Geniculate Neurons and Their Distribution in Binocular and Monocular Segments of Cat Striate Cortex. J Comp Neurol 193:223-236

Updyke BV (1975) The patterns of projection of cortical areas 17, 18 and 19 onto the laminae of the dorsal lateral geniculate nucleus in the cat. J Comp Neurol 163:377-396

Vidyasagar TR (1984) Contribution of Inhibitory Mechanisms to the orientation sensitivity of cat dLGN neurones. Exp Brain Res 55:192-195

Weber AJ, Kalil RE, Behan M (1989) Synaptic Connections Between Corticogeniculate Axons and Interneurons in the Dorsal Lateral Geniculate Nucleus of the Cat. J Comp Neurol 289:156-164

Wörgötter F, Eysel UT (1989) Axis of Preferred Motion is a Function of Bar Length in Visual Cortical Receptive Fields. Exp Brain Res

Yamane S, Maske R, Bishop PO (1985) Properties of end-zone inhibition of hypercomplex cells in cat striate cortex. Exp Brain Res 60:200-203

Microcircuitry of Cat Visual Cortex

Jürgen Bolz, Mark Hübener, and Cornelius Schwarz

Friedrich-Miescher-Labor der Max-Planck-Gesellschaft, Spemannstr. 37-39, 7400 Tübingen, Germany

Cells in the primary visual cortex operate on the signals coming from the retina and analyze different attributes of the visual scene. To do this, cortical cells have a number of specialized receptive field properties that allow them to respond selectively to the orientation, shape, color or movement of the visual stimulus. Because cortical neurons have more complex functional features than their input cells, many of these properties must be generated within the cortex. Therefore, knowledge of intrinsic cortical connections is a basic prerequisite for understanding the neural mechanisms by which the visual cortex analyses sensory information.

Anatomical investigations have revealed a series of regular connections running perpendicular to the cortical surface, between the cortical layers (Ramón y Cajal 1921; Lorente de Nó 1933; Gilbert and Wiesel 1979; Lund et al. 1979; Martin and Whitteridge 1984). These interlaminar connections form the structural basis of the columnar organization of the cortex. Within a column running from the pia to the white matter, all cells have common functional properties, such as orientation specificity (Hubel and Wiesel 1962). In addition to the pattern of interlaminar connections, a portion of cortical cells have axons that run over long distances parallel to the cortical surface (Rockland et al. 1982; Gilbert and Wiesel 1983; Martin and Whitteridge 1984; Hübener et al. 1990). These horizontal connections have a characteristic pattern of clustered axon collaterals and interconnect cells in different cortical columns.

In this paper we will consider the interrelationships between the functional properties of cortical cells and the internal circuitry of the cortex. One example that will be discussed in detail here is a particular component of the cortical circuitry, the interlaminar connection from layer 5 to layer 6. We will first review our anatomical studies that revealed a population of layer 5 pyramidal cells, which have axon collaterals projecting over long horizontal distances into layer 6. We then describe two approaches that attempted to relate a functional role to this distinct cortical connection. The first, a pharmacological technique, was used for the microdissection of the cortical circuit, and in the other a cross-correlation analysis was used to examine the interaction between source and target cells of this interlaminar connection. Our experiments demonstrate that connections of particular cell classes in the cortex have very specific roles in generating functional properties in their target cells.

Morphological types of pyramidal cells in layer 5

The laminar organization of the cortex provides a basic framework for anatomical and physiological studies of the cortical circuit. When viewed in Nissl stained sections, cells in different cortical layers have a characteristic size, morphology and packing density. Cells in different layers receive different afferent input and they usually project to different areas of the brain. Moreover, physiological studies demonstrated that cells within the same layer share receptive field properties and that the functional properties of cortical cells differ across layers. However, along with their common properties, neurons within each layer also exhibit morphological and physiological differences. For example, in layer 5 there are two functional classes of neurons with different length summation characteristics: special complex cells that respond best to a small stimulus placed anywhere within the receptive field, and standard complex cells that respond best to stimuli that are as long as the receptive field (Palmer and Rosenquist 1974; Gilbert 1977).

Both types of complex cells encountered in layer 5, special complex cells and standard complex cells, project to the superior colliculus, the main target of layer 5 (Harvey 1980; Ferster and Lindström 1985; Weyand et al. 1986). Thus, although both cell types are located within a single cortical layer and project to a common target, they are dissimilar with respect to their length summation properties. We examined whether the functional heterogeneity of corticotectal cells is reflected in the morphology of these cells. For this we injected retrograde

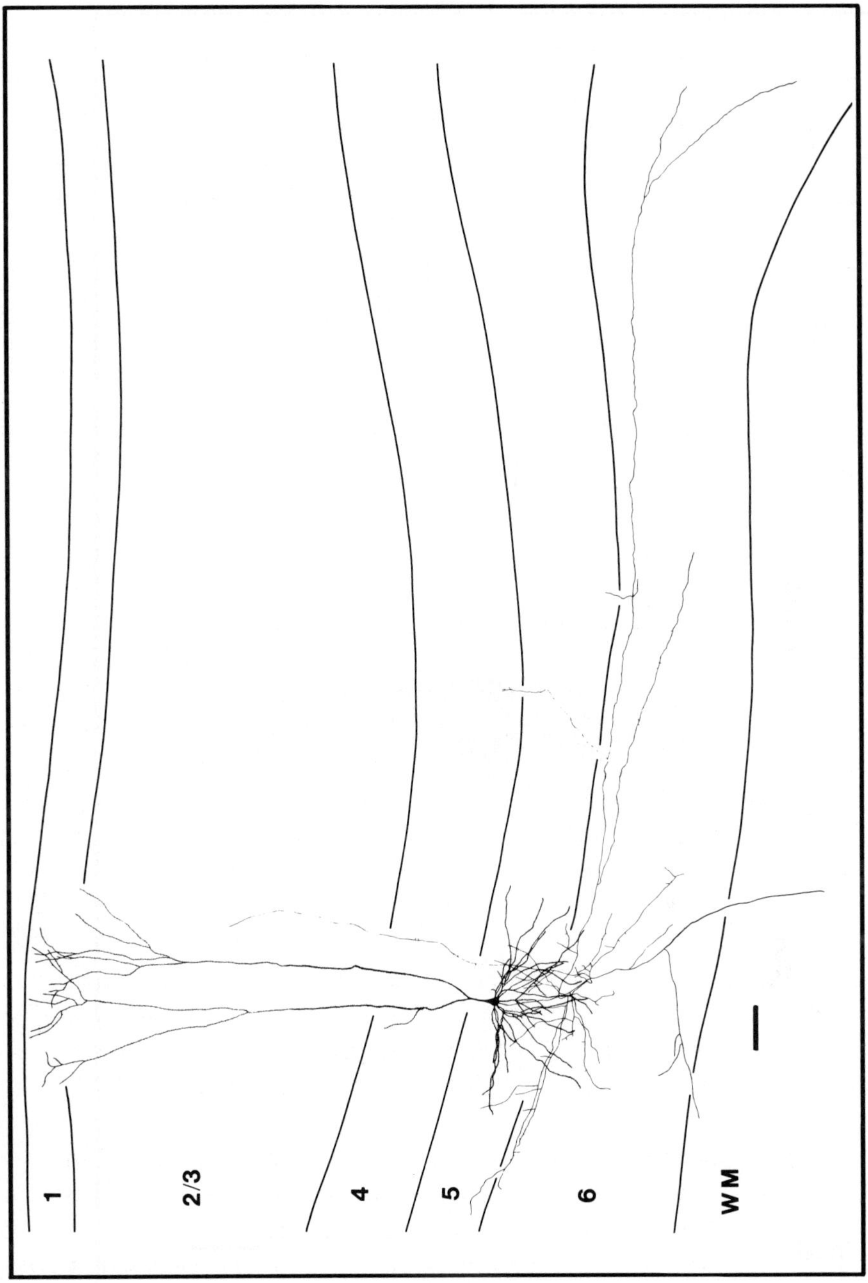

Fig. 1. Drawing of a spiny corticotectal cell. The cell was retrogradely labelled from the superior colliculus and intracellularly stained in a living brain slice. Note the axon collaterals of the cell that run over long distances in layer 6. Scale bar: 100 mm

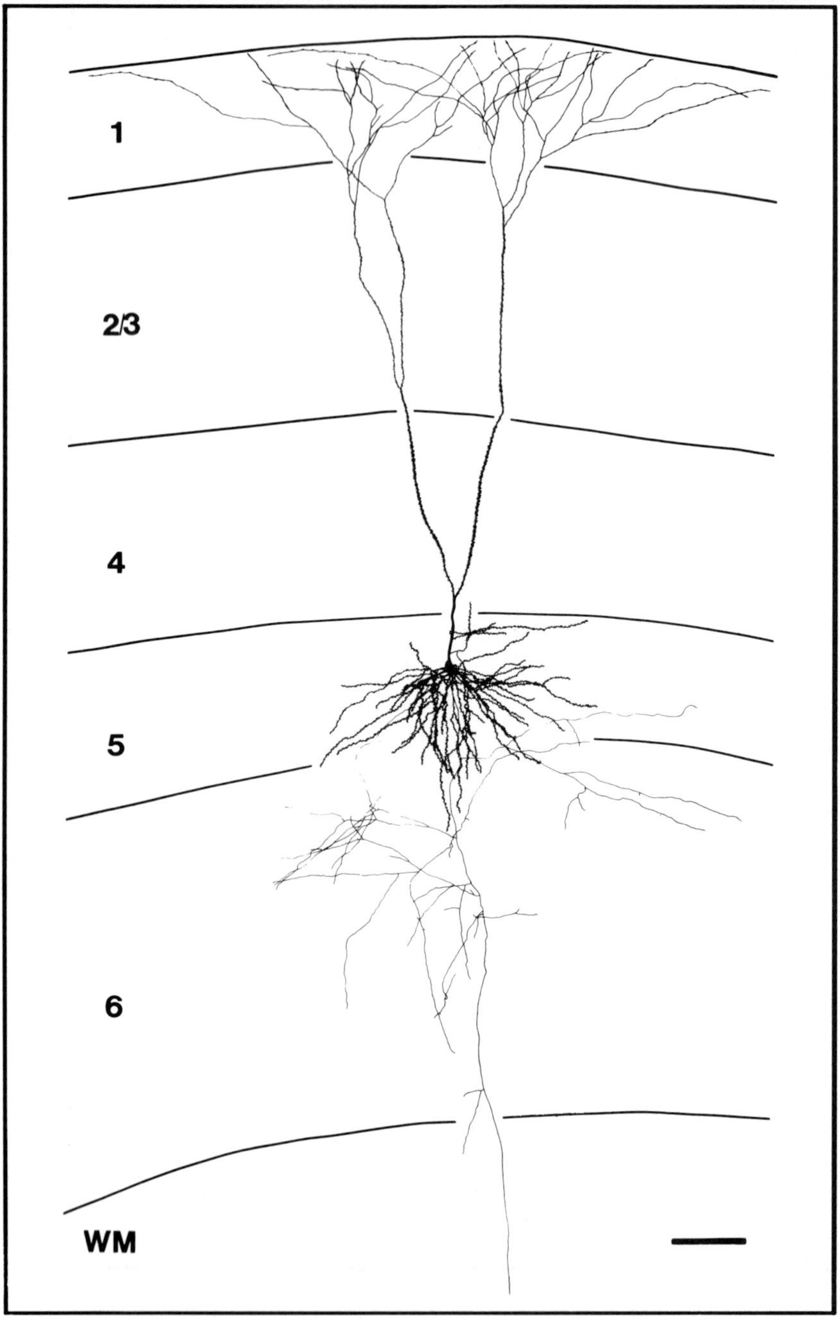

Fig. 2. Spiny corticotectal cell. The efferent axon gives rise to many axon collaterals, most of which are confined to layer 6. Scale bar: 100 mm

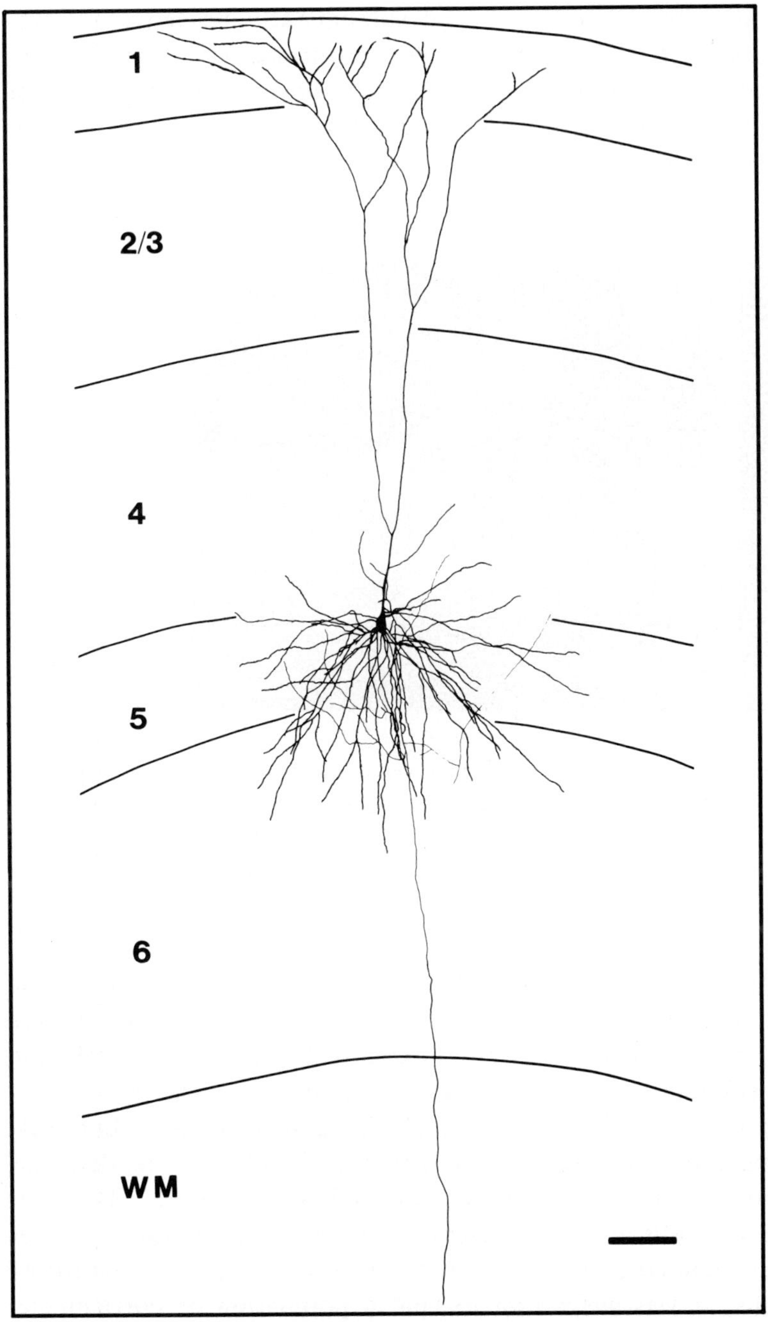

Fig. 3. 'Spinefree' corticotectal cell. The dendritic branching pattern of the cell is similar to spiny corticotectal cells, but the dendrites have extremely few spines. Note that the axon collaterals of the cell do not project into layer 6. Scale bar: 100 mm

tracers into the superior colliculus and subsequently stained individual corticotectal cells in living brain slices intracellularly with Lucifer yellow (Hübener et al. 1990). This approach allows a detailed view of the dendritic branching pattern and local axon collaterals of neurons with identified projection targets.

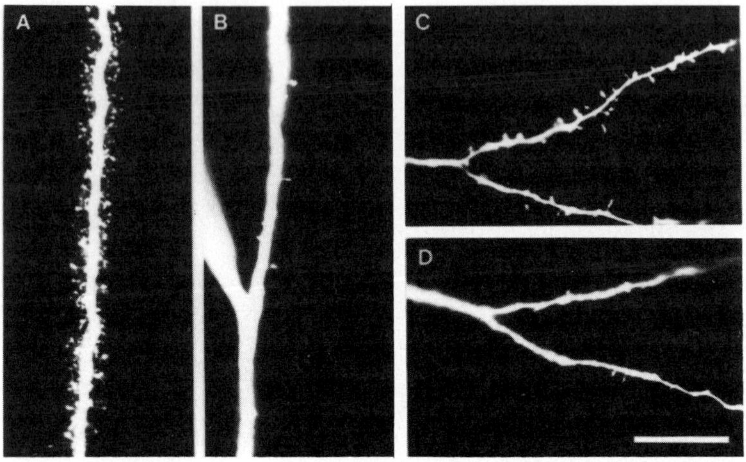

Fig. 4. High-power micrograph of dendrites from corticotectal cells. A, apical dendrite of a spiny and B, of a 'spinefree' corticotectal cell. C, basal dendrites of a spiny and D, of a 'spinefree' corticotectal cell. The dendrites of spiny corticotectal cells are densely covered with spines, the spine density on the dendrites of 'spinefree' corticotectal cells is extremely low. Scale bar: 20 μm

Using this technique we found that corticotectal cells have the characteristic morphology of pyramidal cells (Figs. 1-3). All cells have a prominent apical dendrite, which extends through the overlaying layers and terminates in a very large tuft in layer 1. The basal dendrites branch frequently, they form a dense basal dendritic arbor, that is always smaller than the apical tuft. The apical and basal dendrites of most corticotectal cells are densely covered with spines. However, about 10% of the cells are almost completely devoid of dendritic spines (Fig. 4). Since dendritic spines are considered as a general feature of pyramidal cells, it was surprising to find a population of corticotectal cells that possess almost no spines. It is hard to give a figure for the spine density of these cells, since long portions of their dendrites exhibit no spines at all. For one 'spinefree' corticotectal cell we counted

29 spines, compared to an estimated 10,000 to 20,000 spines on spiny corticotectal cells. The reduction in spine number is always accompanied by other characteristic morphological features. 'Spinefree' corticotectal cells have a larger cell body size and a larger basal dendritic tree than spiny corticotectal cells. There are also differences in their intrinsic axonal arborization. 'Spinefree' cells have only very few axon collaterals that are usually confined to layer 5 (Fig. 3). On the other hand, spiny corticotectal cells exhibit many axon collaterals that arborize extensively in layer 6, and some of these axon collaterals can travel over long distances in this layer (Figs. 1 and 2).

Spinefree pyramidal cells: speculations about their function

The majority of all synaptic contacts on pyramidal cells are made on spines (Colonnier 1968). The pattern of synaptic contacts on 'spinefree' pyramidal cells is therefore very different from the majority of pyramidal cells, and one would assume this to have consequences on how the synaptic input is integrated by these cells. The depolarization at the cell body after an excitatory synaptic input on the spines depends critically on the electrical resistance of the spines and therefore on the geometrical dimensions of the spines. Theoretical studies demonstrated that the shorter and wider the spine neck, the larger the depolarization at the soma and thus at the site of spike initiation (Rall and Segev 1987). Of course, the strongest depolarization would occur if there is no spine at all. Thus, compared to spiny corticotectal cells, a smaller number of active input fibers is sufficient to fire a 'spinefree' corticotectal cell.

One might speculate that the differences in spine density could be related to the different physiological classes of corticotectal cells. One of the principal inputs to layer 5 is the projection from the superficial layers (Gilbert and Wiesel 1979; Martin and Whitteridge 1984). Since the receptive fields of layer 5 cells are much larger than those in the superficial layers, one would expect that cells in layer 5 receive their input from many cells in the superficial layers with spatially displaced receptive fields. As discussed above, a smaller number of presynaptic cells is required to drive a 'spinefree' cell. Thus a short bar stimulating only a few superficial cells might suffice to vigorously drive 'spinefree' corticotectal cells. These cells might therefore posses the receptive field properties of special complex cells, which respond as well to a short bar as to a bar that extends over the full width of the receptive field. On the other hand, a long bar stimulating many superficial cells might be needed to elicit an optimal response in spiny cells, therefore these cells might exhibit the length summation properties of standard complex cells. At least in principle, such a scheme could account for the different receptive field properties of special and standard complex cells in layer 5. Thus one has to consider both the connectivity and the biophysical properties of cortical neurons in order to understand the mechanisms by which receptive field features are generated in the cortex.

If our speculation is correct, that spiny and 'spinefree' corticotectal cells correspond to standard complex cells and special complex cells respectively, then these two classes of complex cells would participate in different intrinsic cortical circuits, since spiny, and not 'spinefree' corticotectal cells have axon collaterals that project heavily into layer 6. One might then expect that layer 6 cells receive their layer 5 input predominantly from standard complex cells. As will be described below, this is consistent with the results from our cross-correlation experiments which suggest that in layer 5 mainly standard complex cells, but very few special complex cells, are interconnected with layer 6 cells.

Pharmacological analysis of cortical circuitry

The findings described in the previous sections showed that a population of pyramidal cells in layer 5 have axon collaterals that can extend for several millimeters in layer 6. A characteristic feature of cells in layer 6 are their long receptive fields (Gilbert 1977). In order to generate these fields, it is necessary to integrate input over a wide area of the cortex, since cells in all other cortical layers have much smaller receptive fields. The interlaminar connection from layer 5 to layer 6 is suitable for performing this function, since this long-ranging projection enables layer 6 cells to obtain input from regions of cortex representing large parts of the visual field. To test this idea, we inactivated layer 5 locally and recorded activity from layer 6 cells displaced horizontally from the inactivated area (Bolz and Gilbert 1989; Bolz et al. 1989). This experimental approach is shown schematically in Fig. 5: We recorded from a cell in layer 6 and inserted a second recording electrode in a glass micropipette into layer 5, 1-3 mm horizontally displaced from the electrode in layer 6. The micropipette contained the inhibitory transmitter GABA, which could be injected by pressure. Since GABA inhibits all cell types in the cortex, we were able to completely block the activity of layer 5 cells in a restricted area about 600 μm in diameter. The inactivation by GABA is reversible, it is therefore possible to examine the response properties of layer 6 cells before, during, and after inactivation of layer 5.

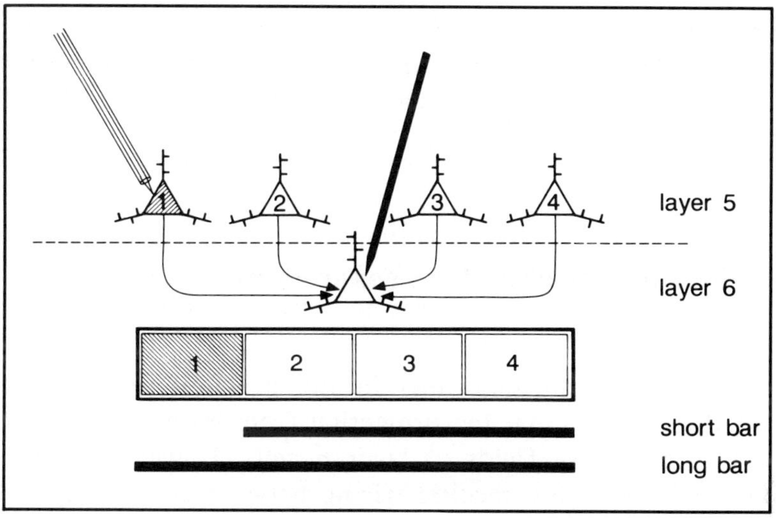

Fig. 5. Schematic diagram indicating the functional role of the layer 5 to layer 6 projection. The layer 5 neurons have long axon collaterals in layer 6. This allows their target cells in layer 6 to integrate input over an extensive region of the cortex, representing a large visual field area. By concatenating the receptive fields of a number of layer 5 cells (small rectangles), long receptive fields are generated in layer 6 (bold outline). This model was tested by focal inactivation of a restricted region of layer 5. An electrode within a GABA pipette recorded the activity of neuron 1 in layer 5 (left). A second electrode (center), horizontally displaced from the GABA pipette, monitored the activity of the layer 6 cell. The layer 6 cell responded better to a long bar stimulating the full receptive field than to a short bar, which does not cover the receptive field of neuron 1. When neuron 1 was inactivated by GABA (indicated by shading), the responses to the long and short bar were equivalent. Each of the layer 5 cells drawn in the diagram represents a cluster of cells with similar functional properties, such that a number of layer 5 cells with overlapping receptive fields provide input to the layer 6 cell

Figure 6 shows response histograms of a layer 6 complex cell. As is characteristic of cells in this layer, the response to a 10° long bar was greater than the response to a 7° long bar. A second electrode within the GABA pipette recorded the activity of a cell in layer 5. The receptive field of the layer 5 cell overlapped with the distal portion of the layer 6 cell receptive field. The long bar stimulus covered the receptive field of the layer 5 cell, and the short bar excluded it. When GABA was injected from the pipette in layer 5, the short bar was unaffected. However the long bar response of the layer 6 cell was reduced, reaching the level of the short bar response. When the activity returned at the injection site in layer 5, the long bar response recovered to its original level. This confirmed the idea that layer 5 cells at the injection site provided the input for the layer 6 cell. Similar effects were seen with layer 6 simple cells. In some cases, after the cells' long bar response recovered, the GABA pipette was advanced from layer 5 into layer 6. At this location GABA injections had no effect on the response of layer 6 cells.

Cross-correlation analysis of cortical connections

The inactivation experiments described in the previous sections are consistent with the proposal that the projection from layer 5 to layer 6 generates the long receptive fields of layer 6 cells. However, such a scheme would require a highly specific wiring between cells in layer 5 and layer 6: layer 5 cells would have to project to layer 6 cells with matching orientation preference and visuotopically aligned receptive fields. With the inactivation method, it is difficult to characterize the presynaptic site of a cortical connection, since all neurons within a region of layer 5 are silenced. We therefore recorded simultaneously from individual neurons in layer 5 and layer 6 and used cross-correlation analysis to study the interaction between source and target cells of this interlaminar connection (Schwarz and Bolz 1991). Cross-correlation analysis is a statistical technique, it compares the firing pattern of two cells and gives an estimate of the probability that one cell fires a spike, given that there is a spike in the second cell. A plot of the frequency of coincident firing as a function of the time delay between the spikes of the two cells is called a cross-correlogram. Figure 7

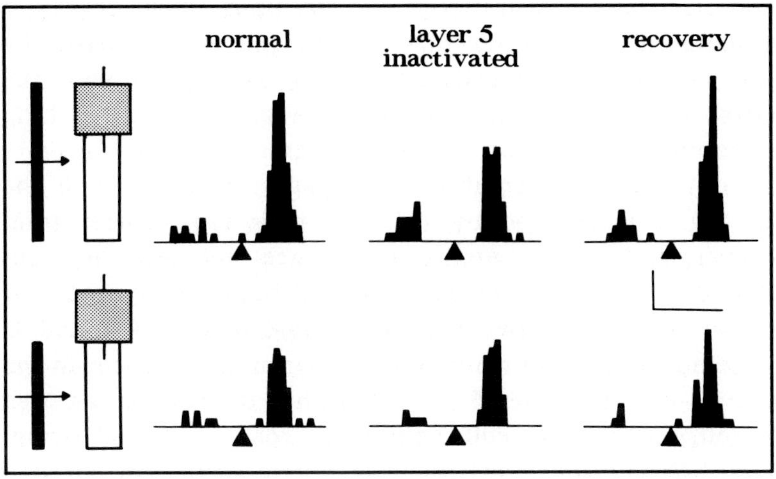

Fig. 6. Effect of local inactivation of layer 5 on a cell in layer 6. The receptive field of the cell recorded with the GABA pipette in layer 5 (shaded rectangles on the left) covered the receptive field of the cell recorded in layer 6 (open rectangles). Response histograms were made for a 10° long bar covering the full length of the receptive field of the layer 6 cell (upper histograms), and for a bar shortened to 7°, excluding the receptive field of the layer 5 cell (lower histograms). The bar stimuli moved backwards and forwards through the receptive fields, the triangles under each histogram indicate the points were the bars changed direction. Before layer 5 inactivation, the response of the layer 5 cell was greater to the long bar than to the short bar that did not stimulate the layer 5 cells near the GABA injection site (left histograms). During local inactivation of layer 5 the long and short bar responses were virtually identical (middle histograms). When the activity returned to layer 5, the layer 6 cell regained its initial length summation characteristics (right histograms). Calibration: vertical mark, 5 spikes per bin; horizontal mark, 1 sec

shows examples of cross-correlograms obtained from different cell pairs, each with one cell in layer 5 and one cell in layer 6. The cross-correlograms on the right are flat, in these cases the cells in layer 5 and layer 6 were firing independently. The correlograms on the left show a peak, indicating that the cells in each pair were connected or received common input from other cells.

Using the cross-correlation technique, we looked to see if there is a relationship in the functional properties of the cells in layer 5 and layer 6 that showed correlated firing. We found that the occurrence of correlated firing depended on the functional properties and on the topographic position of the cells. This is illustrated in Fig. 7. Each layer 5 cell and each layer 6 cell of the two cell pairs shown in Fig. 7 A and B had standard complex receptive fields, and in both pairs the receptive fields of the layer 5 cells completely overlapped with the receptive field of the layer 6 cell. The cells in Fig. 7 A had matching orientation preferences, and their cross-correlogram showed a prominent peak. In contrast, the orientation preferences of the cells in the pair shown in Fig. 7 B differed by 74°, and their cross-correlogram was flat. However, matched orientation preference is a necessary, but not a sufficient condition for correlated firing between layer 5 and layer 6 cells. The cells in the two pairs illustrated in Fig. 7 C and D were standard complex and had matching orientation preference. In the pair shown in Fig. 7 C, the layer 5 cell lay within the summation area of the layer 6 cell, and the two cells exhibited strong correlated firing. The pair in Fig. 7 D had non-overlapping receptive fields, and no sign of correlated firing could be detected in the cross-correlogram. Finally, the occurrence of correlated firing between the layer 5 and layer 6 cells also depended on the receptive field type of the layer 5 cells, that is, whether the layer 5 cell was a standard or a special complex cell. The two cell pairs in Fig. 7 E and F had overlapping receptive fields and similar orientation preference, but the layer 5 cell in one pair (Fig. 7 E) was standard complex, and in the other pair special complex (Fig. 7 F). Only the standard complex cell, and not the special complex cell showed correlated firing with the layer 6 cell.

While the type of the receptive field of layer 5 cells appeared to be critical for the correlated firing, this was not the case for layer 6 neurons. We found that both simple and complex cells in layer 6 fired coherently with neurons in layer 5. A layer 6 simple cell firing in synchrony with a standard complex cell is shown in Fig. 8. In addition, these examples illustrate that the occurrence of coherent firing between layer 5 and layer 6 neurons did not depend on the stimulus patterns which were used to activate the cells.

Our cross-correlation analysis revealed the rules for the occurrence of peaked correlograms between cells in layer 5 and layer 6. Interactions were only observed if the cells had matching orientation preference and if the layer 5 cells lay within the summation area of the layer 6 cells. Moreover, in layer 5 mainly standard complex cells, but very few special complex cells, participated in correlated firing with layer 6 cells. This suggests that cells in layer 6 receive their input from cooriented, coaxially aligned standard complex cells in layer 5. These topographic arrangements and the length summation properties

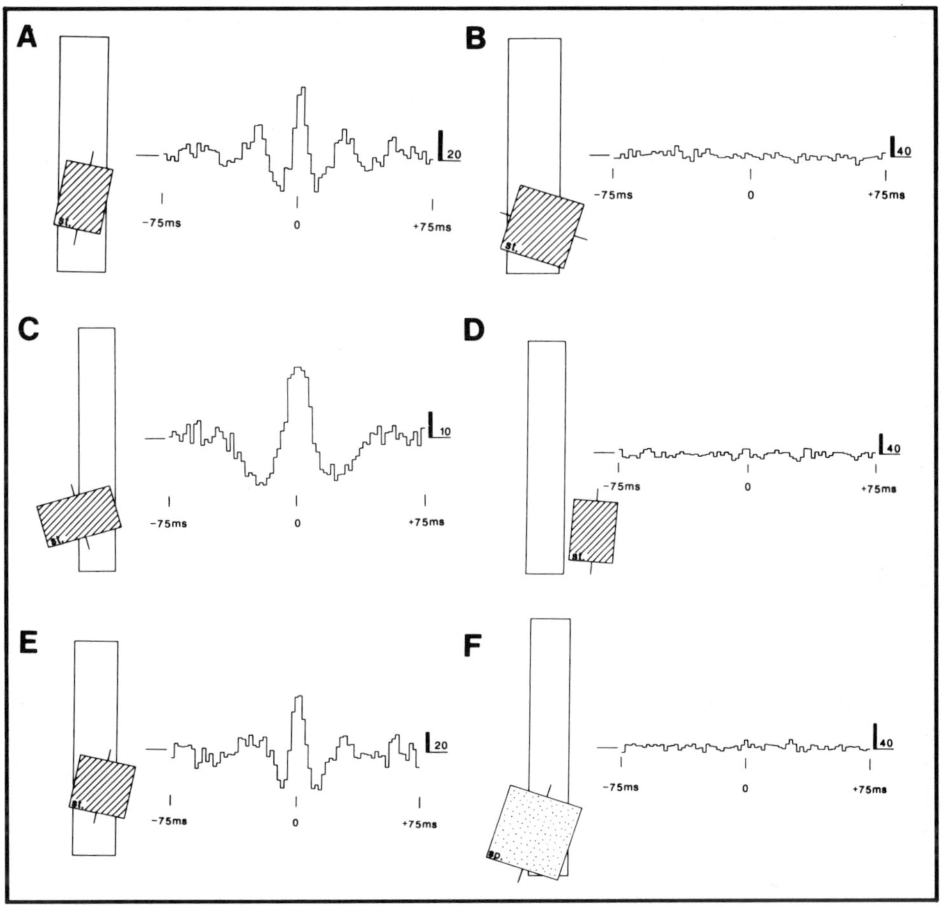

Fig. 7. Cross-correlograms between layer 5 and layer 6 cells illustrating the dependency of coherent firing on matching orientation preference (A, B), on receptive field topography (C, D), and on receptive field type of the layer 5 cell (E, F). The orientation preferences of the layer 5 cells are indicated by the small lines at the rectangles representing the receptive fields (hatched rectangles: standard complex cells; dotted rectangle: special complex cell). For simplification, the receptive fields were always drawn such that the receptive fields of the layer 6 cells (open rectangles) were vertically oriented. Peaked correlograms were only observed (i) if the cells had matching orientation tuning, (ii) if the cells had overlapping receptive fields, and (iii) if the layer 5 cell was a standard complex cell. Calibration: bin-width, 2.1 msec; vertical scale bars indicate number of counts

of standard complex cells are well suited to generate long receptive fields in layer 6.

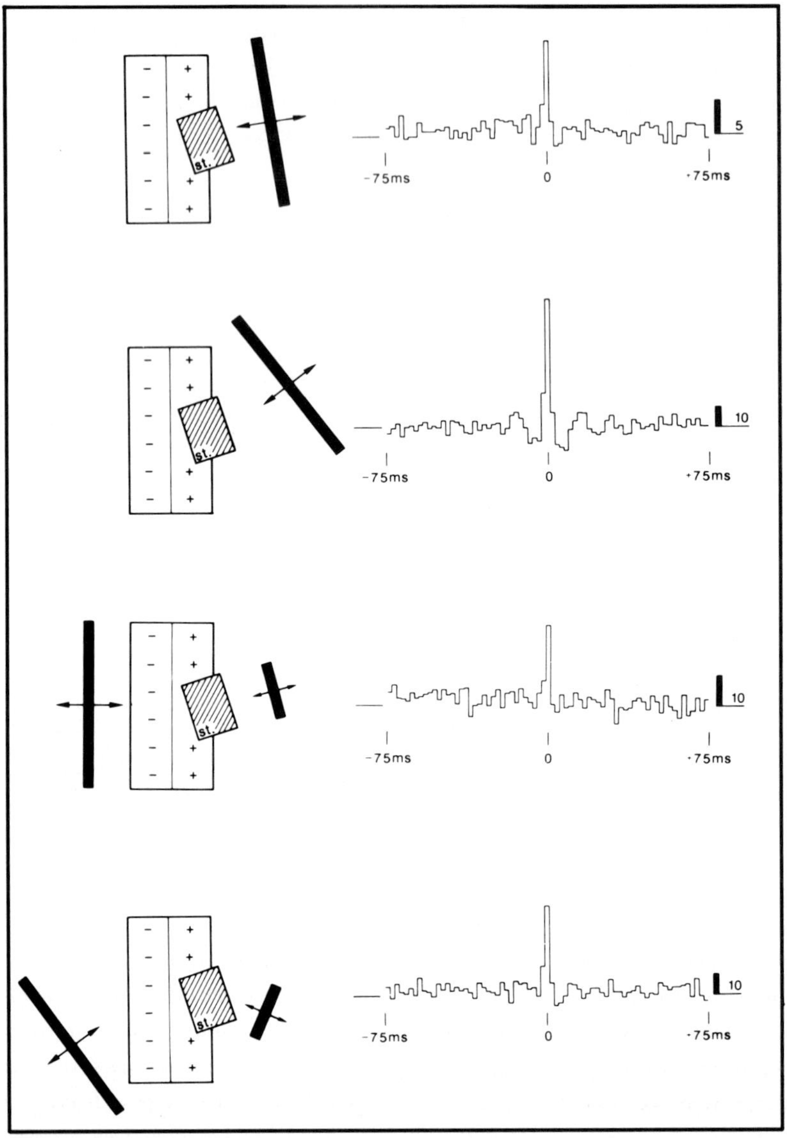

Fig. 8. Peaked correlograms between a standard complex cell in layer 5 and a simple cell in layer 6 with overlapping receptive fields and slightly different orientation preference. Because of the low spontaneous firing rate of cortical neurons, the cells were visually stimulated in order to collect enough spikes to calculate a cross-correlogram. In this case optimal and suboptimal oriented stimuli were applied, using either one or two bars. The increase in the firing rate of the cells in response to these stimuli produced broad peaks in the correlograms. In the correlograms displayed here and in

All cross-correlograms between layer 5 and layer 6 cells that showed any sign of interactions had peaks symmetrical around the zero bin, indicating that the two neurons fired at about the same time. Such correlograms are interpreted to reflect common synaptic input from other neurons (Perkel et al. 1967; Moore et al. 1970). How is this consistent with the idea that the interlaminar projection from layer 5 to layer 6 accounts for the correlated firing of the cells? The anatomical studies have shown that cells in layer 5 have axon collaterals near their own dendritic tree, which allows these cells to contact many other cells in their immediate vicinity. Indeed, electrical stimulation experiments demonstrated that neighboring cells in layer 5 are synaptically connected (Thalluri and Henry 1989). One might therefore expect from such a highly interconnected system, that the contribution of an individual cell to the response of their postsynaptic neurons is rather weak. Thus, even if the cell recorded in layer 5 directly contacts the cell recorded in layer 6, this monosynaptic connection would be occluded by the vast common input from many other layer 5 cells. This explains why all peaks in the correlograms were symmetrical around the zero bin. However, if the correlated firing between two single cells reflects the influence of so many other neurons, then why is the occurrence of correlated firing related to the functional features of only these two neurons? The columnar and topographic organization of the cortex implies that neighboring cells have similar orientation properties and overlapping receptive fields (Hubel and Wiesel 1974). We found another example for this characteristic organizing principle of the cortex, the grouping of functionally related neurons. As illustrated in Fig. 9, standard and special complex cells have a clustered distribution in layer 5. Therefore, if the common input arises from a group of adjacent, highly interconnected cells in layer 5, then these cells have similar orientation preference, similar length summation characteristics and overlapping receptive fields. Thus it might not be unexpected to find relationships between these properties and shared input correlations.

Fig. 7, this stimulus coordination artifact was eliminated using published procedures (Perkel et al. 1967). Under all stimulus conditions used, the central peak in the corrected correlograms remained stable

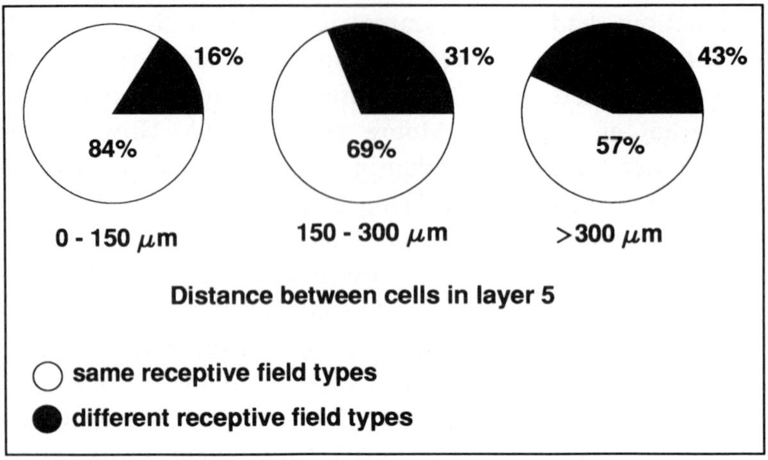

Fig. 9. Clustering of standard and special complex cells in layer 5. The plot shows the probability of two consecutively recorded cells having the same or different receptive field types for various distances between the cells

Concluding remarks

In order to understand the neuronal mechanisms of information processing in the visual cortex, one has to consider both the connectivity and the functional properties of cortical neurons. Here we presented an example of an association between a particular cortical connection and a specific receptive field property. Our experiments suggest that different functional classes of cells participate in different intrinsic connections and have very specific roles in generating functional properties in their target cells. The neuronal interactions observed in the cortex are between groups of cells, rather than between single pre- and postsynaptic cells. This implies that the interrelationships between the cortical circuit and the functional architecture (the spatial distribution of cells with similar functional specificities) are responsible for the functional role of cortical connections. Because of the stereotyped nature of the cortical architecture and the intrinsic cortical connections, it may be possible to generalize the findings in primary visual cortex to other cortical areas serving other functional modalities.

References

Bolz J, Gilbert CD (1989) The role of horizontal connections in generating long receptive fields in the cat visual cortex. Europ J Neurosci 1:263-268

Bolz J, Gilbert CD, Wiesel TN (1989) Pharmacological analysis of cortical circuitry. TINS 12:292-296

Colonnier M, (1968) Synaptic patterns on different cell types in the different laminae of the cat visual cortex. Brain Res. 9:268-287

Ferster D, Lindström S (1985) Synaptic excitation of neurons in area 17 of the cat by intracortical axon collaterals of cortico-geniculate cells. J Physiol 367:233-252

Gilbert CD, (1977) Laminar differences in receptive field properties in cat primary visual cortex. J Physiol 268:391-421

Gilbert CD, Wiesel TN (1979) Morphology and intracortical projections of functionally characterised neurones in the cat visual cortex. Nature 280:120-125

Gilbert CD, Wiesel TN (1983) Clustered intrinsic connections in cat visual cortex. J Neurosci 3:1116-1133

Harvey AR (1980) A physiological analysis of subcortical and commissural projections of areas 17 and 18 of the cat. J Physiol 302:507-534

Hubel DH, Wiesel TN (1962) Receptive fields, binocular interaction and functional architecture in the cat's visual cortex. J Physiol 160:106-154

Hubel DH, Wiesel TN (1974) Sequence regularity and geometry of orientation columns in the monkey striate cortex. J Comp Neurol 158:267-294

Hübener M, Schwarz C, Bolz J (1990) Morphological types of projection neurons in layer 5 of cat visual cortex. J Comp Neurol 301:655-674

Lorente de Nó R (1933) Studies on the structure of the cerebral cortex. J Psychol Neur 45:382-438

Lund JS, Henry GH, Macqueen CL, Harvey AR (1979) Anatomical organization of the primary visual cortex (area 17) of the cat. A comparison with area 17 of the macaque monkey. J Comp Neurol 184:599-618

Martin KAC, Whitteridge D (1984) Form, function and intracortical projections of spiny neurons in the striate cortex of the cat. J Physiol 353:463-504

Moore GP, Perkel DH, Segundo JP (1970) Statistical signs of synaptic interaction in neurons. Biophys J 10:876-900

Palmer LA, Rosenquist AC (1974) Visual receptive fields of single striate cortical units projecting to the superior colliculus in the cat. Brain Res 67:27-42

Perkel DH, Gerstein GL, Moore GP (1967) Neuronal spike trains and stochastic point processes. II. Simultaneous spike trains. Biophys J 7:419-440

Rall W, Segev I (1987) Functional possibilities for synapses on dendrites and dendritic spines. In: Edelman GM, Gall WE, Cowan WM (eds) Synaptic function, pp. 605-636, John Wiley & Sons, New York

Ramón y Cajal, S (1921) Textura de la corteza visual del gato. Arch Neurobiol 2:338-362

Rockland KS, Lund JS, Humphrey AL (1982) Anatomical banding of intrinsic connections in striate cortex of tree shrews (Tupaia glis). J Comp Neurol 209:41-58

Schwarz C, Bolz J (1991) Functional specificity of a long-range horizontal connection in cat visual cortex: a cross-correlation study. J Neurosci (in press)

Thalluri J, Henry GH (1989) Neurons of the striate cortex driven transsynaptically by electrical stimulation of the superior colliculus. Vision Res 29:1319-1323

Weyand TG, Malpeli JG, Lee C, Schwark HD (1986a) Cat area 17. III. Response properties and orientation anisotropies of corticotectal cells. J Neurophysiol 56:1088-1101

Principles of Global Visual Processing of Local Features can be Investigated with Parallel Single-Cell- and Group-Recordings from the Visual Cortex

Reinhard Eckhorn

Philipps-University, Biophysics Department, Renthof 7, 3550 Marburg, Germany

Goals, results and conclusions

In order to investigate *cortical mechanisms of visual integration*, we analyzed relations between feature coding by single neurons and groups of neurons in cat visual cortex (Eckhorn et al. 1988). Local visual coding in the primary cortical areas is well understood and can be characterized by the receptive field (RF) properties of single neurons. RF-properties are due to relatively invariant (though non-linear) spatio-temporal filter properties of the network between receptors and the neuron in question. Neurons with similar RFs are retinotopically organized in a number of interconnected "feature maps" (visual cortical areas; Hubel and Wiesel 1962, 1963). The constant relations between retinal surface, retinotopic cortical maps and RF-properties probably form *invariant frames of reference* between outer visual world and perception. However, in order to cope with the immense variety of local feature combinations in natural scenes, *flexible mechanisms of feature association* are required. To date flexible principles of global visual processing are barely understood and there are no proven theories of how local coding properties of single cortical neurons are flexibly linked into a coherent global percept.

We follow the hypothesis that *stimulus-related synchronizations support the definition of global visual relations*: it was stated that the activities of those visual neurons become synchronized that are activated by a coherent "visual object" (Eckhorn et al. 1988; Gray et al. 1989). In order to substantiate this hypothesis we recorded single cell and mass activities in cat visual cortex in parallel with multiple microelectrodes. Our recordings revealed stimulus specific synchronizations between visual cortical assemblies in the same and in different visual cortex areas of the same and different cortical hemispheres. Two types of synchronizations were encountered: 1. *Stimulus-locked synchronizations* are evoked by fast stimulus transients, they are generally not rhythmic and are already present in the retina. 2. *Stimulus-induced oscillatory synchronizations* (35-80 Hz) occur preferentially with sustained stimuli and are probably of cortical origin (Eckhorn et al. 1989). We found that stimulus-locked responses can inhibit stimulus-induced oscillations (Eckhorn and Schanze 1991). This effect is interesting, because during natural vision slow retinal image drifts that induce oscillatory activities (during fixation) alternate with sudden shifts that evoke fast transient activities (in response to saccades or sudden object movements).

Our investigations of synchronized cortical activities were facilitated by the fact that cells with similar receptive field properties are grouped in clusters *(local assemblies)* in the visual cortex. Neurons in such clusters are therefore simultaneously activated by the same stimulus. A rough estimate of the synchronized components of an assembly's activity can be obtained by extracellular recordings of neural "mass" signals with micro- or semi-microelectrodes positioned within such an assembly. From the point of experimental effort, isolation of synchronized signal components by means of extracellular mass signal recording is simple and effective and it extracts just those signal components that are relevant for testing our "linking-by-synchronization" hypothesis.

It was argued that the stimulus related synchronizations, observed by us in cat visual cortex, are mediated via special intra- and interareal *linking networks* (association fibers systems) that generally include projections to targets beyond the retinotopically correct locations of cortical maps (Eckhorn et al. 1988; 1990a,b,d). Our combined single cell and group activity recordings support this view: We found significantly coupled oscillatory activities also between cortical positions that represent non-corresponding visual locations, besides correlations in retinotopically corresponding positions. Such correlated activities were found in the same and in different cortical areas of the same and different hemispheres of cat visual cortical areas 17, 18 and 19. We modelled these results by "biologically inspired" neural networks and found that a variety of the observed cortical synchronization effects could be explained if two different types of model synapses are used, "standard synapses" for the feeding connections and "modulatory synapses" for the linking connections (Eckhorn et al. 1990b). The feeding networks in our models mainly generate the receptive field properties of the neurons (local coding) while the signals delivered via the linking network modulate the "postsynaptic" signals of the feeding "synapses" and by this means simultaneously active neurons can mutually synchronize their activities.

Our results from parallel recordings of single cell and mass activities from cat visual cortex and the modelling of the observed synchronization effects can explain some neural mechanisms of *perceptual feature linking*, such as mutual enhancement among similar, spatially and temporally dispersed features, definitions of spatial and temporal continuity, scene segmentation, figure-ground discrimination and other related phenomena. We further assume that mutual enhancement and synchronization of cell activities are general principles of temporal coding by assemblies, that are also used within other sensory modalities and among different modalities.

At what resolution in space and time does cortical activity make sense?

The above question cannot be answered by us in general, because the special functional architecture and the electrical properties of cortical tissue have to be taken into account. In addition, our particular interests in cortical processing and the experimental techniques available requires reformulation of the question: At what level of neural organization should we look for relations between local and global principles of visual cortical sensory processing? In experimental terms this means: where should we record what types of signals and how should we analyze them?

Precisely timed interactions between separate cortical assemblies are rare and weak

One important cortical property is that monosynaptic lateral interactions between single cortical neurons are rare and weak, at least within the range of our electrode separations of minimally 250 μm. The probability of finding significantly coupled single cell spike trains of neurons in the visual cortex, manifesting monosynaptic connections and, hence, narrow peaks in cross-correlograms, is low under our (and comparable) experimental conditions (Fig. 1), (Eckhorn and Reitboeck 1988, Eckhorn et al. 1989: cat A17,18; Krüger 1983; Aertsen et al. 1987: monkey, V1). It is, therefore, experimentally not efficient to search exclusively for just these rare interactions, if global coding principles are of primary interest as is the case in our investigations.

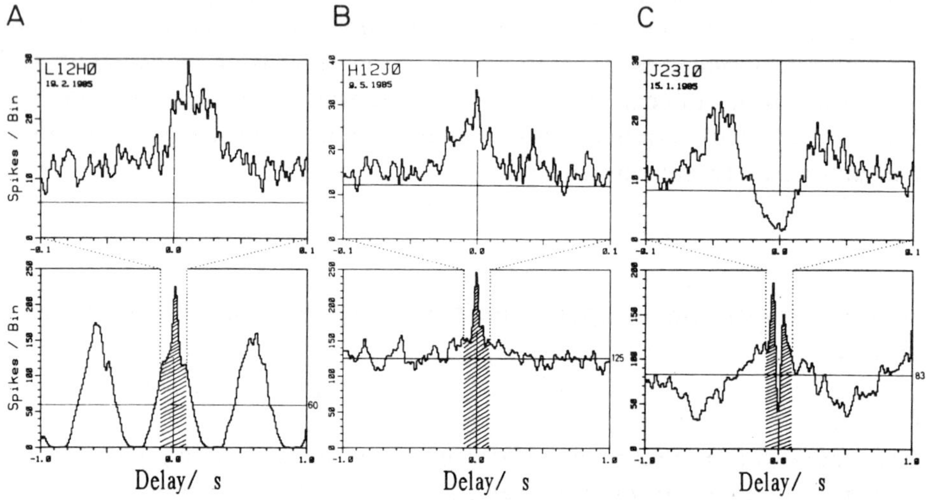

Fig. 1. Precisely timed single cell correlations are rare in the visual cortex. Cross-coincidence correlograms of spike trains from three pairs of visual cortex neurons with overlapping RFs. **A**: Two simple cells with similar orientation preferences, one in A17, the other in A18. **B**: Two complex cells in A18, horizontal separation 2.5 mm. **C**: Simple and complex cell in A18, horizontal separation about 2 mm. The upper cross-correlograms are expanded from the lower by a factor of 10. Stimulation: **A**: Random dot pattern that moved randomly across the RFs (two-dimensional Gaussian white noise movement during repetitive periods of 300 ms movement and 300 ms of stationary position). Note the large broad periodical correlation peaks at 600 ms delay that are due to the rhythmic start/stop movement cycle. Note also the narrower peaks that appear only at the center (upper panel) and not at the side peaks. The 35 ms broad peak is due to the common stimulation by the randomly moving dot pattern while the very narrow one (at a delay of 12 ms) is due to an internal A18-to-A17 projection (stimulus and internal influences on correlogram were estimated by calculation of a simple type of "shift-predictor" (e.g. Aertsen and Gerstein 1985). **B**: Stimulation by a continuously and randomly moving disk of light (of half the RF width). **C**: Same stimulus as in A, with the difference that the duration of a start/stop movement cycle was 1 s in this case. The broad peak is again due to the movement cycle

Our rare observations of precisely coupled cortical neurons correspond with anatomical data. The probability of more than a single monosynaptic connection between cortical neurons of more than 100 μm separation is negligibly small (Braitenberg and Schüz 1990). A single connection (if really present) will in general not exert strong and precisely timed signal correlations. Less precise couplings are, however, found relatively often (peakwidths of cross-correlograms: 20-500 ms; Eckhorn 1991). The rare observations of precise correlations is not astonishing if we consider the thousands of synaptic contacts on each cortical neuron (that mask effects of single monosynaptic connections (Abeles 1982; Krüger 1983; Eckhorn and Reitboeck 1988; Krüger and Aiple 1988, 1989). Many of these inputs contain weak signal components that are influenced by neighboring (and remote) neurons via multi-synaptic pathways. Correlated components that arrive via multiple delay pathways, however, summate and may result in strong (though temporally "broader") correlations, even without direct connections. Temporal dispersion of correlated signals is reflected in correspondingly broad peaks of cross-correlograms. As we are interested just in the correlated components of cortical assemblies we decided to adapt the temporal scale of our data analyses to the peak widths of cross-correlograms and choose a spatial scale adapted to the diameters of cortical cell clusters (in which neurons have similar RF-properties; Hubel and Wiesel 1962, 1963). We will argue below that temporal resolutions in the order of few milliseconds and electrode spacings of about 250 μm are a good compromise for tackling our questions with the recording and data evaluation methods available in our laboratory.

Multiple-resolution recording in the visual cortex makes sense because neurons with similar RF-properties are locally clustered

Evidence for clustering of single cell receptive field (RF) properties in sensory cortex was provided already many years ago (e.g. Mountcastle 1957, 1978; Hubel and Wiesel 1962, 1963). RF-clustering means that cortical neurons with like RF-properties are locally grouped and that

---

while the two narrower peaks and the trough at the center are due to a common neural input, possibly modulated by the random components of the stimulus movement. (Fig. from Eckhorn and Reitboeck 1988)

many neurons in such a local cluster are, therefore, activated in parallel by a single stimulus. In cat visual cortex (A17,18) we consistently found cells with similar RF-properties over 200-700 μm of electrode advancement, both in perpendicular and tangential recording tracks. At the borders of such clusters the RF-properties generally change considerably over short cortical distances of few tens of micrometers (e.g., orientation and direction specificities change to perpendicular values; Bauer et al. 1989; Eckhorn et al. 1989; Eckhorn 1991). Functional clustering in the visual cortex is obvious with respect to stimulus orientation and movement direction but also the functional types of neurons seem to be grouped (including simple and complex). Clustering has been reported by many other investigators using a variety of methods: by long recording tracks in A17 (e.g. Payne et al. 1981); by silencing certain A17 layers while recording from others (Weyand et al. 1987); by double electrode recordings and cross-correlation of SUA in A17 (Ts'o et al. 1986) and by direct sampling with multiple penetrations in A18 (Matsubara et al. 1985). The spatial sampling of 250 μm, chosen most often by us, is a reasonable compromise between the few electrodes (7-19) available and the demand of sampling over long cortical distances. This compromise makes sense, because we recorded local group signals (next to single cell spike trains) with each of the microelectrodes. In particular, local slow wave field potentials (LFPs, 12-120 Hz) are spatially dispersed due to the extent of dendritic structures and due to volume conduction by the extracellular media, so that the 250 μm sampling distance is well "bridged" by volume conducted LFP components (more details below).

Clustering of cortical RF-properties provides a simple means for obtaining an estimate of the synchronized components from clusters by simply recording extracellular group signals (mass activities). Such mass activities are a linear superposition of signals from neural components of the neighborhood (e.g. Mitzdorf 1985, 1987; for the required linear behavior of extracellular media in the interesting frequency range from zero to above 10 kHz see: Hoeltzell and Dykes (1979). The spatial dispersion of mass signals in cortical tissue is typically dependent on temporal frequencies. In the neocortex estimates of the average "field of view" of our microelectrodes are roughly 500 μm at frequencies of 40-80 Hz (reduction by 80% amplitude; LFP oscillation spindles), and about 50 μm at frequencies of 1-10 kHz (MUA, spikes; for specifications of our fiber electrodes see following Section).

In view of our "linking-by-synchronization" hypothesis we are interested in just the synchronized components. Synchronization in a certain state will generally depend on "exogenous" correlations (evoked by a common stimulus) and by "endogenous" correlations (mediated via neural coupling pathways) (e.g. Johannesma et al. 1986). Local couplings leading to endogenous correlations within local groups of neurons (assembly) can be due to various mechanisms including 1) general ("diffuse") couplings via local gradients in electric fields near correspondingly sensitive membranes (Schwartzkroin 1983), 2) special coupling arrangements like those among bundled apical dendrites in certain subgroups of cortical pyramidal cells (Fleischhauer 1974), and/or 3) couplings via chemical synaptic transmission. Any type of coupling can increase the coherence of signals that are generated by members of local assemblies (e.g. Aertsen and Gerstein 1985; Palm et al. 1988). During states of increased "cooperativity" we therefore expect that average group signals occur with high amplitudes while uncorrelated signal components are "averaged out" largely. During states of reduced cooperativity correlated group signals of lower average amplitudes are expected while signal variability will increase due to reduced couplings between the assembly members. Both expectations were confirmed by our recordings of local slow wave field potentials (LFPs, 12-120 Hz) and multiple unit spike activities (MUA, 1-10 kHz) in cat visual cortex. Flexible involvement of single cortical neurons in synchronized states of local assemblies was estimated in some detail by calculating cross-correlations between the single cell spike trains and the LFPs/MUAs that were recorded with the same microelectrode (results presented in Figs. 6 and 7).

From the point of experimental effort, isolation of synchronized signal components by means of extracellular mass signal recordings is a simple and effective means of extracting just those signal components that are probably relevant for the understanding of neural cooperation processes in general, and that are interesting in particular for our questions regarding coding mechanisms of global visual aspects.

Multiple microelectrode recordings of single-cell and group-activities

We made multiple microelectrode recordings from visual cortical areas 17, 18 and 19 in chronically prepared, lightly anesthetized and paralyzed cats (e.g. Eckhorn et al. 1988; Eckhorn et al., in press) from up to 19 independently drivable fiber electrodes (Reitboeck 1983a,b). From each microelectrode we derived 1) an estimate of the synchronized components of the postsynaptic potentials on dendritic and somatic structures near the electrode tip by recording the local extracellular field potentials (LFPs; 12-120 Hz), 2) an estimate of the somatic spike activities of the assembly near the electrode tip by recording multiple unit activities (MUAs; 1-10 kHz, transformed to 0-120 Hz by envelope demodulation), and 3) single neuron spikes (SUA). Special fiber electrodes were fabricated in order to keep tissue damage as small as possible (Reitboeck 1983b). The electrodes have thin shafts (70 μm diameter; Pt-Wo core, quartz insulation; 3-7 Megohms at 1 kHz), they are coated with an anti-adhesive film to minimize tissue displacements during electrode movements, and they can penetrate the intact dura of cat (Eckhorn and Reitboeck 1988) and monkey (Mountcastle et al. 1991). Our fiber electrodes pick up extracellular field

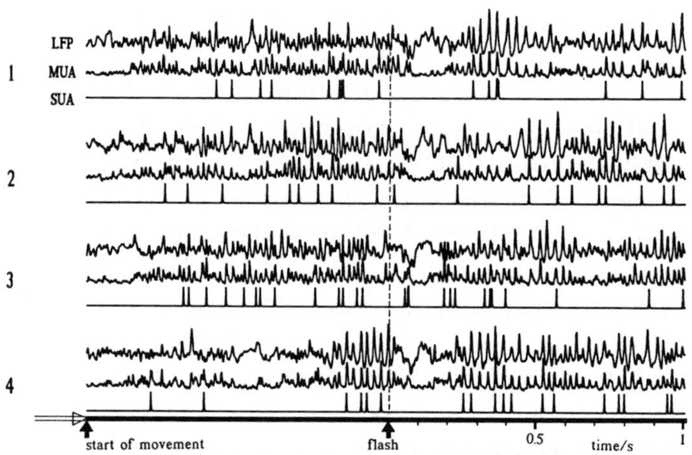

Fig. 2. Single cell spike trains and local group signals, recorded with multiple microelectrodes. Responses to 4 identical stimulus repetitions of three types of neuronal signals recorded in parallel with the same microelectrode: local field potentials (*LFPs*; 12-120 Hz); multiple unit activities (*MUA*; derived by filtering (1-10 kHz) and subsequent envelope demodulation (0-120 Hz); single unit spike activity (*SUA*). Stimulus: grating of 0.25 cycl/deg, moving at v = 4.5 deg/s. Arrows below mark beginning of stimulus movement (left) and instance of a light flash (middle) that was given while the grating continued to move. Note the 200 ms post flash evoked potentials in the LFPs during which gamma activity is reduced in amplitude; note also the reduced MUA activity during this period. (Fig. from Eckhorn and Schanze 1990)

potentials down to less than 1 Hz as well as fast extracellular action potentials. This broadband recording capability opens up a wide range of possibilities for studies of the interactions of single cells with local group activities (MUA and LFPs). The electrode spacings in our manipulators were either 250 or 330 μm center-to-center, although of course the electrode tips were not always at the same depth (electrodes were singly advanceable in micron steps). This electrode separation combined with the recording of mass activities is a suitable compromise for the sampling of the discrete cortical patch structures that generally extend over 200-700 μm (e.g. Hubel and Wiesel 1962, 1963; Gilbert 1985; Payne et al. 1981; Bauer et al. 1989; Eckhorn et al. 1989; Eckhorn et al. 1990a).

The ease of finding cooperating neural assemblies was dramatically increased by recording neural mass signals such as MUA and LFPs in parallel with single unit spike trains. This "triple recording" from each electrode offered us the opportunity to investigate neural couplings on different levels of organization and specificity by analyzing all possible combinations of interactions between the different signal types.

Stimulus-induced oscillations in the visual cortex of the cat

Overview

Our parallel "multiple-level recordings" provided new results that could not have been discovered with conventional single cell techniques. The discovery of stimulus-induced oscillatory synchronizations at functionally close but spatially distant locations of cat visual cortex is considered by us as the most important result of our recent investigations. We showed experimentally the occurrence of stimulus-induced transient groupings between spatially separated assemblies, assessed by increased signal correlations (Eckhorn et al. 1988).

Stimulus-response characteristics of oscillation-spindles (LFPs and MUA) were found to have specific correlations with classical single cell receptive field properties (Gray and Singer 1989; Eckhorn et al. 1988). This means that the generation of oscillation-spindles can specifically be correlated with tuning properties of local cell assemblies, including RF-position, ocularity, binocular disparity, orientation, contrast, movement direction and velocity of contrast borders and textures (Eckhorn 1991).

Stimulus-induced synchronizations were found throughout all layers of vertical columns of the iso- as well as of the cross-orientation type (Bauer et al. 1989). Synchronizations were induced among separate vertical columns of the same cortical area (Eckhorn et al. 1988; Gray et al. 1989) and even among assemblies of different cortical areas and different hemispheres at those positions where the neurons had some of their receptive field properties in common (A17, 18, 19: Eckhorn et al. 1988, Eckhorn et al., in press; A17, LS-areas: Engel et al. 1990b). These observations from the visual cortex are essential prerequisites for our model of global visual coding, in which correlated activity can act as a label to link related features in a visual scene and to signalize a momentary association.

The internal temporal structure of stimulus-induced oscillations is not stimulus-correlated

Oscillatory activities of LFPs and MUA show up in a waxing and waning fashion during specific stimulation (Fig. 3). They appear as *oscillation spindles* (35-80 Hz) of about 50-300 ms duration, separated by intervals of more irregular activity, and they generally occur after transient visually evoked cortical potential (VECPs) have declined. This means that delays of oscillation spindles were found to be significantly longer than the fast components of the averaged event related visually evoked cortical responses. Oscillation spindles occur with considerable temporal jitter in response to identical stimuli and their "momentary frequencies" are highly variant (Gray and Singer 1987a,b; Eckhorn et al. 1988; Eckhorn and Schanze 1991; see also following Section). It is not astonishing, therefore, that the "micro-timing", as revealed by the phases of the oscillations, was generally not coupled with the stimuli. Independence from stimulus events is demonstrated in Fig. 3, where single LFP response sweeps are shown in the upper part and response averages to identical stimulus repetitions below. Averaging, obviously, uncovers the stimulus-locked VECPs at short delays, but averages out the oscillatory components. This seeming lack of stimulus-response coupling of the oscillations' frequencies and phases, in combination with the predominance of signal averaging techniques, might be one of the reasons why we as well as other groups have been unaware of oscillatory activities in the visual cortex until recently.

Despite the lack of correlation of the oscillations' frequencies / phases to the stimulus phase, strong stimulus couplings can often be found with the *envelope* of the oscillatory neural response. This means that the occurrence of spindles is itself stimulus coupled, even though their phases are not (Eckhorn 1991). "Envelope-coupling" of spindles with visual stimuli is, however, a basic requirement for our hypothesis of global sensory coding via oscillatory synchronizations.

Synchronization statistics of stimulus-specific oscillatory events

We are interested in the statistical evaluation of stimulus-induced oscillations and their synchronizations in order to get indications of their underlying mechanisms. Oscillatory activities occurred as *oscillation spindles* (35-80 Hz) of LFPs and MUAs (average durations 120 ms;

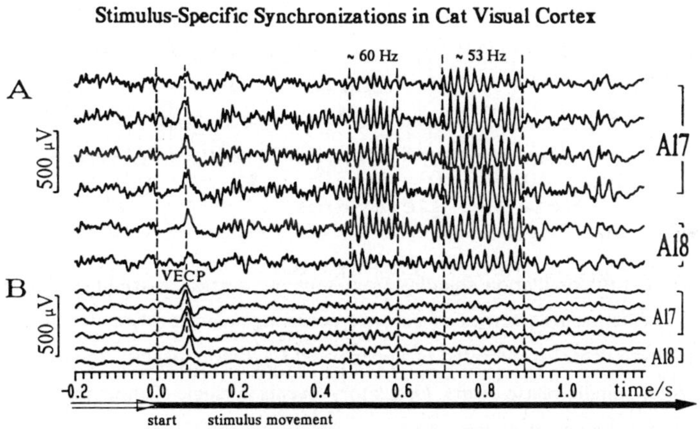

Fig. 3. Two types of stimulus-related synchronizations among visual cortical areas A17 and A18 of the cat: 1. primary, visually evoked (event-locked) field potentials (*VECP*) and 2. stimulus-induced oscillatory potentials. **A**: Single-sweep local field potential (LFP) responses (bandpass: 12-120 Hz). **B**: Averages of 18 LFP-responses to identical stimuli. Note that the oscillatory components (480-900 ms post stimulus) are averaged out, while averaging pronounces the primary evoked potentials (50-120 ms). Binocular stimulation (drifting grating; 0.7 cycles/deg swept at 4 deg/s; movement starts at t=0 and continues for 3.4 s). Simultaneous recordings with linear array of 7 microelectrodes from layers II/III; the RFs of A17- and A18-neurons overlapped partially. (Fig. from Eckhorn et al. 1990b)

Schanze et al. 1990). We evaluated for single-channels and pairs of channels (correlations) the following statistical parameters of spindles (Schanze and Eckhorn 1991): probabilities of amplitudes, durations, frequencies and stimulus-response latencies; for pairs of recordings: cross-spectral PSTHs, relative temporal delays, phase differences, and oscillation frequency scatter-diagrams. These measures were derived in a variety of stimulus and recording configurations (same or different cortical area/hemisphere; overlapping and non-overlapping receptive fields).

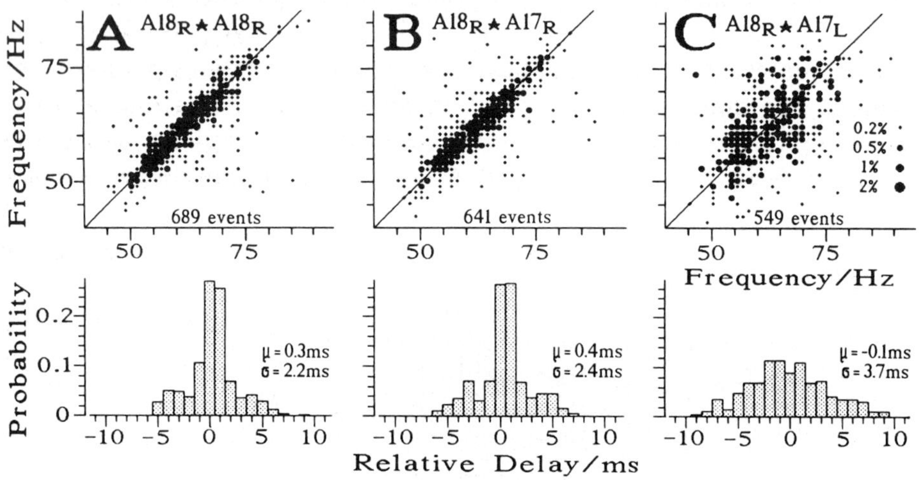

Fig. 4. Correlation statistics of LFP oscillation spindles from separate cortical assemblies. Upper panels: Scatter diagrams of oscillation frequencies of pairwise occurring spindles (diameter of dots indicate percentage of respective events, as indicated in upper panel C). Lower panels: Relative frequencies ("probability") of inter-spindle phase delays. Oscillatory events in single channel recordings were isolated from the other remaining signal components by digital filtering (30-90 Hz, Blackman-Harris window) and a "spindle search algorithm" (Eckhorn and Schanze 1991). **A**: Both recordings from upper layers of A18 (1 mm electrode separation). **B**: A18-A17 recordings; overlapping RFs with similar directional preferences. **C**: A18-A17 recordings from different hemispheres; RFs partly overlapped; similar directional preferences. Stimulation: Whole field grating of 0.4 cycl/deg moving at 4 deg/s in the prefered direction. The data are from the same multiple electrode recording. Note the strong covariance of spindle frequencies and their tight phase couplings in A and B. Broad (weak) correlations as in C were typical for our interhemispheric recordings. Note also the typical broad distributions of spindle frequencies in all three recordings. (Fig. from Schanze and Eckhorn 1991)

The statistical analyses revealed that oscillations occur seldomly earlier than 50 ms after the first cortical responses; typical response delays of single channel and correlated spindles are 130 ± 50 ms post stimulus onset. Average phase differences and average delays between oscillations at separate cortical positions were generally near zero, in most cases not significantly depending on the type of stimulation. (Larger average phase differences were frequently found). In pairs of spatially separate parallel recordings the distributions of oscillation phase differences vary over a broad range depending on stimulus and recording configurations (same area: σ = 1 ms at 1 mm distance; different hemispheres: σ up to 4 ms with neighboring RFs; see lower panels of Fig. 4). Examples of scatter diagrams of oscillation frequencies (pair recordings) are shown in the upper panels of Figure 4. Pair recordings of oscillation spindles were from a single cortical area (Fig. 4A), from different areas (Fig. 4B), and from the same cortical area in different hemispheres (Fig. 4C). The scatter diagrams indicate a high degree of covariance of the oscillation frequencies of simultaneously occurring spindles if pair events cluster near the diagonal over a large frequency range. This is the case in Figs. 4A and 4B, where the spindle frequencies of a single recording of 2 minutes are broadly distributed between 35 and 85 Hz. High covariances of momentaneous spindle frequencies are another expression for phase lock of oscillatory processes. The distributions of spindle amplitudes versus oscillation frequencies in Figure 5 indicate in addition, that spindle occurrences, amplitudes, frequencies and correlations between A17 and A18 recording positions are clearly stimulus depending.

The strong correlations often found between specific single cell stimulus preferences and the occurrence probability and amplitude of LFP oscillation spindles at the same recording positions are indications for a cortical generation of oscillations in local assemblies (instead of a supply from a common subcortical source). For these reasons and some other ones we assume that stimulus-induced oscillations and synchronizations are cooperative phenomena among local cortical "oscillation units" (see Eckhorn 1991; Eckhorn et al. in press).

Single neurons are differently involved in oscillatory group activities

We stated in our "linking hypothesis" that the receptive field properties of those neurons are linked into a perceptual entity that develop a

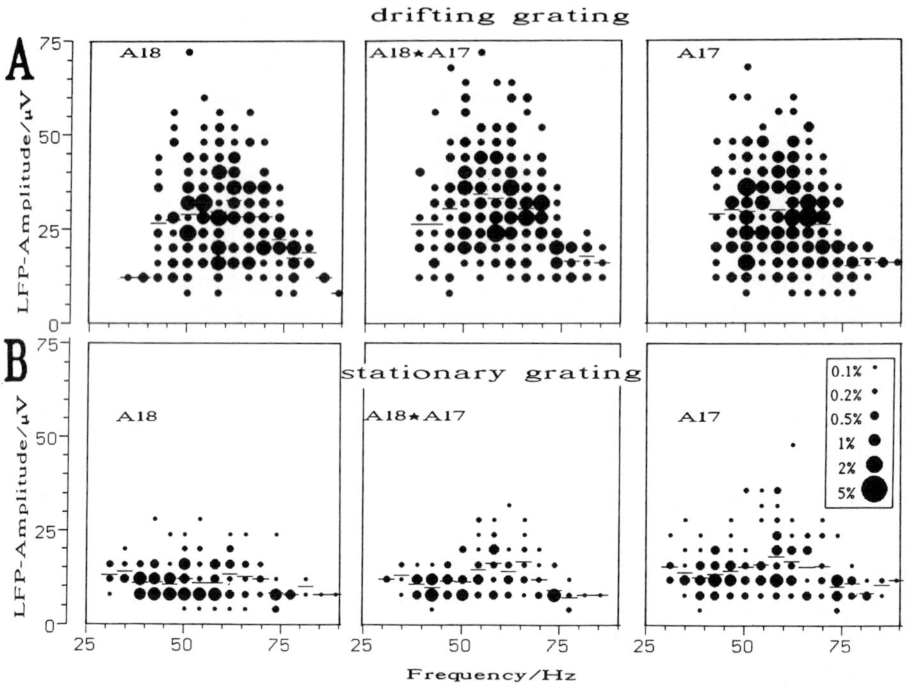

Fig. 5. Distributions of occurrence frequencies of LFP oscillation-spindle amplitudes versus their oscillation frequencies. Simultaneous LFP recordings from visual cortex areas A17 and A18. Oscillatory events in single channel recordings were isolated from the other remaining signal components by digital filtering (30-90 Hz, Blackman-Harris window) and a "spindle search algorithm" (Eckhorn and Schanze 1991). "Correlation-spindles" were searched for by the same algorithm, but instead of original records here short-epoch cross-correlograms (128 ms) were taken for the spindle search procedure. Search for correlation spindles was carried out on temporally overlapping parts in intervals of 32 ms. Dot size indicates relative spindle occurrence frequency, normalized to the data where the stimulus grating remained stationary; (calibrations in the insert of the lower right panel). Spindle occurrence frequencies are shown for data recorded during stimulation with a drifting grating (**A**) and while the grating remained stationary (**B**). A18 and A17 (outer panels) denote that single channel data were analyzed, while A18 * A17 (center panels) denotes that "correlation spindles" of the two channels are shown. Note the wide "spread" in the direction of large oscillation amplitudes and the higher occurrence frequencies of oscillation-spindles in the data obtained during stimulation (**A**) compared with those obtained while the grating stimulus remained stationary. Note also, that during stationary stimuli low frequency spindles appear that are absent during drift stimulation. (Fig. from Eckhorn and Schanze 1991)

common synchronized state in response to a common coherent stimulus. We were interested in how and when single cortical neurons participate in such synchronized group activities.

The stimuli used consisted of gratings or bars of light that drifted with constant velocities across the receptive fields such that the resulting temporal modulation (in a fixed stimulus position) was always below 10 Hz (i.e. the stimulus contained no frequency component in the oscillation range of 35-80 Hz; in addition, phases of oscillation spindles were never phase-locked to stimulus events). Participation of single neurons in group oscillations was quantified by cross-correlations between SUA and LFP or MUA at the same electrode and between different electrodes (same and different cortex areas). We characterized three types of neurons with respect to their participation in oscillatory group activities (Obermüller et al. 1991):

1. *Rhythmically discharging neurons* (Fig. 6A) show significant stimulus-specific rythmicities in their discharge patterns (quantified in their auto-coincidence correlograms). The rhythmicities of spike patterns are in general strongly correlated with oscillatory group activities at the same electrode (LFPs: Fig. 7A and MUA: Fig. 7C), and are often (65%) significantly correlated with those at other electrodes in the same and different cortical areas (A17,18,19) where neurons have similar tuning preferences (max. recording distance: 7 mm). During "spontaneous" activities and when non-preferred stimuli are applied, rhythmic correlations with group activities are only weak or even absent (Fig. 7B and D). The auto-coincidence histograms of rhythmically discharging neurons show that rhythmicity is generally reduced in such non driven states.
2. *Lock-in neurons* (Fig. 6B) do not contain significant rhythmic components in their spike patterns. However, the stimulus-driven spikes of lock-in neurons can be strongly phase-locked with oscillations of group activities on the same electrode (LFPs: Fig. 7A and MUA: Fig. 7C) and at separate positions of the same and different cortical areas.
3. *Non-participating neurons* had neither oscillatory components in their spike trains nor were they coupled with "spontaneous" or stimulus-induced group oscillations under our experimental conditions.

We assume that rhythmically discharging neurons are directly involved in the generation of group oscillations due to intrinsic single-cell mechanisms and/or due to local feedback circuits via inhibitory interneurons. We further assume that they are mutually coupled via linking connections (Eckhorn et al. 1990c; in press). Rhythmically discharging neurons might belong to the group of cortical pyramidal cells that were found to respond with repetitive bursts in the range 30-80 Hz in slice preparations when current is injected into their soma ("intrinsically bursting cells" (Chagnac-Amitai and Connors 1989).

Lock-in neurons probably receive subthreshold rhythmic inputs via synaptic connections or via dendro-dendritic coupling in bundles of apical dendrites. If afferent visual (or other) inputs fire the cell's spike encoder a fast and strong acting inhibition blocks the generation of series of rhythmic spikes at the oscillation frequency of a present spindle event. This is in line with our observation that lock-in neurons discharge only a single spike or a very short burst during a single cycle of an oscillation spindle. The lack of oscillatory components in the spike trains of lock-in neurons can be explained by the observation that intervals between consecutive oscillation spindles are stochastic on

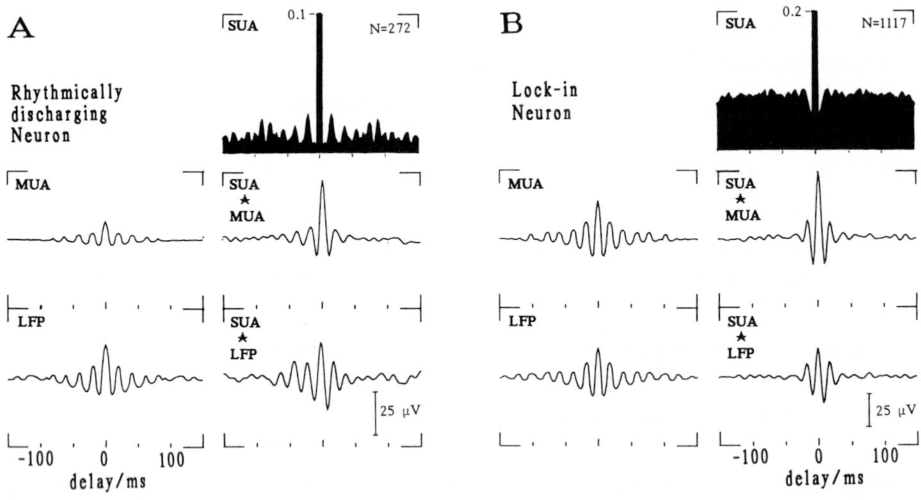

Fig. 6. Single neurons participate differently in stimulus-specific oscillations of the surrounding assembly. SUA: Auto-coincidence histograms of single unit activities. MUA (or LFP): Autocorrelation histograms of MUA (or LFPs). SUA * MUA (or SUA * LFP): cross-correlograms between single cell spiketrain and MUA (or LFPs), calculated as spike-triggered averaging of MUA (or LFPs). **A**: Rhythmically discharging neuron. **B**: Lock-in neuron

a temporal scale of a single oscillation cycle (i.e., inter spindle intervals are not multiple integers of oscillation periods; consecutive discharges of lock-in neurons are therefore mainly determined by these inter-spindle intervals). It is possible, however, that lock-in neurons contribute well to the amplitudes of the extracellularly recorded oscillation spindles (of LFP and MUA). If we assume that locally a larger number of them is activated (temporally dispersed across a spindle) their subthreshold membrane oscillations and action potentials can, as a group, massively support the oscillatory process without being involved in it during every period of a spindle. When a lock-in neuron is not driven by a visual stimulus, (because that stimulus has no overlap with the neurons' RF-properties), its "spontaneously" discharging spikes are in general not significantly coupled to stimulus-induced oscillations in groups of other neurons (see Fig. 7B,D).

We found that the three cell classes (characterized above) are present in relative close vicinity (their cortical distribution has, however not been investigated in detail). This is interesting, because it shows that non participating neurons can have their cell bodies at cortical locations where high amplitude oscillatory LFPs are present. This means that extracellular field potentials are not able to directly influ-

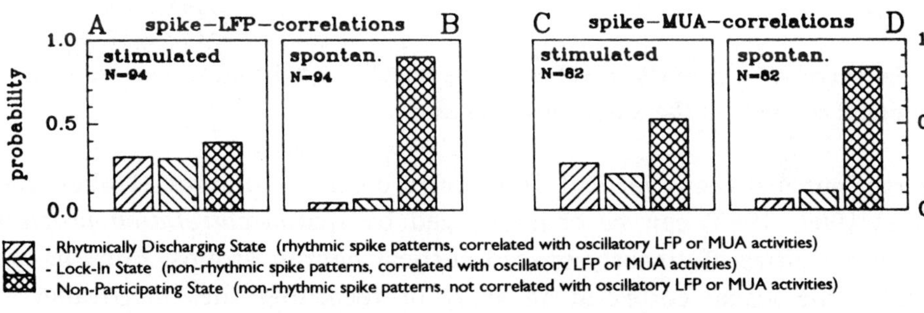

Fig. 7. Coupling "probabilities" between single unit activities (SUA, spikes) and oscillatory group signals (LFPs, MUA) at the same recording location in A17, A18 and A19. Relative occurrence frequencies of the conditions indicated below the Figure. Stimuli (**A** and **C**) were gratings or bars, moving at constant velocity in the prefered direction at speeds between about 1 and 10 deg/s. **B** and **D** are results obtained with stationary stimuli ("spontaneous" activity). Note the spike-to-oscillation coupling during stimulation in 60% (LFPs) and 50% (MUA) of the single neurons encountered, while these numbers were 10% (LFPs) and 15% (MUA) without stimulus movement. (Fig. from Obermüller et al. 1991)

ence such neurons significantly. Other reasons why non-participating neurons are not influenced by oscillations in nearby neural structures can include the following: 1) The neurons have no effective synaptic supply of oscillations, which means that there is no supply or it is weak. 2) We might have used the wrong stimuli - other stimuli perhaps could induce oscillations in these neurons due to a stimulus related change in the efficacies of the local coupling network (however, our drifting bar and grating stimuli were applied with various spatial frequency contents and movement velocities and non-participating neurons were well activated by these stimuli). 3) Non-participating neurons have no tight electrical couplings with other neurons that are involved in oscillatory group activities (or existing connections are not activated by our stimuli). It is not probable, therefore, that non-participating neurons do belong to the layer-III or -IV pyramide cells that form tight bundles of apical dendrites (Fleischhauer 1974). 4) Non-participating neurons might have either relatively small dendritic trees, or, if their dendritic trees are larger, they are confined to cortical regions where oscillatory extracellular fields have no significant gradients that could lead to effective modulations of membrane currents at the oscillation frequencies.

Further work will be needed in order to bring the three present cell classifications in register with known cell classes.

Spatial correlation profiles reveal stimulus specific synchronizations between functional columns of the same cortex area

Interactions between vertical functional cortical columns (Hubel and Wiesel 1962, 1963) can be characterized by spatial *correlation profiles* among activities of linearly spaced cortical neuron groups. For this we sampled the visual cortex at an array of recording sites in parallel to the cortical surface. The obtained correlation profiles depend specifically on visual stimulation, as is shown in the example (Fig. 8): Different stimulus movement directions, for example, reveal coupling maxima between different cortical columns. In Fig. 8A the stimulus moved in the preferred direction of the neurons near electrodes 2, 3 and 7, while in Fig. 8B the perpendicular direction was preferred by neurons near el. 5 and 6. It can be seen that oscillatory activities of cell groups with similar orientation/direction specificities are more strongly correlated (el. 3 and 7) than oscillations in neighboring cell

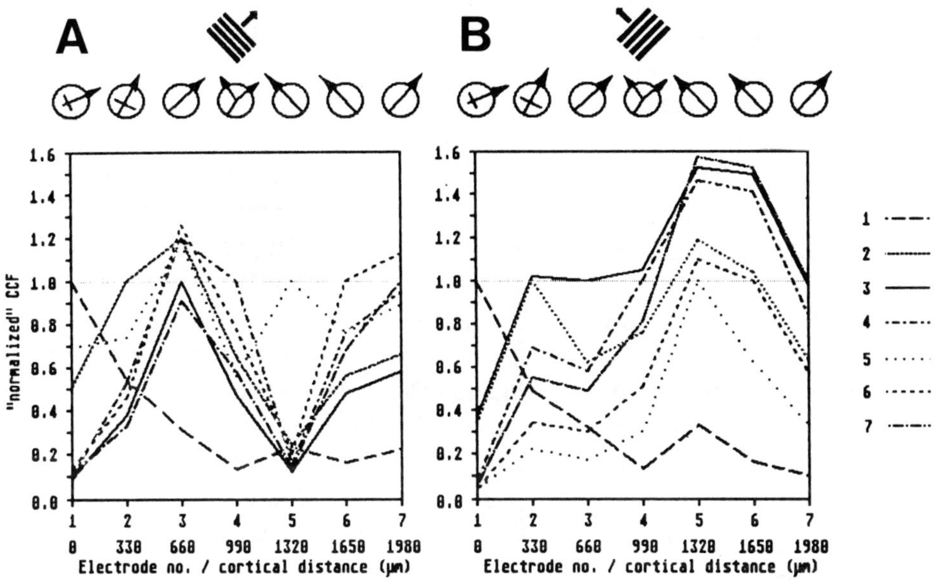

Fig. 8. Spatial correlation profiles of stimulus-specific synchronizations within and between orientation-columns of the same cortical area (A17). Simultaneous recordings of LFPs from layers II/III with a linear array of 7 microelectrodes. Stimulus: as in Fig. 5 (8 **A** and **B** in orthogonal directions, as indicated above). RFs of neighboring recording positions overlapped. Ordinates: peak amplitudes of "normalized" cross-correlograms were plotted over cortical distance (normalization to RMS-values during stimulus pause). Different profiles were obtained by taking signals from each electrode as reference for cross-correlations with those on the remaining electrodes. Orientation/ direction specificities of single neurons at each recording position are indicated above. (Fig. from Eckhorn et al. 1990c)

groups with different orientation/direction properties (about orthogonal; el. 3, 4, and 5).

Correlations between different cortical areas

Stimulus-specific oscillations occurred also correlated in different cortical areas (A17,18,19). Correlation strengths between assemblies in different cortex areas (positions with RF-overlap) were as strong as those between neighboring "Iso-RF-Columns" in the same area (up to 70% linearly correlated LFP amplitudes, e.g., between two assemblies

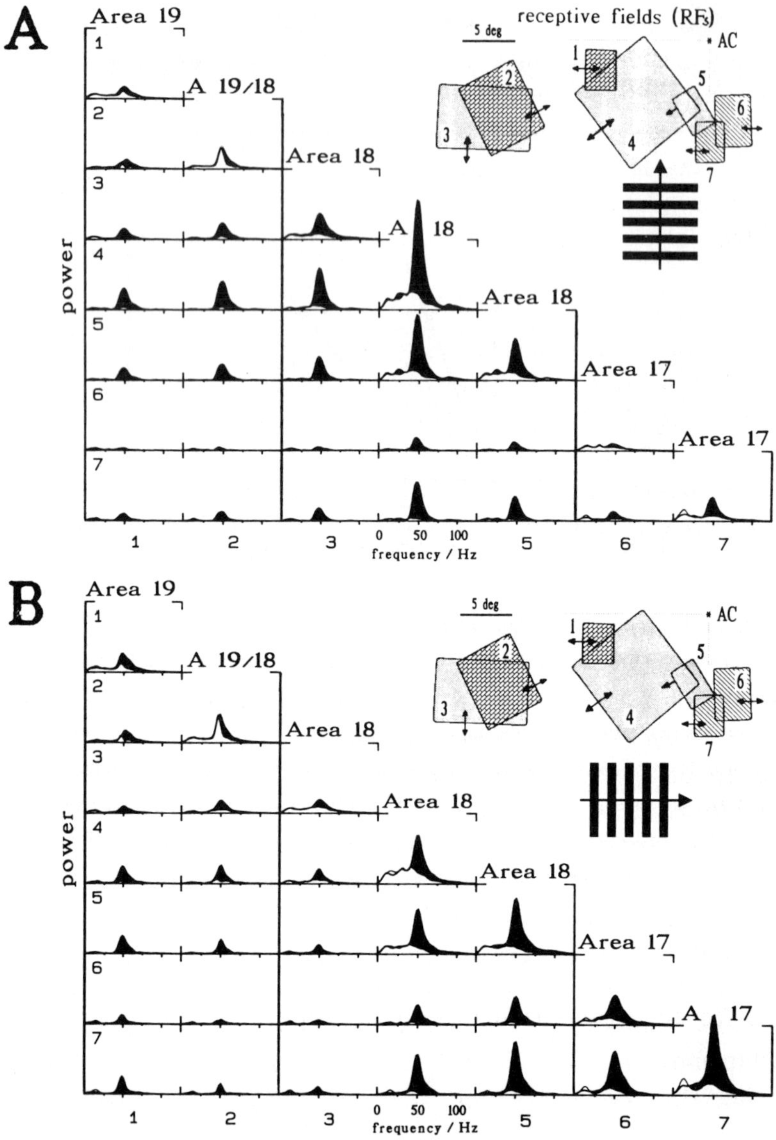

Fig. 9. Stimulus-induced correlations among gamma-rhythms of three different visual cortex areas (A17,18,19): Auto- (diagonals) and cross-power spectra (off-diagonals) were calculated for upward movement of a drifting grating (**A**), and movement to the right (**B**). Black areas indicate the difference between the spectral power determined during the 3.45 s of stimulus movement and those obtained during the 2.45 s inter-stimulus pauses (blank areas below thin curves). Simultaneous recordings of LFPs from layers II/III with a linear array of 7 microelectrodes (1 mm inter-electrode

that "prefer" the same stimulus orientation). With appropriate stimulation (that could activate the neurons in parallel) significant correlations of LFP spindles were present in almost all cortical positions where RFs overlapped (corresponding positions of visual representations), while significant correlations between MUA spindles were found only in those subareas of the RF-overlap regions, where we could find directly projecting neurons from the other cortex areas (proved with microinjections of the retrogradely transported tracer HRP (Eckhorn et al. 1990a,c).

Simultaneous activation is a general requirement for the occurrence of synchronized oscillation spindles. This means that sufficient "coding overlap" (in RF-properties) is required in order that the same stimulus can induce correlated oscillation-spindles in separated cortical assemblies. The latter statement holds also for non-overlapping RF-positions, as we found: oscillation-spindles (MUA and LFP) that are correlated in two visual cortex areas were observed in those positions where the neurons have some other RF-properties in common (i.e., other than RF-position; for example directional preferences for stimulus motion within a range of ± 30 degrees).

Correlation time courses of oscillations in two different cortical areas were evaluated by calculating the spectral coherence of LFPs at the oscillation frequencies. In order to obtain reliable estimates for short response epochs, we repeated the stimulus cyclically and calculated an ensemble average of the coherence values of equivalent "time slices" of the stimulus cycle (Fig. 10: N = 12; each of 250 ms duration; frequency resolution: 2 Hz). The significance of these short-duration coherence values was estimated by subtracting the average coherence during the stimulation pauses from them (n = 12; each of 2s duration). Figure 10 shows a time course of such A17-18 coherence at the respective average oscillation frequencies. Shortly after the grating stimulus starts to move (t = 0, Fig. 10), coherence increases from 0.1 to about 0.6 during the movement and goes down again to low values

---

spacing). Stimulus: Grating, 0.2 cycl/deg, drifting at 4 deg/s in the directions indicated by the arrows in the inserts at the upper rights, where grating and receptive fields are plotted to the same scale. Numbers in rows and columns of power-spectra and on receptive fields denote the electrodes' numbers. Note the stimulus specific oscillatory coupling among the different areas, depending on stimulus movement direction and the neurons' preferred stimulus directions (small arrows at RF borders). (Fig. from Eckhorn et al., in press)

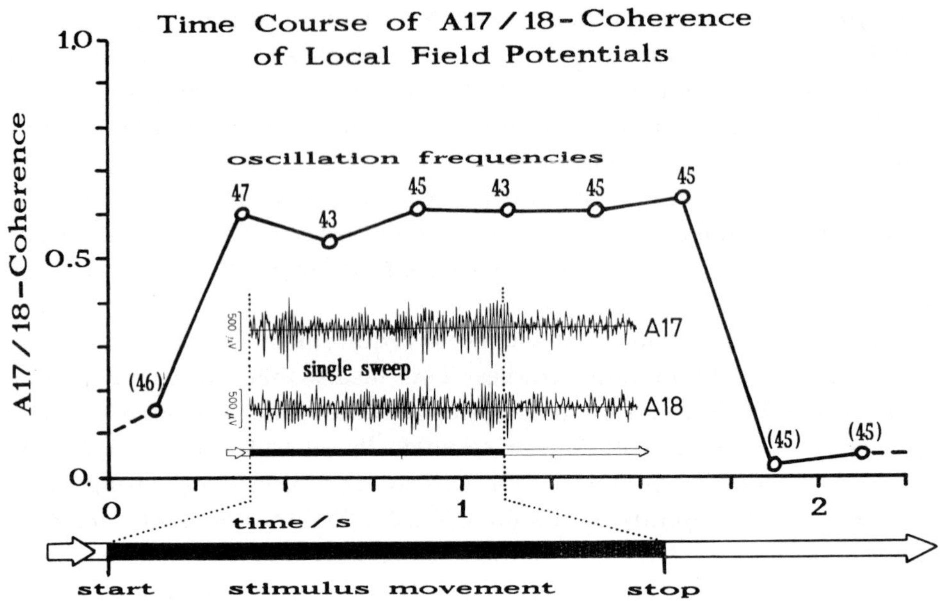

Fig. 10. Temporal course of gamma-spindle coherence in two different cortex areas in response to a moving stimulus. Coherence values were determined as averages from short-epoch (250 ms) LFP-responses to 10 identical stimulus repetitions. Recordings were from A17 and A18 positions with overlapping RFs. A single sweep response pair is shown as insert. More details are in the text. (Fig. from Eckhorn 1991)

after the stimulus stopped. This example (together with other results from our laboratory) shows, that the coupling strength between two visual cortical areas (its "efficacy") is highly "modulated" under stimulus control. More detailed analyses of simultaneously occurring spindle pairs from two areas revealed, that coupling can increase from near zero to full strength (e.g. 0.6) within a single cycle of an oscillation spindle.

Feeding and linking connections

We propose that the experimentally discovered synchronizations are due to special cortical *linking networks* that are likely to involve translaminar connections within vertical cortex columns as well as "patchwise" projecting intra- and inter-areal recurrent connections (anatomists call them association fiber systems (e.g. Creutzfeldt et al. 1966). Such long range connections are assumed to mediate phase coupling and to act "modulatory" on the afferent visual *feeding signals* (Eckhorn et al. 1990b). If association connections between neurons with different RF-properties (e.g. with different RF-positions) were not modulatory but additive (superimposing), then the RF-properties of the connected neurons would "smear out" their specificities during simultaneous activations. However, such RF-smearings have not been observed to date. Consequently, we were led to the following extensions of our working hypothesis by the simple assumption that convergent summation of signals from cells with different RF-coding properties would generate response properties in the convergence cell that resemble the superposition of the RFs of its input cells. We therefore assume:

- Visuotopically arranged projections (RF overlap) of cells with similar RF-properties from lower visual stages to higher ones (relative to the retina) are generally of the *feeding type*, leading to a superposition of their RF-properties at higher cortical stages.
- Connections in forward, lateral or backward directions among cells with different coding properties are generally of the *linking type* (association connections; e.g., among cells with non-overlapping RF positions, or with differently preferred movement directions and overlapping RFs).

This simplifying view of two general types of connections is schematically illustrated in Fig. 11.

Flexible stimulus representations by local cortical assemblies: "interpolation coding"

In the following paragraph some elaborations about flexible stimulus representations by local cortical assemblies will be made along our working hypothesis ("linking-by-synchronization"). Assembly coding has been discussed by various groups under a variety of assumptions, several are interesting with respect to our proposal (e.g. Abeles 1982;

Aertsen and Gerstein 1985; Aertsen et al. 1986; Johannesma et al. 1986; Palm 1982; Gerstein et al. 1989).

We assume that a local cortical assembly can represent transitorily a part of a visual scene by an interactive process of mutual facilitation and synchronization of those activities that are evoked by that part of the scene. It is further assumed that an individual neuron contributes to the momentary stimulus representation of a local assembly according to its (dynamic, spatio-temporal) RF-properties, weighted by the degree of its momentary activation, e.g. its spike density (for dynamic visual RFs see: Krause and Eckhorn 1983; Krause et al. 1987; Eckhorn and Reitboeck 1988; Lohmann et al. 1988 ; Dinse et al. 1990). In more detail, each assembly member that discharges an action potential contributes, at that moment, its RF-properties to the current stimulus representation. An assembly's current stimulus representation, hence, is assumed to be defined by some interpolation process among contributions of the individual member neurons. The simplest assumption for such interpolation would be averaging by linear superposition. This concept for *sensory interpolation coding* corresponds to that of the population vector proposed by Georgopoulos for the motor system (e.g. Georgopoulos et al. 1989). If a local visual assembly has, for example, two groups of neurons that prefer orthogonal stimulus orientations, and their synchronized activities are at about the same firing rates, this would indicate (represent) a local stimulus orientation that is in the middle of the "prefered" main orientations of the subpopulations. Any local orientation could be "interpolated" by such an assembly in a graded way. The resolution would depend on the tuning widths of the RF-properties, on the variability in the stimulus-response activities, on the degree of the current correlation among these activities, and on the number of cells that contribute. (Note that an RF representation is projected into visual space (Krause and Eckhorn 1983; Krause et al. 1987; Eckhorn and Reitboeck 1988; Lohmann et al. 1988; for general RF-concepts see also Johannesma et al. 1986).

The assumed stimulus representations by local assemblies will, in the following, be termed *"interpolation coding"*. The linear interpolation, proposed above, is mathematically the simplest form, but physiologically and perceptually more plausible are non-linear "context dependent" interpolations in order to explain, for example, the high degree of context dependence for perceptions of the same visual objects.

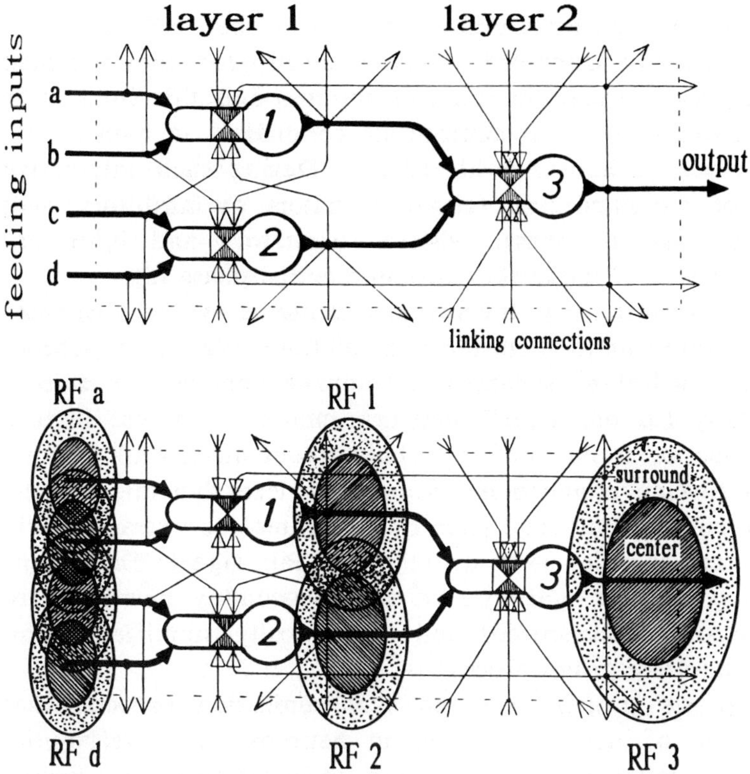

Fig. 11. Scheme of two different types of connections in sensory systems. Top: *1*, *2* and *3* denote three schematic neurons with feeding and linking inputs. Feeding connections (thick lines) converge in retinotopic order from lower onto higher layer neurons. They can activate the neurons directly and by this means the next layer's receptive fields (*RF*, with center and surround, shown in bottom diagram) are formed by the superposition of the lower layer RFs. Linking connections (thin lines) are much more numerous; they project in forward, lateral and backward directions (not in strict topographic order) and terminate on linking synapses that facilitate (modulate, multiply) the feeding signals and by this means provide mutual synchronizations among the neurons without deterioration of their RF properties (Fig. from Eckhorn et al., in press)

Interpolation coding, as defined above, requires the parallel activation of the neurons involved in such a dynamic coding process. In general, activation is stimulus related and it may typically proceed in the following phases in a local assembly of the visual cortex. Initial activation by a stimulus is mediated mainly by the afferent visual feeding inputs, and many "members" of a local assembly are generally activated together (though differently strong) since their RF-properties are similar, as already discussed. It is assumed that the activated neurons interact via mutual linking connections, and this interactive process might culminate, under appropriate conditions, in highly synchronized activities (Eckhorn et al. 1990b). During such interactive states neurons of the same class (either excitatory or inhibitory) will discharge on average in phase, whereas excitatory and inhibitory neurons will be active at relatively constant average phase lags.

It is further assumed, that the primary stimulus-evoked responses are facilitated without major deteriorations of their relative amplitudes (spike densities) via linking synapses that connect members of a local assembly mutually (in our neural network models of visual feature linking such behavior is included: e.g. Eckhorn et al. 1990b). Mutual facilitation via linking connections, if present, is a dynamic process that can occur rhythmically and thereby generates the extracellularly recorded oscillation spindles as an average assembly signal. This means that the stimulus-specific activities of single assembly members are temporally "sorted" (synchronized) and rhythmically amplified in an interactive and iterative group process.

Summarizing, we propose for the synchronization process, that mutual facilitation of neural activities in neurons with overlapping RF-positions and similar RF-properties (i.e. in local assemblies) results in enhancement of correlated components ("signal") and suppression of uncorrelated ones ("noise"). This means that the "signal-to-noise" ratio is improved - the coherent, high amplitude activity of such active assembly "pops out" against uncorrelated activities of other neurons.

We are aware of the problem that the interpolation coding proposed requires continuous "awareness" of the RF-properties by the visual system, e.g. it has to "know" these properties and has to use them, as mentioned above, as reference information between the outer "visual world" and perception. Such an assumption (of a "labelled line code" in lower visual centers) is testable, at least qualitatively, by single cell recordings from behaving animals that are trained to respond to specific visual features which are coded by the RF-properties of the visual cortical neurons recorded from (our present experimental results give no clues to relations between synchronization effects and perception, because they were obtained from anesthetized cats).

For the validity of the "linking-by-synchronization" hypotheses it is essential that local assemblies not only can synchronize their activated members internally, but that synchronously active sub-assemblies (that process local features by interpolation coding) can lock their activities to those other activated sub-assemblies in the same and in other cortical areas that are currently processing the stimulus properties of the same "visual object". The presence of such inter-assembly synchronizations is supported by our experimental results, where we found stimulus-specific synchronized activities in several visual cortex areas of both hemispheres.

There are indirect hints on the implementation of interpolation coding in the visual system: we can, for example, perceive thousands of different colors on the basis of only three different types of color receptors. It is clear that special neural network connections and the dynamic activations within the networks give rise to the specificities of color perception (although the detailed mechanisms are mainly unknown). Whether the flexible mechanism of "color-interpolation" is similar to the "interpolation" mechanism assumed above is largely unknown. However, it seems reasonable to assume that similar neural mechanisms are used for the processing of different visual features, and even for features in and between different sensory modalities in different mammals and in humans.

It is believed, in addition, that interpolation coding is also used in motor systems. A convincing indication is given already by the work of Georgopoulos and coworkers (1989). They showed that a transitory "population vector" can be calculated by an average of the components of several motor neurons, where the components were derived (from a set of cortical motor neurons in a trained monkey) by weighing the main vector of a neuron's "motor field" with its present spike rate. It was shown that such a population vector tightly matches the real motor performance of the monkey. One has to note that the motor neurons were recorded in succession and not in parallel from simultaneously active motor assemblies so that their real degree of synchronization is not known. However, for the calculation of population vectors the activities were temporally "sorted" according to a common motor act on which the monkey was trained (Georgopoulos et al. 1989). In terms of the present paper this might resemble "event-locked" synchronizations (next Section) although it is not clear, whether the degree of correlation in monkey motor units is really of the same order of magnitude as in event locked responses of sensory cortices.

Two modes of processing and their interactions in cat visual cortex: stimulus-induced oscillatory synchronizations and stimulus-locked non-oscillatory synchronizations

In addition to stimulus-induced oscillatory synchronizations we further suggested that stimulus-locked cortical responses play a role in sensory integration (Eckhorn et al. 1990c). Recently we found that stimulus-locked cortical synchronizations can suppress oscillatory activities immediately (Eckhorn and Schanze 1991). In order to determine interactions between both types of synchronizations in some detail, we applied stimuli where they occurred simultaneously (Kruse et al. 1991).

Oscillatory synchronizations (40-80 Hz; Fig. 12A,C) of high probability and strength were induced in our experiments preferentially by sustained slowly moving grating or bar stimuli that do not evoke brisk transient responses in cortical neurons. *Stimulus-locked synchronizations* occurred in the range 1-40 Hz (Fig. 12B,D) and they were evoked in our experiments by 1) sudden stimulus movements (jerks), 2) stochastic Gaussian movements with variable standard deviations, and 3) light flashes. During phases of sustained oscillatory activations (that were induced by continuously drifting stimuli) gradual increases in the stimulus-locked response amplitudes (Fig. 12B) are correlated

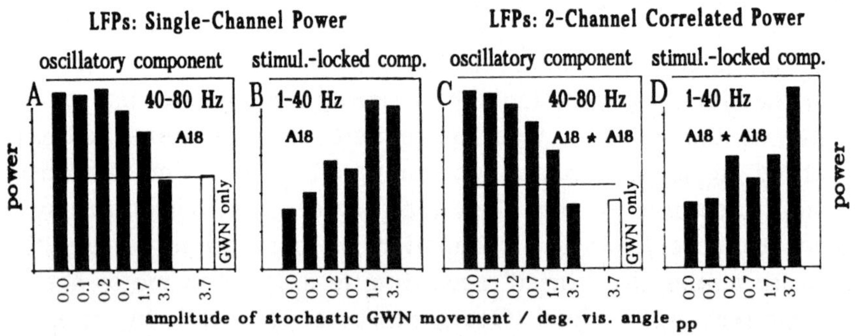

Fig. 12. Interactions between stimulus-induced oscillatory synchronizations and stimulus-locked non-rhythmic synchronizations. Spectral power (arbitrary units) of internally generated oscillatory components (A and C) and stimulus-locked non-oscillatory components (B and D) of LFP-recordings from cat A18. **A, B**: single electrode data ("auto" spectral power), **C, D**: pair recording ("cross" spectral power). (Fig. from Kruse et al. 1991)

with gradual decreases in amplitudes and occurrence probabilities of oscillatory events (Fig. 12A,C) and a slight increase in oscillation frequencies (10%). The larger the stimulus-locked responses, the longer they inhibited the generation of oscillatory events (up to 250 ms after jerks and flashes). After inhibitory periods, oscillation spindles can, however, occur with enhanced amplitudes and probabilities compared with situations where no stimulus-locked responses interfered with spindle generation (Eckhorn and Schanze 1991).

Sudden positional jerks in a slowly drifting grating could evoke strong stimulus-locked responses in the cortical neurons we recorded from. Such jerks affected the generation of oscillation spindles considerably: Jerks superimposed on the continuous drift of a stimulus led to a reduction of average spindle amplitudes and spindle durations, to an increase in average spindle oscillation frequencies, and to lower oscillation probabilities (Eckhorn and Schanze 1991).

When the jerks were made by an otherwise stationary grating we found a remarkable effect (Fig. 13): after a short stimulus-locked burst and an inhibitory pause oscillation spindles were generated over several hundred milliseconds. The spindles' amplitudes and durations were slightly smaller under these conditions, while oscillation frequencies and probabilities did not change significantly compared with the values obtained with drifting stimuli. The possible significance of these findings for feature linking in natural vision will be discussed below.

Explanations why response latencies of stimulus-locked activities are shorter and more precise than those of oscillation spindles could be as follows: Stimulus-locked responses dominate cortical activities and thereby generate essentially different spike patterns in individual neurons. This heterogenous response of cortical neurons is probably one of the reasons why mutual oscillatory synchronizations are not present during transient visual drive. After strong visual activations a certain "relaxation" time is required for the dominating stimulus influence to wear off until a process of self organization can lead to oscillatory synchronizations. Under the assumption that individual intra- and inter-cortical linking connections are weak, the release from dominating visual drive is essential for the generation of oscillations. There is evidence from our neural network models, that the larger the differences in the neurones' responses, the less probable is the formation of a common phase-locked oscillatory state.

Periods of strong stimulus-locked and oscillatory stimulus-induced synchronizations might characterize extreme processing states of the

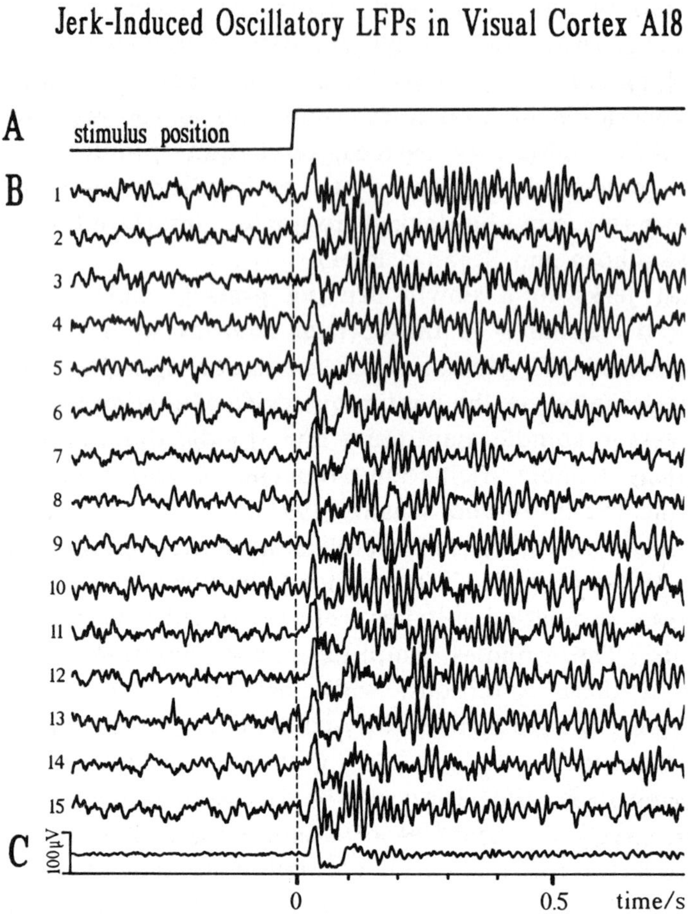

Fig. 13. Jerk-induced oscillatory LFPs in visual cortex (A18). **A**: At $t = 0$ a previously stationary grating jerks by half a spatial cycle; orientation and jerk direction correspond with the preferences of the neurons at the recording position in visual cortex area 18. **B**: 15 consecutively recorded LFP epochs from the same electrode in response to identical jerk stimuli (upward is negative). **C**: Stimulus-locked ensemble average of LFP epochs in B. Amplitudes in B and C are calibrated to the same scale. Note the high amplitude oscillation spindles after the primary "jerk potential" in B and the suppression of oscillatory components in C due to stimulus-locked averaging (Fig. from Eckhorn and Schanze 1991)

visual cortex. In natural vision, short stimulus shifts are often followed by phases with more stationary retinal images, for example during saccade-fixation sequences or when a visual object suddenly moves and stops again. In both visual situations the primary stimulus-locked responses, that occur synchronized in many cortical neurons, might help to signal in a relatively crude but fast way the "When", "Where" and "What" of the current visual events. The following silent phase of partial inhibition may play a role for perceptual suppression of the fast retinal image shifts during saccades, and/or it may transitorily put the system into a state of fast responses, but relative insensitivity during which stimulus-locked signals can precisely be transmitted with high signal-to-noise ratios, while internally generated signals, including cortical oscillations, are largely suppressed. Post inhibitory rebound activations after sudden shifts of an object or after saccades, might be useful for the sensitive generation of oscillatory synchronizations in just those parts of the cortical network in which the linking connections are still sensitized by the fast stimulus-locked response components (Eckhorn et al. 1990b). During conditions of natural vision oscillatory signal processing, however, is time consuming (20 ms per cycle at 50 Hz; average spindle duration is about 100 ms). In temporally critical situations it is, therefore, of advantage, that stimulus-induced oscillatory states can quickly be suppressed by sudden stimulus transients.

We propose, *in conclusion*, that strong stimulus-locked and oscillatory synchronizations occur in alternation during natural vision in the cat and that they are superimposed if the stimulus-locked responses are of lower amplitudes. Oscillatory synchronizations are supported during post-inhibitory rebound states (e.g. after a strong post-saccadic response) and with slow retinal image movements. It is known from behavioral and psychophysical investigations with cats, monkeys and humans that sustained and transient phases of stimulation both can lead to specific visual perceptions. This means that oscillatory modes of activation in the visual cortex are probably not a prerequisite for visual perception, at least not in the cat, in which the oscillatory activities (of 35-80 Hz, as observed by us experimentally) are suppressed by stimulus-locked responses. We are convinced, that it is the simultaneity of neural activities in coupled networks of cortical assemblies that supports perceptual binding, irrespective of how it is generated. Such a view is in line with basic neurophysiological knowledge of spatial and temporal integrating capabilities of single neurons: synchronized activities of equal type (e.g., excitatory) are enhanced in their action on the spike encoder while temporally dispersed inputs of different types are mainly "averaged out" by the low pass properties of dendrites and soma. This means that each neuron can acts as a "covariance detector", independent on how the covariances were generated. Covariances on a more global scale of cortical activation, however, depend significantly on the different extrinsic and intrinsic sources and mechanisms that lead to different spatio-temporal patterns of correlated firings and which probably lead to qualitatively different percepts: *Stimulus locked synchronizations* may mainly support crude "instantaneous" percepts", and *stimulus-induced oscillatory synchronizations* may support more complex percepts that require iterative interactions among different processing levels and memory.

Acknowledgements

I am especially thankful to Prof. H. J. Reitboeck, the head of our Biophysics Department, for his continuous support in developing both concepts and the multiple-electrode instrumentation. This article could not have been written without the numerous discussions with my colleagues Dr. R. Bauer, M. Brosch, W. Jordan, W. Kruse, M. Munk, A. Obermüller, and T. Schanze, and without their extensive help in experiments, data acquisition and processing, as partly credited in the Figure captions. Expert help in care and preparation of our cats and help in experimental techniques were supplied by U. Thomas, J.H. Wagner and W. Lenz. Thanks also to Ad Aertsen for his helpful comments on this manuscript and for improving the English. The financial support for this project is greatly acknowledged: from Deutsche Forschungsgemeinschaft Re 547/2-1,2 (to H.J. Reitboeck and R. Eckhorn), Ec 53/4-1 (to R. Eckhorn and J.I. Nelson), Ja 475 (to P. Janich, R. Bauer, R. Eckhorn, H.J. Reitboeck), Ec 53/6-2 (to R. Eckhorn and R. Bauer).

References

Abeles M (1982) Local Cortical Circuits. Springer, Berlin Heidelberg New York

Aertsen AMHJ, Gerstein GL (1985) Evaluation of neuronal connectivity: sensitivity of cross correlation. Brain Res 340:341-354

Aertsen AMHJ, Gerstein GL, Johannesma PIM (1986) From neuron to assembly: neuronal organization and stimulus representation. In: Palm G, Aertsen AMHJ (eds) Brain Theory, Springer, Berlin Heidelberg New York, pp 7-24

Aertsen AMHJ, Bonhoeffer T, Krüger J (1987) Coherent activity in neuronal populations: analysis and interpretation. In: Caianiello E (ed) Physics of Cognitive Processes, World Scientific Publishing, Singapore, pp 1-34

Bauer R, Eckhorn R, Jordan W (1989) Iso- and Cross-orientation columns in cat striate cortex: A reexamination with simultaneous single- and multi-unit recordings. Neurosci 30:733-740

Braitenberg V, Schüz A (1990) Anatomy of the Cortex, statistics and geometry. Studies of Brain Function. Springer, Berlin Heidelberg New York

Chagnac-Amitai Y, Connors BW (1989) Horizontal spread of snchronized activity in neocortex and its control by GABA-mediated inhibition. J Neurophysiol 62:1149-1162

Creutzfeldt OD, Watanabe S, Lux HD (1966) Relation between EEG-phenomena and potentials of single cells. Part I and II. Electroencephalogr Clin Neurophysiol 20:1-37

Dinse HR, Krüger K, Best J (1990) A temporal structure of cortical information processing. Concepts Brain Sci 1:199-238

Eckhorn R, Reitboeck HJ (1988) Assessment of cooperative firing in groups of neurons. In: Basar E (ed) Springer Series in Brain Dynamics, vol I, Springer, Berlin Heidelberg, pp 219-227

Eckhorn R, Bauer R, Jordan W, Brosch M, Kruse W, Munk M, Reitboeck HJ (1988) Coherent oscillations: A mechanism of feature linking in the visual cortex? Multiple electrode and correlation analysis in the cat. Biol Cybern 60:121-130

Eckhorn R, Bauer R, Reitboeck HJ (1989) Discontinuities in visual cortex and possible functional implications: Relating cortical structure and function with multi-electrode/correlation techniques. In: Basar E, Bullock TH (eds) Springer Series in Brain Dynamics, vol II, Springer, Berlin Heidelberg New York, pp 267-278

Eckhorn R, Brosch M, Salem W, Bauer R (1990a) Cooperativity between cat area 17 and 18 revealed with signal correlations and HRP. In: Elsner N, Roth G (eds) Brain - Perception - Cognition. Thieme, Stuttgart New York, p 237

Eckhorn R, Reitboeck HJ, Arndt M, Dicke P (1990b) Feature linking via synchronization among distributed assemblies: Results from cat visual cortex and from simulations. Neural Computation 2:293-307

Eckhorn R, Dicke P, Arndt M, Reitboeck HJ (1990c) Temporal linking between remote sensory representations simulated with a neural network. In: Elsner N, Roth G (eds) Brain - Perception - Cognition. Thieme, Stuttgart New York, p 17

Eckhorn R, Brosch M, Salem W, Bauer R (1990d) Cooperativity between cat area 17 and 18 revealed with signal correlations and HRP. In: Elsner N, Roth G (eds) Brain - Perception - Cognition. Thieme, Stuttgart New York, p 237

Eckhorn R, Schanze T (1991) Possible neural mechanisms of feature linking in the visual system: Stimulus-locked and stimulus-induced synchronizations. In: Babloyantz A (ed) Self-Organization, Emerging Properties and Learning. Plenum, New York

Eckhorn R (1991) Stimulus-evoked synchronizations in the visual cortex: Linking of local features into global figures? In: Krüger J (ed) Neural Cooperativity Springer, Berlin Heidelberg New York, pp 184-224

Eckhorn R, Schanze T, Brosch M, Salem W, Bauer R (in press) Stimulus-specific synchronizations in cat visual cortex: Multiple microelectrode and correlation studies from several cortical areas. In: Bullock TH, Basar E (eds) Induced Rhythms in the Brain. Springer Series in Brain Dynamics. Springer, Heidelberg Berlin New York

Engel AK, König P, Gray CM, Singer W (1990a) Stimulus-dependent neuronal oscillations in cat visual cortex: Inter-columnar interaction as determined by cross-correlation analysis. Europ J Neurosci 2:588-606

Engel AK, König P, Kreiter AK, Singer W (1990b) Inter-areal and inter-hemispheric synchronization of oscillatory responses in cat visual cortex. Soc Neurosci Abstr 16:1269

Fleischhauer K (1974) On different patterns of dendritic bundling in the cerebral cortex of the cat. Z Anat Entwickl Gesch 143:115-126

Freeman WJ (1975) Mass action in the nervous system. Academic Press, New York

Freeman WJ, Skarda C A (1985) Spatial EEG patterns, non-linear dynamics and perception: the Neo-Sherringtonian view. Brain Res Rev 10:147-175

Georgopoulos AP, Lurito JT, Petrides M, Schwartz AB, Massey JT (1989) Mental rotation of the neuronal population vector. Science 243:234-236

Gerstein GL, Bedenbaugh P, Aertsen AMHJ (1989) Neuronal assemblies. IEEE Trans Biomed Engin 36:4-14

Gilbert CD (1985) Horizontal integrations in the neocortex. Trends Neurosci 8:160-165

Gray CM, Singer W (1987a) Stimulus-dependent neuronal oscillations in the cat visual cortex area 17. 2nd IBRO-Congrs, Neurosci Suppl, 1301P

Gray CM, Singer W (1987b) Stimulus specific neuronal oscillations in the cat visual cortex: a cortical functional unit. Soc Neurosci Abstr 404.3

Gray CM, König P, Engel AK, Singer W (1989). Oscillatory responses in cat visual cortex exhibit inter-columnar synchronization which reflects global stimulus properties. Nature 338:334-337

Gray CM, Singer W (1989) Stimulus-specific neuronal oscillations in orientation columns of cat visual cortex. Proc Nat Acad Sci (USA) 86:1698

Hoeltzell PB, Dykes RW (1979) Conductivity in the somatosensory cortex of the cat-evidence for cortical anisotropy. Brain Res 177:61-82

Hubel DH, Wiesel TN (1962) Receptive fields, binocular interaction, and functional architecture in the cat's visual cortex. J Physiol 160:106-154

Hubel DH, Wiesel TN (1963) Shape and arrangement of columns in cat's striate cortex. J Physiol 165:559-568

Johannesma P, Aertsen A, van den Boogaard H, Eggermont J, Epping W (1986) From synchrony to harmony: ideas on the function of neural assemblies and on the interpretation of neural synchrony. In: Palm G, Aertsen A (eds) Brain Theory. Springer, Berlin Heidelberg, pp 25-47

Krause F, Eckhorn R (1983) Receptive fields for motion stimuli (RFM) determined for different types of cat visual neurons. Neurosci Lett (Suppl) 14:209

Krause F, Gonzalez F, Nelson JI, Eckhorn R (1987) A fast method for predicting coding properties of visual cortical simple cells. Perception 16, Suppl:262

Krüger J (1983) Simultaneous individual recordings from many cerebral neurons: techniques and results. Rev Physiol Biochem Pharmacol 98:177-233

Krüger J, Aiple F (1988) Multimicroelectrode investigation of monkey striate cortex: spike train correlations in the infragranular layers. J Neurophysiol 60:798-828

Krüger J, Aiple F (1989) The connectivity underlying the orientation selectivity in the infragranular layers of monkey striate cortex. Brain Res 477:57-65

Kruse W, Eckhorn R, Schanze T (1991) Two modes of processing and their interactions in cat visual cortex: Stimulus-induced oscillatory and stimulus-locked synchronizations. In: Elsner N, Penzlin H (eds) Synapse - Transmission - Modulation. Thieme, Stuttgart New York

Lohmann H, Eckhorn R, Reitboeck HJ (1988) Visual receptive fields of local intracortical potentials. J Neurosci Meth 25:29-44

Mitzdorf U (1985) Current source density method and application in cat cerebral cortex: investigation of evoked potentials and EEG phenomena. Physiol Rev 65:37-100

Mitzdorf U (1987) Properties of the evoked potential generators: current source-density analysis of visually evoked potentials in the cat cortex. Intern J Neurosci 33:33-59

Mountcastle VB (1957) Modality and topographic properties of single neurons of cat's somatic sensory cortex. J Neurophysiol 20:408-434

Mountcastle VB (1978) An organizing principle for cerebral function: The unit module and the distributed system. In: Edelman GM, Mountcastle VB (eds) The Mindful Brain. MIT Press, Cambridge, Massachusetts

Mountcastle VB, Reitboeck HJ, Poggio GF, Steinmetz MA (1991) Adaptation of the Reitboeck method of multiple microelectrode recording to the neocortex of the waking monkey. J Neurosci Meth 36:77-84

Obermüller A, Eckhorn R, Kruse W (1991) Stimulus-induced oscillatory synchronizations in cat visual cortex: single neurons are differently involved. In: Elsner N, Penzlin H (eds) Synapse - Transmission - Modulation. Thieme, Stuttgart New York

Palm G (1982) Neural Assemblies. Studies of Brain Function vol 7. Springer, Berlin Heidelberg New York

Palm G, Aertsen AMHJ, Gerstein GL (1988) On the significance of correlations among neuronal spike trains. Biol Cybern 59:1-11

Payne BR, Berman N, Murphy EH (1981) Organization of direction preferences in cat visual cortex. Brain Res 211:445-450

Reitboeck HJ (1983a) A 19-channel matrix drive with individually controllable fiber microelectrodes for neurophysiological applications. IEEE SMC 13:676-682

Reitboeck HJ (1983b) Fiber microelectrodes for electrophysiological recordings. J Neurosci Meth 8:249-262

Reitboeck HJ (1988) Neural mechanisms of pattern recognition. In: Sensory Processing in the Mammalian Brain: Neural Substrates and Experimental Strategies. Lund J (ed) Oxford University Press, pp 420-465

Schanze T, Eckhorn R, Baumgarten H (1990) Properties of stimulus-induced oscillatory events in cat visual cortex. In: Elsner N, Roth G (eds) Brain - Perception - Cognition. Thieme, Stuttgart New York, p 238

Schanze T, Eckhorn R (1991) Synchronization statistics of stimulus-specific oscillatory events in cat visual cortex. In: Elsner N, Penzlin H (eds) Synapse - Transmission - Modulation. Thieme, Stuttgart New York

Ts'o DY, Gilbert CD, Wiesel TN (1986) Relationships between horizontal interactions and functional architecture in cat striate cortex as revealed by cross-correlation analysis. J Neurosci 6:1160-1170

Van Kan PLE, Scobey RP, Gabor AJ (1985) Response covariance in cat visual cortex. Exp Brain Res 60:559-563

Weyand TG, Malpeli JG, Lee C, Schwark HD (1987) Cat area 17: IV. Two types of corticotectal cells defined by controlling geniculate inputs. J Neurophysiol 56:1102-1108

Imaging the Functional Architecture of Cat Area 18 in vivo

Tobias Bonhoeffer[1] and Amiram Grinvald

The Rockefeller University, New York, NY 10021, USA; IBM Research Division, Yorktown Heights, NY 10598, USA; The Weizmann Institute of Science, Rehovot, Israel

Introduction

The mammalian cerebral cortex in general and the visual cortex in particular is organized in a columnar fashion (Mountcastle 1957; Hubel and Wiesel 1965). Thus, despite some lamina-dependent differences, neurons lying below each other, from the pia to the white matter, share important functional properties. A method which has proven to be very useful for investigating the functional architecture across a cortical area is the 2-Deoxyglucose (2-DG) technique (Sokoloff 1977). It takes advantage of the fact that neuronal activity is associated with enhanced metabolic activity, which can be autoradiographically visualized with a radioactive glucose analog.

There are only two ways, however, to label 2-Deoxyglucose radioactively. This presents a severe experimental restriction since it limits the number of activity maps which can be recorded from a piece of cortical tissue. This hampers obtaining clear answers to the outstanding questions concerning the spatial relationships between different functional components in the cortex (for example, the relationship between columns of different orientation preference or between orientation and ocular dominance columns in the visual cortex). Additionally, these results can only be obtained post mortem and it is therefore impossible to use the acquired information to guide further in vivo experiments on the same animal.

---

[1] present address: Max-Planck-Institut für Hirnforschung, Deutschordenstrasse 36, 6000 Frankfurt a. M. 71, Germany

Recently our lab has developed a new technique which allows visualization of metabolic activity in vivo (Grinvald et al. 1986; Ts'o et al. 1990). This new technique, optical imaging of intrinsic signals, therefore has the advantage that one can obtain multiple activity maps from a single cortical area by presenting the animal with many different stimuli. The resulting data thus provide a far more complete picture of the functional architecture of the cortex.

Optical imaging of intrinsic signals makes use of the fact that the optical properties of cortical tissue change with electrical activity. There are various sources for the optical signal which conveys information about cortical activity (Frostig et al. 1990). The major component of the intrinsic signal is related to oximetry. In active regions of the tissue oxy-hemoglobin is converted into hemoglobin in response to the metabolic demand for oxygen. Oxy-hemoglobin and hemoglobin have different absorption-spectra and thus oxygen delivery is easily detectable optically. Other sources of the intrinsic signal include changes in blood volume (due to activity-dependent dilation of capillaries), cytochrome-absorption and light scattering. Utilizing these intrinsic signals, we can image cortical activity with a resolution of approximately 100 μm.

In the first set of experiments we took advantage of the fact that one can obtain multiple maps from one cortical region to examine whether "directionality columns" exist in cat visual cortex. Such columns have been reported in cat area 17 (Tolhurst et al. 1981; Payne et al. 1980) and area 18 (Swindale et al. 1987) but these results remained somewhat controversial. By directly comparing high-resolution activity maps obtained with a grating moving in one direction with those obtained with the same grating moving in the opposite direction, we could determine whether cells are sorted into columns according to preferred direction of motion.

Besides our interest in directionality columns, we also wanted to clarify the detailed organization of orientation preference. There has been a great deal of debate about how orientation columns are spatially organized in cat visual cortex. Hubel and Wiesel originally described them as "swirling stripes with many bifurcations and endings" (Hubel et al. 1977; Hubel et al. 1978). On the other hand, von Seelen (1970) and Braitenberg and Braitenberg (1979) showed that many of the data obtained by Hubel and Wiesel could also be explained by centers around which the different orientation domains were organized in a pinwheel-like fashion (each orientation appearing around the center twice). Löwel et al. (1987) challenged this interpretation by performing an extensive 2-DG study of area 17 and 18 in the cat from which they concluded that orientation was organized in stripes rather than pinwheels. Subsequent data from monkey V1 (Blasdel and Salama 1986) and area 18 of the cat (Swindale et al. 1987) again revived the idea of orientation being organized around centers. These data prompted several authors (Linsker 1986; Götz 1987) to suggest that instead of orientation centers around which every orientation appears twice (as suggested by Braitenberg and Braitenberg) the actual organization might rather be one with every orientation appearing only once in the circle. These studies were based on work with monkeys, but work on cat area 18 (Swindale et al. 1987) suggested that the organization there might be similar. The latter experiments had, however, the disadvantage that the maps obtained had a resolution of only 300-400 μm. Consequently the orientations between these data points could only be interpolated and were thus burdened with some uncertainty.

Since all the previously performed experiments lacked either sufficient resolution (electrode recordings) or the benefit of having data from many different orientations (2-DG experiments), we used our new method to take a closer look at the organization of orientation preference in cat area 18. In particular we aimed to distinguish between the three proposed models for the organization of orientation preference. (1) Parallel bands of orientation preference (Hubel et al. 1977; Hubel et al. 1978), (2) orientation centers with every orientation appearing twice around the center (Braitenberg and Braitenberg 1980) or (3) orientation centers (appearing with two different handednesses, clockwise and counterclockwise) with every orientation appearing around the center singularity only once (Swindale 1982; Linsker 1986; Götz 1987).

Material and methods

Animals

Cats were initially anesthetized with ketamine HCl (20 mg/kg, IM) followed by sodium pentothal (20 mg/kg, IV) and further injections as needed. A tracheotomy was performed and after paralysis (succinylcholine HCl, 20 mg/kg/h, IV) the animal was artificially respirated.

EEG, ECG, expired CO2 and rectal temperature were monitored throughout the experiment.

A retinoscope was used to determine the correct refractive power for the contact lenses which were put in the cat's eyes.

Optical chamber

The skull of the cat was opened above area 18 by drilling two elongated holes whose centers lay at Horsley-Clarke A5 and 0.5 mm lateral to the mid-line. After a stainless steel chamber was cemented onto the skull, the dura was removed, the chamber filled with silicone oil and sealed with a round glass coverslip. This arrangement minimized the movement of the cortex due to heartbeat and respiration which otherwise severely hampered satisfactory optical imaging.

CCD camera and optics

The basic experimental setup is shown in Figure 1. The surface of the cortex was illuminated by two adjustable light guides. These guides were attached to a Zeiss tungsten-halogen lamp. The light was passed through interference filters of different wavelengths. The filter most often used for visualizing the surface of the cortex and its blood vessels had a transmission maximum at 540 ± 15 nm whereas the filter for the optical imaging proper was a 630 ± 5 nm filter.

A slow scan CCD camera (Photometrics) recorded pictures from the exposed parts of the cortex. The pictures which in the current arrangement have a spatial resolution of 192 x 144 pixels were digitized and fed into a DEC Microvax II computer.

We used two different kinds of lenses for our experiments. In some of the experiments standard 35 mm camera lenses were used; in most cases this was a 2.8/135 macro-lens (Pentax); in a few cases we additionally used a 2x converter in order to achieve a two-fold higher magnification. With these lenses the size of the imaged area was 8.8 x 6.6 mm^2 or 4.4 x 3.3 mm^2. Thus each pixel monitored activity of a 46 x 46 μm^2 or 23 x 23 μm^2 area of cortex. In this case the aperture of the lens was always set to 2.8 which provided us with a depth of field of several hundred microns.

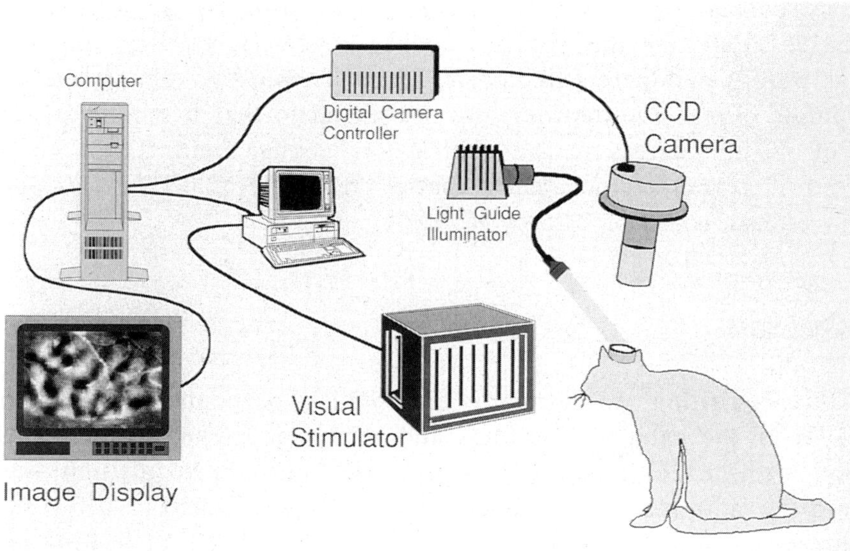

Fig. 1. Setup for an optical recording experiment. The cat is visually stimulated with gratings moving on a CRT screen (visual stimulator). The brain is illuminated with light of 630 nm wavelength. A CCD camera is used to take high resolution images from the exposed brain region. These pictures carrying information about neural activity are digitized and sent to a computer where they are processed. The resulting activity maps are then displayed on a video display

In other experiments we used a "tandem-lens" arrangement which was developed in our laboratory (Ratzlaff and Grinvald 1991). This device is in essence a microscope (with a rather low magnification) built out of two photographic lenses which together provide an unusually high numerical aperture. This system consequently has a very low depth of field (approximately 50 μm). It allowed us to eliminate virtually all artifacts caused by blood vessels on the surface of the cortex (Malonek et al. 1990). The largest magnification used was 2.7x. With this magnification each pixel recorded activity from a 17 x 17 μm^2 "column" of cortex.

Visual stimuli

Visual stimuli were displayed on a CRT screen (Mitsubishi) in 60 Hz non-interlaced mode at a distance of 25-45 cm from the animal's eyes. The stimuli were generated by an IBM PC/AT with a Number Nine

Graphics board. This powerful system, developed by K. Christian, allowed us to specify the stimulus quality (e.g. bars, gratings, random dots) as well as parameters like color, spatial frequency, velocity etc. in very simple terms. The monitor was positioned so that it stimulated an angle of 40-60 degrees in the contralateral visual field. The stimuli consisted of gratings which had a spatial frequency of 0.15 cycles/deg and moved at a speed of 2.25 cycles/sec.

Data acquisition

For data acquisition we normally presented a particular stimulus to both eyes of the cat for 3 seconds and recorded 5 frames of 600 ms duration with the CCD camera. This period of data acquisition was followed by a 6 sec inter-stimulus interval after which a different stimulus was shown. We presented every stimulus 10 to 100 times randomizing the order of appearance in order to average out any stimulus dependent after-effects.

Data analysis

The first step for data analysis was to add the frames acquired for every visual stimulus. These pictures were then divided by a "blank" trial in order to correct for uneven illumination. This blank trial was obtained by two different procedures. In some experiments the pictures for all different stimuli were summed together ("combination-blank"), in others we used the frames acquired during a trial in which the cat saw a blank screen. The resulting blank-adjusted pictures represented the activity map for the corresponding stimulus.

For complete analysis of the organization of orientation preference we calculated orientation maps in which the responses to all four (or eight) gratings were summed vectorially. The angle of the resulting vector was then displayed using a discrete pseudocolor code.

Results

All our experiments were performed in area 18 of anesthetized and paralyzed cats.

The first step in analysis of our data was to look at the activity maps that were produced by dividing the pictures acquired during one stimulus condition (e.g. a moving grating of oblique orientation) by the blank stimulus. These maps were produced for all the stimulus conditions and served us as a first indication of the quality of the experiment. Figure 2 shows two such maps. Figure 2A shows the cortical region from which the optical signals were recorded. In Figure 2 B and C two activity maps are displayed which were obtained with two oblique, moving gratings. High activity leads to strong absorption of the red illuminating light; thus these regions reflect less light and appear darker in the picture. The strong intensity differences between the light and the dark areas in the Figure are deceptive. They are only obtained by appropriate scaling. The difference in reflected light intensity between the lighter and the darker areas is minute; it is only in the order of 10^{-4} to 10^{3} of the absolute reflected light intensity. By comparing Figure 2 B and C one notices that the cortical regions activated by the two different stimuli are interdigitating; regions strongly activated by one grating are weakly activated by the orthogonal one and vice versa. This confirms what is well-known from electrophysiological studies: cells in one location of the cortex respond very well to a moving grating of a particular orientation but hardly to a grating of the orthogonal orientation. This emphasizes once more the point that all the data gathered in optical experiments are in good agreement with conventional electrophysiological data. In some of our experiments we confirmed the optically obtained maps with conventional single unit recordings. In every case we found an excellent agreement between the optical and the electrophysiological data.

We first investigated whether cells were clustered into direction columns (Payne et al. 1980; Tolhurst et al. 1981; Swindale et al. 1987). To this end we stimulated the eyes with a grating moving in one direction and recorded the activity map from area 18. We then compared this map with the activity map obtained for a grating of the same orientation but the opposite direction of motion. This comparison revealed whether the two gratings stimulate distinct cortical regions (implying that cells are grouped into separate directionality columns)

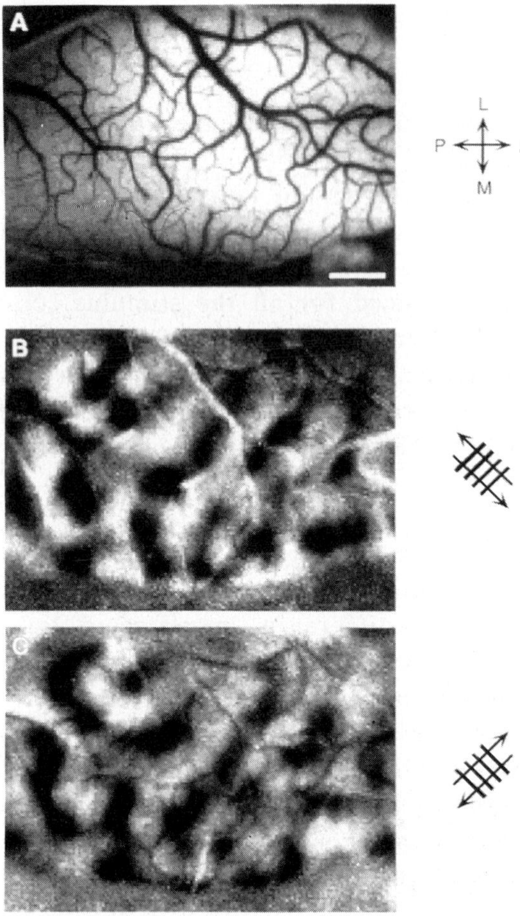

Fig. 2. Activity maps obtained from a 6 by 9 mm piece of visual cortex (area 18). **A**: Bloodvessel pattern of the recorded region. **B**: Activity map recorded with an oblique moving grating as stimulus. Dark areas in the map denote areas of stronger absorption and hence higher activity. **C**: Activity map obtained with the orthogonal stimulus. By comparing part B to part C of this figure one can see how regions strongly activated by one stimulus are only weakly activated by the orthogonal one. Scale bar is 1 mm

or whether the same cortical area is activated by the two stimuli (implying that there are no directionality columns). Our data displayed in Figure 3 indicate that the latter is the case. The activity map for a vertical grating moving to the left is shown in Figure 3A, the map for the same grating moving to the right in Figure 3B. Examination of

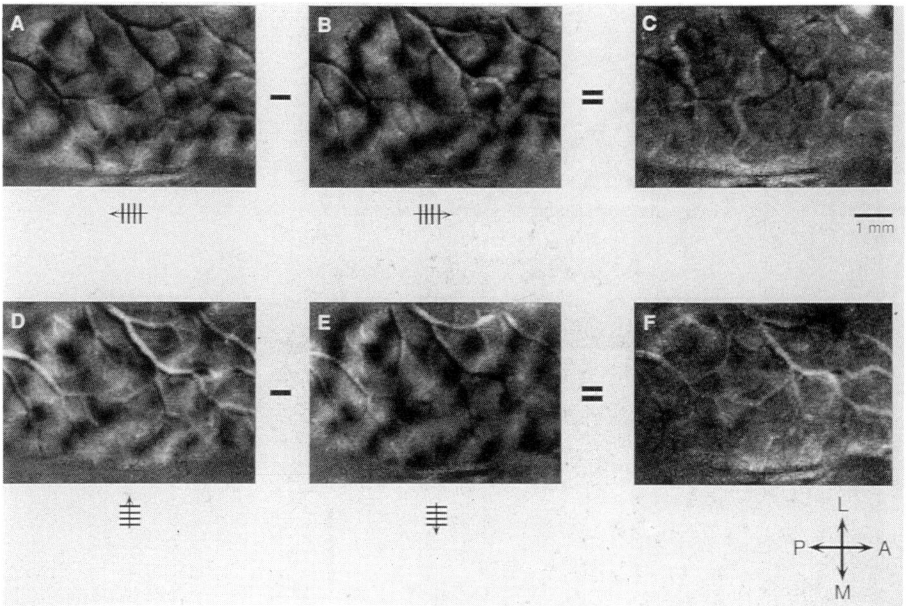

Fig. 3. Activity maps obtained with two gratings having the same orientation but moving in two different directions. The area from which these data are obtained is shown in Fig. 2A. **A**: activity map produced by a vertical grating moving to the left. **B**: activity map produced by the same vertical grating moving to the right. **C**: Subtraction of the two maps results in a patternless picture. **D, E, F**: Similar data for horizontal gratings moving either upward (D) or downward (E). These data suggest that cells in area 18 are not clustered in "directionality columns". Scale bar is 1 mm

these two images indicates that the two maps are very similar: if one subtracts the two maps one is left with a patternless picture shown in Figure 3C. Figure 3D,E,F show similar data for a horizontal grating moving upward (resp. downward). Also in this case the two maps are very similar, and subtraction results in an image with no signs of significant clustering. We performed similar experiments in 16 hemispheres of 9 cats (with 4 or 8 orientations per experiment) and invariably found that maps obtained for a grating moving in one direction were indistinguishable from those obtained with the same grating moving in the opposite direction. These data strongly suggest that cells in area 18 are not grouped into directionality columns, but rather that cells preferring the same orientation but different directions of motion are intermingled.

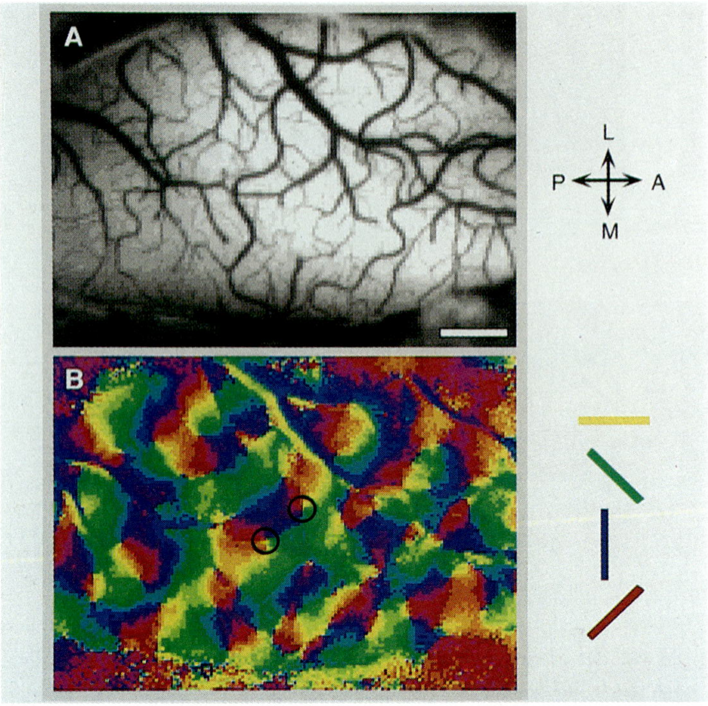

Fig. 4

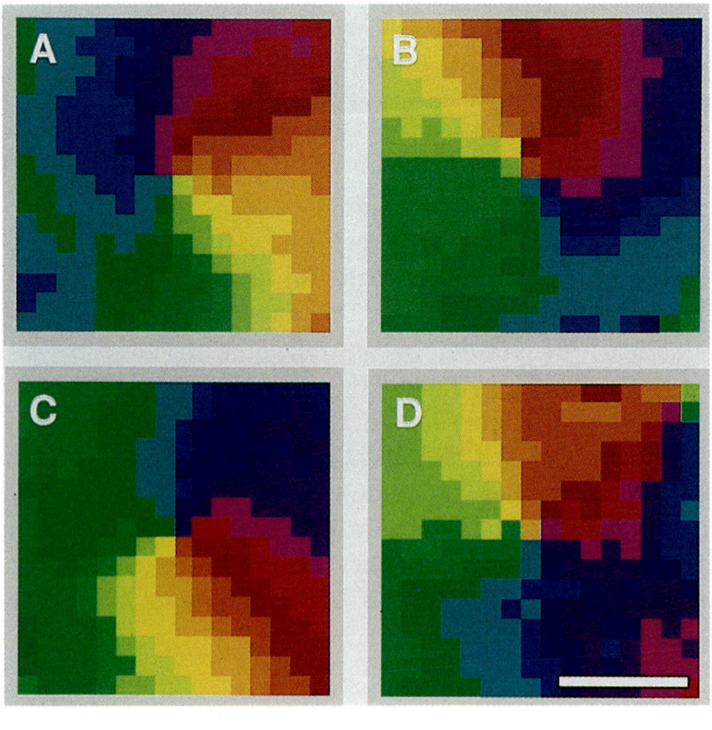

Fig. 5

Data like those presented in Figure 2 are equivalent to 2-DG pictures and - since they only provide information about one orientation - give a very incomplete picture of the organization of orientation in area 18. The unique advantage of optical imaging of intrinsic signals is that one can obtain many maps from one piece of tissue. We made use of this fact and combined the data from eight different orientations to derive a much more complete picture of the overall organization of orientation preference. We took the eight different activity maps and (after multiplying the angles by two (cf. Batschelet 1981; Blasdel and Salama 1986) added them vectorially and coded the resulting angle (again divided by two) in color. Data of this kind are presented in Figure 4 which then give a complete orientation map.

A closer look at these orientation maps reveals a number of noteworthy features. First, the overall appearance of this map is certainly patchy as opposed to banded as one might have expected from 2-DG studies and from Figure 2 of the present work. We found that in 10 out of the 12 hemispheres in which we did this kind of analysis the appearance of orientation columns was clearly patchy. Only in two of the hemispheres did we find the appearance of the map to be banded (both of those experiments were performed in a relatively posterior part of area 18 close to the vertical meridian).

A prominent feature of these maps is that orientation preferences seem to be organized around points which we termed "orientation centers" (two of them are marked with black circles in Figure 4). Areas with different preferred orientation are ordered in a pinwheel-like fashion around the orientation centers. We found on the average 1.2 of these orientation centers per mm^2. In Figure 5 four typical orientation centers are shown at a higher magnification. Different orientation domains encircle the orientation centers. Every orientation appears around an orientation center once. In our experiments we found alto-

---

Fig. 4. Pseudo-color-coded map of orientation preference. **A**: Cortical area from which this orientation map was imaged. **B**: Organization of orientation preference across this cortical area. Preferred orientations are color-coded according to the scheme to the right of the picture (regions preferring moving gratings of vertical orientation are coded in blue, those preferring horizontal gratings are coded in yellow, etc.). Two typical orientation centers are marked with a circle. Scale bar is 1 mm

Fig. 5. Close-up pictures of four "pinwheels" around orientation centers from Fig. 4. Two "clockwise" (**A,C**) and two "counterclockwise" (**B,D**) pinwheels are shown. Scale bar is 300 mm

gether 120 orientation centers and in all of them we found that every orientation appears around the center once. Figure 5 also shows that the "pinwheels" appear in two different forms. One in which the sequence of the colors (and thus orientations) blue, red, yellow and green is clockwise (Fig. 5A,C) and the other one having a counter-clockwise sequence (Fig. 5B,D).

In some of our experiments we observed that gratings of eight different orientations did not activate the cortex in a uniform fashion but produced a distinct pattern of strongly and weakly activated patches of cortex. Figure 6 shows such a result. Part A of the Figure shows the area of cortex that we imaged in this experiment. Part B shows a map which was obtained by adding all the activity maps obtained with 8 different orientations (covering the full range between 0 and 180 degrees). Clearly, not all regions of the cortex are uniformly activated. The dark spots in this picture indicate that certain regions on average were stimulated more strongly than the rest of the field. The magnitude of these differences is much smaller than that observed in a map like the one displayed in Figure 2. In typical cases the dynamic range between the strongest and the weakest activation of such a picture is about 30% of the values obtained for instance in Figure 2. Nevertheless, the activity map obtained with this kind of analysis is quite strong and clearly discernible. We conclude from these data that moving gratings of different orientations do not activate all of the cortex and that there are likely to be other stimulus parameters which are required to stimulate the entire cortical area. There are various possible candidates for these stimulus parameters as will be discussed below.

Discussion

"Direction maps"

Our experiments showed that the maps obtained with a grating moving in one direction were very similar to the ones obtained with a grating moving in the opposite direction. In fact, when subtracting two images acquired with opposing directions a patternless picture resulted (Fig. 3). This suggests that cells in area 18 of the cat are not arranged in directionality columns. However, two alternative possibilities remain to

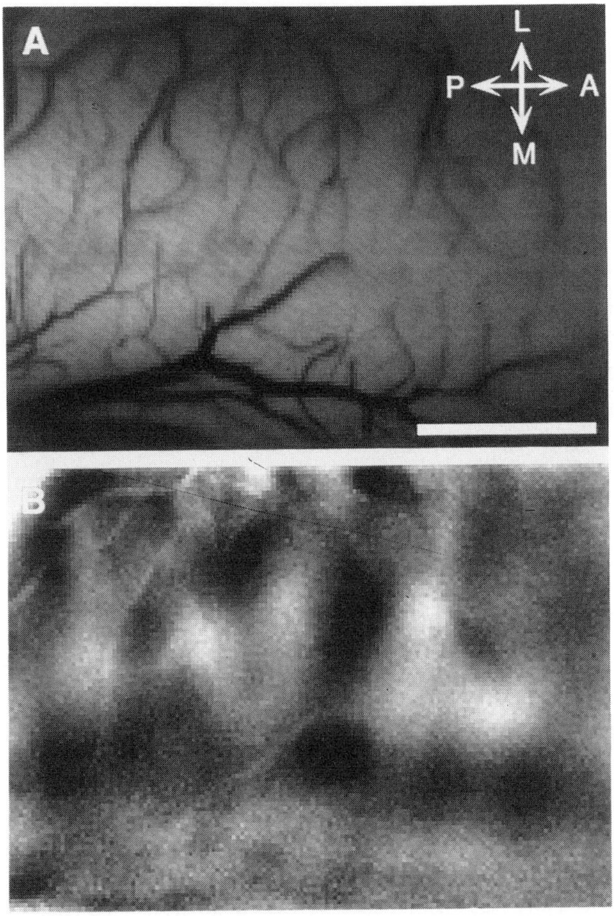

Fig. 6. Not all regions in the cortex are activated evenly with stimuli comprising eight different orientations. A: Region of cortex from which these data were imaged. B: Map obtained by combining activity maps from all eight orientations. Some areas of the cortex appear darker meaning that they are activated more strongly than others. This shows that these moving gratings of eight different orientations do not form a complete set of stimuli which activates area 18 evenly

be ruled out. (1) The directionality clusters could be so small that they lie below our technique's resolution of approximately 100 μm. (2) If there were clusters of direction preference which had opposite preferred direction of motion and they were to lie above each other in the cortex our method would not be able to tell the different clusters apart.

In area 17 Payne et al. (1980) and in area 18 Swindale et al. (1987) reported clusters of cells which all had similar direction preferences. The clusters described by both these groups had a size which was in the order of 500 μm and should thus be easily resolvable with intrinsic imaging. In none of our experiments were we able to find such areas in the cortex.

The only remaining explanation for these contradicting results is then the above mentioned possibility that there are clusters of cells having opposite direction preference lying above each other. This explanation, however, would contradict the findings of Tolhurst et al. (1981) who reported similar direction preference for cells across one whole cortical column reaching from the pia to the white matter.

We are currently working on improvements of our experimental setup which will allow three-dimensional imaging of the functional architecture of the cortex. With this apparatus we performed preliminary experiments (D. Malonek, T. Bonhoeffer, A. Grinvald, unpublished results) which seem to refute the above mentioned explanation of our results, at least for the upper 500 μm.

Altogether we find it unlikely that our results would be due to one of the two alternative explanations and we propose that there are indeed no direction columns in area 18 of cat visual cortex.

"Stripes" or "Patches" ?

In most of the experiments that we analyzed for the global organization of orientation we found that the distribution of iso-orientation domains was "patchy" rather than banded as one might have expected from 2-DG pictures (see e.g. Löwel, this volume). Only in two out of twelve hemispheres that we analyzed in such a fashion we observed a banded appearance. It is interesting to note that both of those recordings happened to be taken from a posterior part of area 18 relatively close to the vertical meridian. In view of the small number of recordings from the posterior part of area 18 we are presently not able to determine whether it is a consistent finding that areas closer to the vertical meridian have a more banded appearance. In this context it should also be noted that all the information we gather in our experiments is collected from a very restricted part of area 18, a narrow strip of the lateral gyrus which is exposed to the surface. We can thus not rule out the possibility that in other regions and at other eccentricities the functional organization might be different.

2-Deoxyglucose pictures published in the literature seem to suggest that a region preferring the same orientation should be a band or slab rather than a patch (Hubel et al. 1977; Hubel et al. 1978; Löwel et al. 1987). And indeed also Figure 2 of our data seems to support such an interpretation. If one looks, however, at the organization of orientation preferences for all the orientations (which is not possible with the 2-DG technique) the picture is very different. The grey regions connecting the dark beads (Löwel et al. 1987) in the "band" for one particular orientation turn out to respond very vigorously to another orientation and should thus not be considered belonging to the same orientation "band" but to a patch of different orientation preference. We would therefore like to point out that the data that lead us to conclude that iso-orientation domains are patchy and not banded are not at variance with data from 2-DG studies. It is rather that richer data enable us to gain a more complete picture of the overall cortical organization.

"Pinwheels" around orientation centers

In our experiments we observed that the patches of orientation preference seem to be organized around points which we called "orientation centers". In these points regions of all orientation preferences border one another. The orientation preferences are distributed around the centers either clockwise or counterclockwise in a pinwheel-like fashion. Centers of this sort have also been observed by Swindale et al. (1987) using maps obtained from interpolation between multiple electrode recordings.

In the monkey cortex it seems natural to assume that the orientation centers would come to lie in the cytochromeoxidase-rich "blobs" (Horton and Hubel 1981) which are known to contain many orientationally unresponsive cells (Livingstone and Hubel 1984). In the cat, however, nothing is known about regions of poor orientation response. Our optical imaging studies indicate that there are regions in which the orientation tuning was poor. In these regions cells could either have poor orientation tuning, or, alternatively, single, well tuned cells of different orientation preference are intermingled. In both cases it will be very interesting to investigate the properties of the cells in these regions. If all the cells were unoriented one would assume that there is some other visual attribute which these cells are processing. If on the other hand all the cells were sharply tuned but cells of different orientation were intermingled, cells in these regions might be particularly apt to do certain kinds of computations since they have information from many cells with different orientation tuning easily accessible. Our preliminary studies using conventional electrophysiological recordings suggest that single cells in close neighborhood of the orientation centers are sharply tuned.

One or two orientation cycles?

It has been suggested (e.g. von Seelen 1970; Braitenberg and Braitenberg 1979) that the visual cortex could be organized around orientation centers instead of being a banded structure as originally proposed by Hubel and Wiesel. Braitenberg and Braitenberg (1979) showed that many of the data obtained by Hubel and Wiesel could be very well fit by a scheme of circular organization. Braitenberg and Braitenberg proposed that these centers should be spaced at a distance of approximately 0.5 mm and that every orientation should appear twice around an orientation center. More recently different groups have - mostly on theoretical grounds - proposed an organization with orientation centers around which every orientation appears once. Most recently Götz (1987), based on data obtained by Blasdel and Salama (1986) in the monkey cortex, proposed that V1 of the monkey cortex might be constructed in such a way. Götz also introduced the notion of chirality or handedness in order to describe the different kinds of singularities. Singularities around which every orientation between 0 and 180 degrees appears twice (i.e. 360 degrees orientation change appear *once* in the 360 degrees around the singularity) have a chirality of 1 or -1 whereas orientation centers around which every orientation appears once consequently have a chirality of +1/2 or -1/2.

The measure of chirality is the crucial distinction between the different models. We therefore inspected our data very closely with respect to the question whether the orientation centers have a chirality of +1/2 or -1/2, or whether it rather is +1 or -1. We found that by far the most of the singularities that we observed were of the type ± 1/2. Only in very few instances we found centers around which every orientation appeared twice and even in those centers the interpretation was - due to noise - not unequivocal. We conclude that our data obtained in area 18 of the cat lend experimental support to theories which propose orientation centers with only one representation of all orientations around the center singularity.

Emergence of orientation centers

There are several models in the literature which predict the emergence of orientation centers for different reasons. Durbin et al. (1990) and Obermayer et al. (1990) show that the "principle of continuous mapping" leads to orientation centers. Swindale (1982), Linsker (1986) and Götz (1988) use different models of self-organization to achieve a pattern of orientation preference which looks similar to the experimentally observed orientation maps. Götz's model is particularly interesting since it predicts (Götz, personal communication) that in early stages of the cats postnatal development there should be more centers of chirality 1 or -1 (which means that one should be able to find orientation centers around which every orientation appears twice) and only subsequently, through the self-organizing process, these centers each break up into two centers of chirality +1/2 or -1/2. In order to experimentally test this theory it would thus be interesting to see whether in very young kittens (or other mammals in which orientation tuning develops mostly postnatally) one indeed finds the centers around which every orientation appears twice which we rarely found in adult cats.

Are there additional columnar systems in area 18?

In Figure 6 we showed that moving gratings of eight different orientations are not the complete set of stimuli required to uniformly activate area 18. Some regions are activated much stronger than others. One possibility would, of course, be that the nonuniformity of these images simply reflects a corresponding nonuniformity of the sources of the intrinsic signal. Assuming that this is not the primary source of our observation, the interesting question arises: What are the missing stimuli that would activate the whole cortex more evenly? The first possibility is, of course, that 8 orientations are insufficient and that the white spots in the Figure represent the regions that would have been activated by intermediate orientations. To rule out this possibility we compared maps obtained by adding four orientations to maps of eight orientations and found that the two resulting maps are very similar. This suggests that the lack of stimuli of a certain orientation cannot explain the non-uniformity we observed. This is not surprising in view of the fact that the average orientation tuning width of a population of neurons at given cortical site is certainly larger than steps of 22.5 degrees we have used.

The second possibility is that these irregularities in the map are caused by "spatial-frequency" columns. Tootell et al. (1981) reported that in area 17 of the cat neurons responding to gratings of different spatial frequencies are arranged in columns. Although this result was obtained in area 17 it is conceivable that this organization extends into area 18 and explains our results. In a few experiments we have tried to visualize spatial frequency columns in cat visual cortex (Doron Shoham, unpublished results) and have so far not obtained a clear cut result. In order to elucidate whether the result presented here is really caused by the grouping of cells into spatial frequency columns more experiments are needed. In addition one should investigate whether the regions we found to be less activated by oriented stimuli might be dedicated to the processing of other - perhaps more complicated - stimulus attributes.

Acknowledgements

We thank Larry Katz for his critical comments on the manuscript and Eyal Bartfeld for the cream cheese bagels in the middle of the night.

References

Batschelet E (1981) Circular statistics in biology. Academic Press, New York

Blasdel GG, Salama G (1986) Voltage-sensitive dyes reveal a modular organization in monkey striate cortex. Nature 321:579-585

Braitenberg V, Braitenberg C (1979) Geometry of orientation columns in the visual cortex. Biol Cybern 33:179-186

Durbin R, Mitchison G (1990) A dimension reduction framework for understanding cortical maps. Nature 343:644-647

Frostig RD, Lieke EE, Ts'o DY, Grinvald A (1990) Cortical functional architecture and local coupling between neuronal activity and the microcirculation revealed by in vivo high-resolution optical imaging of intrinsic signals. Proc Natl Acad Sci USA 87:6082-6086

Grinvald A, Lieke E, Frostig RD, Gilbert CD, Wiesel TN (1986) Functional architecture of cortex revealed by optical imaging of intrinsic signals. Nature 324:361-364

Götz KG (1987) Do "d-blob" and "l-blob" hypercolumns tessellate the monkey visual cortex?. Biol Cybern 560:107-109

Götz KG (1988) Cortical templates for the self-organization of orientation-specific d- and l-hypercolumns in monkeys and cats. Biol Cybern 58:213-223

Horton JC, Hubel DH (1981) Regular patchy distribution of cytochrome oxidase staining in primary visual cortex of macaque monkey. Nature 292:762-764

Hubel DH, Wiesel TN (1965) Receptive fields and functional architecture in two non-striate visual areas (18 and 19) of the cat. J Neurophysiol 28:229-289

Hubel DH, Wiesel TN, Stryker MP (1977) Orientation columns in macaque monkey visual cortex demonstrated by the 2-deoxyglucose autoradiographic technique. Nature 269:328-330

Hubel DH, Wiesel TN, Stryker MP (1978) Anatomical demonstration of orientation columns in macaque monkey. J Comp Neurol 177:361-380

Linsker R (1986) From basic network principles to neural architecture: Emergence of orientation columns. Proc Natl Acad Sci USA 83:8779-8783

Livingstone MS, Hubel DH (1984) Anatomy and physiology of a color system in the primate visual cortex. J Neurosci 4:309-356

Löwel S, Freeman B, Singer W (1987) Topographic organization of the orientation column system in large flat-mounts of the cat visual cortex: a 2-deoxyglucose study. J Comp Neurol 255:401-415

Malonek D, Shoham D, Ratzlaff E, Grinvald A (1990) In vivo three dimensional optical imaging of functional architecture in primate visual cortex. Soc Neurosci Abstr 130.4

Mountcastle VB (1957) Modality and topographic properties of single neurons of cat's somatic sensory cortex. J Neurophysiol 20:408-434

Payne BR, Berman N, Murphy EH (1980) Organization of direction preferences in cat visual cortex. Brain Res 211:445-450

Ratzlaff EH, Grinvald A (1991) A Tandem-lens epifluorescence macroscope: hundred-fold brightness advantage for wide field imaging. J Neurosci Meth (to be published)

Sokoloff L (1977) Relation between physiological function and energy metabolism in the central nervous system. J Neurochem 19:13-26

Swindale NV (1982) A model for the formation of orientation columns. Proc R Soc Lond B 215:211-230

Swindale NV, Matsubara JA, Cynader MS (1987) Surface organization of orientation and direction selectivity in cat area 18. J Neurosci 7(5):1414-1427

Tolhurst DJ, Dean AF, Thompson ID (1981) Preferred direction of movement as an element in the organization of cat visual cortex. Exp Brain Res 44:340-342

Tootell RB, Silverman MS, De Valois RL (1981) Spatial frequency columns in primary visual cortex. Science 214:813-815

Ts'o, DY, Frostig RD, Lieke EE, Grinvald A (1990) Functional organization of primate visual cortex revealed by high resolution optical imaging. Science 249:417-420

von Seelen W (1970) Zur Informationsverarbeitung im visuellen System der Wirbeltiere. Kybernetik 7:89-106

Blobs or Slabs - is that the Question?

Siegrid Löwel

Max-Planck-Institut für Hirnforschung, Deutschordenstr. 46, 6000 Frankfurt a. M. 71, Germany

Theoretical models and hypotheses are the basis of any experimental work. Their predictive value has to be tested by appropriate experiments in order to select those concepts that are more viable than others.

It is a well established phenomenon of cortical organization that neurones are not scattered randomly but clustered together according to specific response properties. In visual cortex, cells recorded along electrode penetrations perpendicular to the cortical layers were found to respond to similarly oriented lines whereas a gradual shift of orientation preference was observed along tangential penetrations (Hubel and Wiesel 1959, 1974; Albus 1975). The development of the 2-deoxyglucose (2-DG) method by Sokoloff et al. (1977) allowed to map the topographical arrangement of iso-orientation columns more comprehensively than with electrophysiological techniques (i.e. Albus 1979; Singer 1981; Hubel et al. 1977; Humphrey et al. 1980). This approach revealed that iso-orientation domains frequently have the shape of slabs and bands rather than of isolated columns. Two mathematical models about the development of orientation selectivity (Swindale 1982; von der Malsburg and Cowan 1982) also inferred that iso-orientation domains should be arranged as *parallel* and regularly spaced slabs with trajectories essentially orthogonal to area boundaries. An alternative geometrical concept has been put forward by Braitenberg and Braitenberg (1979) in which orientations are proposed to be arranged *radially* around centers. A 2-DG study in our laboratory directly tested the validity of the two alternative concepts by comparing activity patterns in the cat visual cortex induced by visual stimulation with gratings of various orientations (Löwel et al. 1987).

If iso-orientation domains are arranged as parallel bands i) the trajectories of the 2-DG bands must be invariant to changes in stimulus orientation and ii) presentation of horizontal and vertical contours should lead to similar patterns except that the spacing of activated bands should be reduced by a factor of 0.5 (doubling of the spatial frequency composition of the 2-DG patterns). If - on the other hand - Braitenbergs' concept is right i) the trajectories of activated iso-orientation domains should change with stimulus orientation and ii) stimulation with orthogonal contours should activate short slabs of cortical tissue that are orthogonal to each other (no change in the spatial frequency composition). Figure 1 summarizes the main results of this study. Visual stimulation with gratings of a single orientation induced highly ordered patterns of increased 2-DG uptake consisting of regularly spaced and beaded stripes (B) with a mean distance of 1.0 - 1.2 mm (C). Stimulation with two orthogonal orientations led to patterns with similar general layout (A) but with "twice as many" stripes: one-dimensional Fourier analyses perpendicular to the main trajectories of the bands revealed an additional peak at the doubled spatial frequency (C). Similar analyses parallel to the iso-orientation bands revealed no major differences in the spectra between the single and double stimulated visual cortices (D). Additional two-dimensional Fourier analyses also confirmed that stimulation with two rather than with one orientation increased the spatial frequency content of the 2-DG patterns along vectors perpendicular to the bands but not along vectors parallel to the bands.

Finally I would like to present some data concerning the ongoing discussion whether iso-orientation domains consist of elongated slabs (which can be assigned a certain trajectory) or isolated columns. Optical density measurements along vectors perpendicular (E) resp. parallel

---

Fig. 1. A, B: After all these theories some "real" cortical maps: 2-DG autoradiographs of flat-mounts of the left (**A**) and right (**B**) visual cortices of a cat. The animal was stimulated in its right visual hemifield with horizontal and vertical gratings that were presented in alternation and in its left visual hemifield with a vertically oriented grating only. **C, D:** The spatial frequency composition of the autoradiographs as determined by one-dimensional Fourier analyses. Average of measurements along vectors perpendicular (**C**) resp. parallel (**D**) to the main trajectories of the iso-orientation bands in the single (solid line) and double (dotted line) stimulated hemispheres. Note that the second peak at doubled spatial frequency occurs only after stimulation with two orientations and only in measurements perpendicular to the iso-orientation bands (dotted line in **C**). **E, F:** Optical density measurements perpendicular (**E**) and parallel (**F**) to the bands. Note that the radioactive labeling along the bands is always higher than between them (dotted area). Abbreviations: *a* = anterior, *p* = posterior

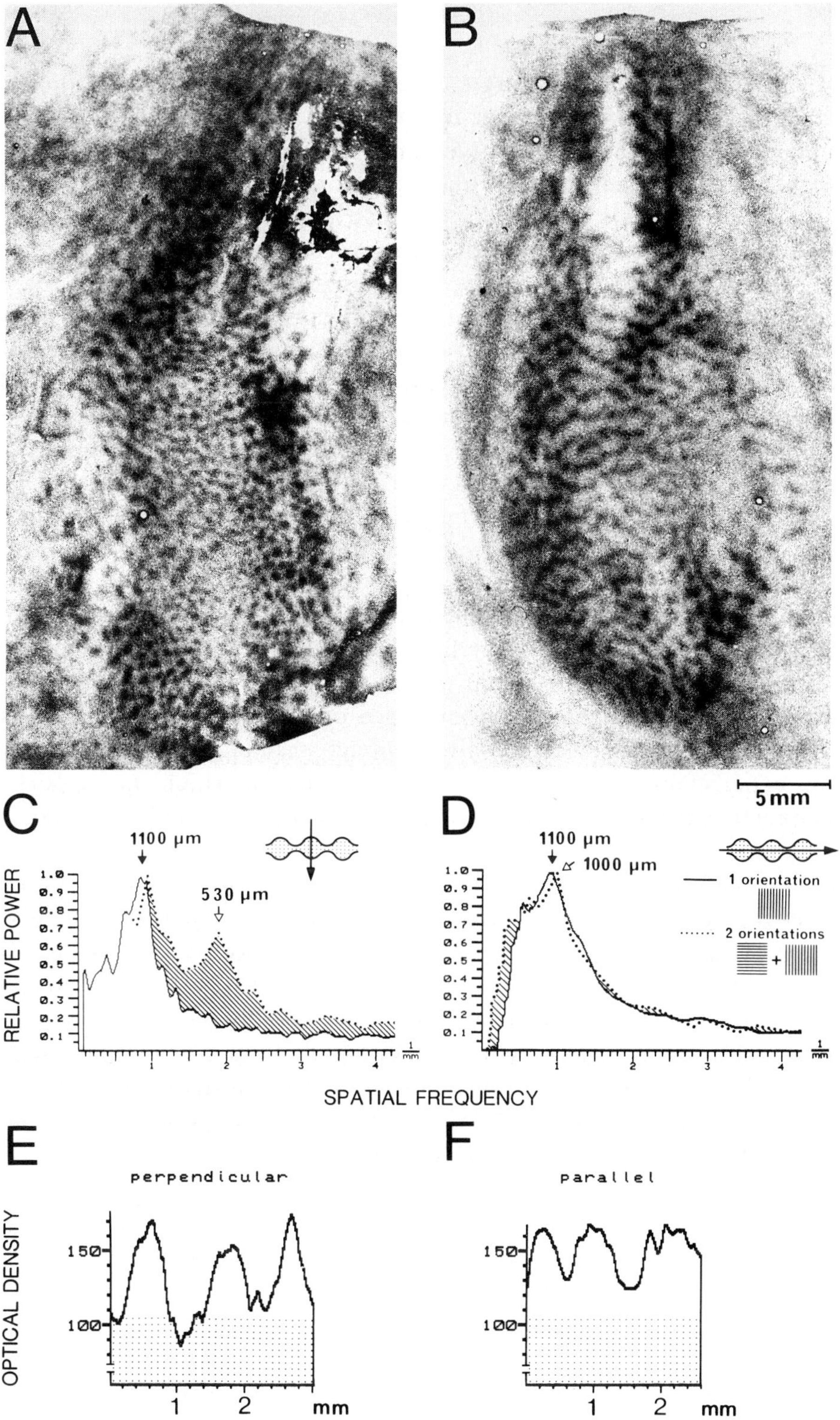
A
B
5mm
C
1100 µm
530 µm
RELATIVE POWER
1.0
0.9
0.8
0.7
0.6
0.5
0.4
0.3
0.2
0.1
1
2
3
4
1/mm
D
1100 µm
1000 µm
1 orientation
2 orientations
SPATIAL FREQUENCY
E
perpendicular
OPTICAL DENSITY
150
100
1
2
mm
F
parallel
150
100
1
2
mm

(F) to the "bands" demonstrate i) a periodic fluctuation in radioactive labeling in both cases (due to the bands (E) resp. beads (F)) and more importantly ii) that radioactive labeling along the "bands" is always higher than between them. Thus the autoradiographs exhibit a specific asymmetry in their optical density distribution which is more suggestive of a parallel than of a radial arrangement of activated regions.

Taken together these results are compatible with the hypothesis that stimulation with two orientations activates twice as many parallel orientation bands than stimulation with a single orientation. Thus, our data indicate that cortical regions containing neurones with similar orientation preference have the form of elongated slabs that run parallel to each other and that interdigitate with iso-orientation slabs encoding different orientations. Our results are definitively *not* compatible with Braitenbergs' hypothesis about the geometry of cortical line detectors because i) trajectories of iso-orientation domains do not change with stimulus orientation and ii) stimulation with orthogonal contours induces activity patterns with doubled spatial frequency content. Our results may however be compatible with a more recent variation of the radial arrangement theme proposed by Götz (1988). In this model, all orientations occur only once on a circular trajectory around the center. Indeed there are already some results from optical recording experiments in monkey V1 and cat area 18 which do support the Götz concept (Blasdel and Salama 1986; Bonhoeffer and Grinvald, this volume).

In the end, the reader may ask what do we learn at all from knowing the exact topography of the orientation domains. Is this all not just "l'art pour l'art" or some meaningless academical dispute? It is our belief that these maps or representations of particular functional properties are the result of an ontogenetic process and are "shaped" by experience. It is hoped that knowledge of their layout may help to elucidate the underlying developmental mechanisms and eventually contribute to the fundamental question why neurones with similar response characteristics are clustered at all.

References

Albus K (1975) A quantitative study of the projection area of the central and the paracentral visual field in area 17 of the cat. II. The spatial organization of the orientation domain. Exp Brain Res 24:181-202

Albus K (1979) ^{14}C-deoxyglucose mapping of orientation subunits in the cat's visual cortical areas. Exp Brain Res 37:609-613

Blasdel GG, Salama G (1986) Voltage-sensitive dyes reveal a modular organization in monkey striate cortex. Nature 321:579-585

Braitenberg V, Braitenberg C (1979) Geometry of orientation columns in the visual cortex. Biol Cybern 33:179-186

Götz KG (1988) Cortical templates for the self-organization of orientation-specific *d*- and *l*-hypercolumns in monkeys and cats. Biol Cybern 58:213-223

Hubel DH, Wiesel TN (1959) Receptive fields of single neurones in the cat's striate cortex. J Physiol (L) 148:574-591

Hubel DH, Wiesel TN (1974) Sequence regularity and geometry of orientation columns in the monkey striate cortex. J Comp Neurol 158:267-294

Hubel DH, Wiesel TN, Stryker MP (1977) Orientation columns in macaque monkey visual cortex demonstrated by the 2-deoxyglucose autoradiographic technique. Nature 269:328-330

Humphrey AL, Skeen LC, Norton TT (1980) Topographic organization of the orientation column system in the striate cortex of the tree shrew (Tupaia glis). II. Deoxyglucose mapping. J Comp Neurol 192:549-566

Löwel S, Freeman B, Singer W (1987) Topographic organization of the orientation column system in large flat-mounts of the cat visual cortex: a 2-deoxyglucose study. J Comp Neurol 255:401-415

Singer W (1981) Topographic organization of orienation columns in the cat visual cortex. Exp Brain Res 44:431-436

Sokoloff L, Reivich M, Kennedy C, Des Rosiers MH, Patlak CS, Pettigrew KD, Sakurada O, Shinohara M (1977) The (^{14}C)deoxyglucose method for the measurement of local cerebral glucose utilization: Theory, procedure, and normal values in the conscious and anesthetized albino rat. J Neurochem 28:897-916

Swindale NV (1982) A model for the formation of orientation columns. Proc R Soc Lond (B) 215:211-230

von der Malsburg C, Cowan JD (1982) Outline of a theory for the ontogenesis of iso-orientation domains in visual cortex. Biol Cybern 45:49-56

How Ideas Survive Evidence to the Contrary: A Comment on Data Display and Modelling

Valentino Braitenberg

Max-Planck-Institut für biologische Kybernetik, Spemannstrasse 38, 7400 Tübingen, Germany

The papers by Löwel and by Bonhoeffer and Grinvald in this volume do me the honour of referring to a model of the visual cortex published some time ago (Braitenberg and Braitenberg 1979). However, both fail to mention a more comprehensive and more explicit proposal which I have made since (Braitenberg 1985). It is the latter model that I want to defend here, the reason being that I still consider it most efficient in terms of the large number of facts explained and minimal number of assumptions made. In fact, in this model the only departure from a general description of cortical structure (Braitenberg and Schüz 1991) is the assumption of inhibitory neurons lumped in certain places of the visual area which probably coincide with cytochrome oxidase "blobs" (Horton and Hubel 1981). Among other things, the variation of orientation sensitivity in different places on the cortical surface is fully explained by this.

There is nothing in the deoxyglucose maps published by Löwel (Löwel et al. 1987; Löwel, this volume) which our model does not predict (Braitenberg and Schüz 1991). This may not be so for some of the false-colour maps displaying the results of optical recording (Blasdel and Salama 1986; Grinvald et al. 1986; Bonhoeffer and Grinvald, this volume), as Götz (1987) pointed out. The latter author notes that our model predicts centers around which loci of different orientation sensitivity are arranged in such a way that each orientation occurs *twice* (like the spokes of a wheel or the tangents of a circle). In contrast Götz, perusing the coloured maps in search of local singularities where regions of different orientation sensitivity meet, only found whirls with each orientation occurring *once* going around the center. There were two kinds of such whirls in Götz' analysis, equal in number but distinguished by their "chirality": in the d-kind, proceeding counterclockwise around the center, the orientations change clockwise, in the l-kind counterclockwise. Götz took this as evidence against our model.

My answer is this. Our model indeed predicts orientations arranged around centers like the tangents of a circle (Fig. 1). It does not predict, however, that these orientations should meet in the center of the hypercolumns (the circles on Fig. 1), for there, according to the mechanism we postulated, and according to Livingstone and Hubel (1984), the neurons should be without orientation specificity.

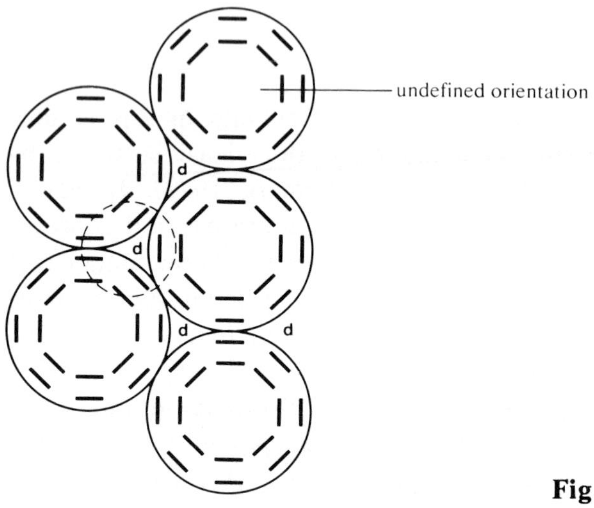

Fig. 1

Thus, I am not surprised if Götz does not find on the published maps the singularities which he expects on the basis of our model, since in reality our model does not predict them. Different orientations should indeed come together in the corners between the hypercolumns (d on Fig. 1) if our model is correct, and there each orientation occurs only once (dashed circle) and the chirality is d. Where do the whirls of the l-kind come from which Götz finds on the coloured maps?

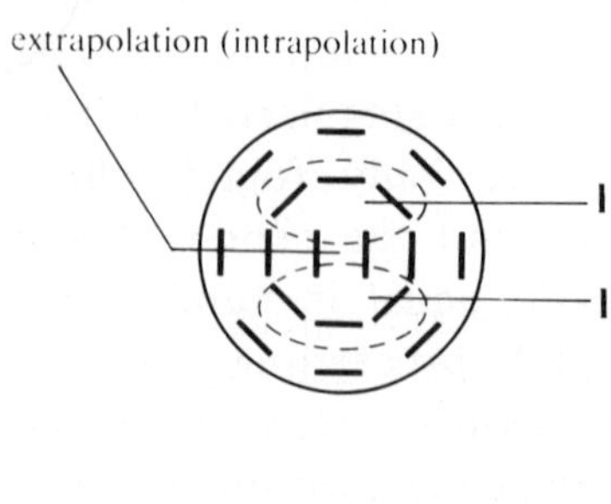

Fig. 2

They are a consequence of the fact that these maps (Blasdel and Salama 1986; Grinvald et al. 1986; Bonhoeffer and Grinvald, this volume) do not show the regions with undefined orientation in the center of the hypercolumns (Fig. 1). I surmise that these centers, which should be grey, are filled in by extrapolation from one of the peripheral colours thereby producing in each hypercolumn a spurious bar of one and the same orientation crossing it (Fig. 2). This will give

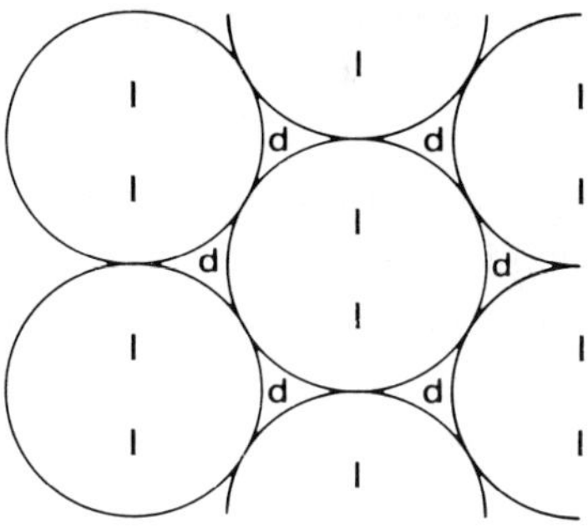

n hypercolumns

$$N_d = \frac{6}{3} n = 2n$$

$$N_l = 2n$$

$$N_l = N_d = 2n$$

Fig. 3

each hypercolumn two regions (dashed ellipses on Fig. 2) in which the orientations seem to whirl around with chirality l. The number of these (fictitious) l-whirls is equal to the number of (real) d-whirls if the hypercolumns are arranged in a hexagonal array (Fig. 3), since there are six corners surrounding a hypercolumn, each shared by three hypercolumns. Q. e. d.

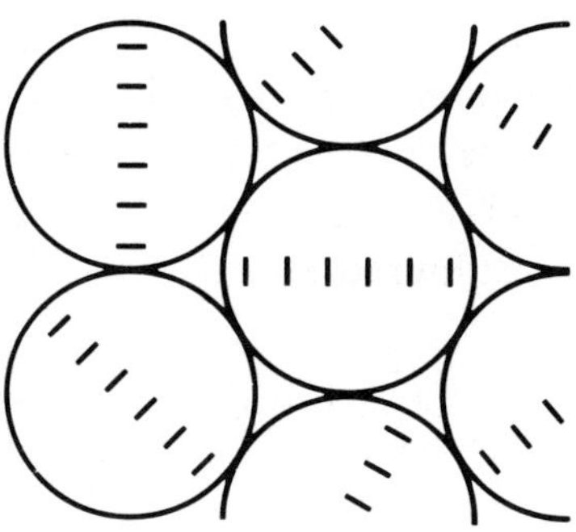

Fig. 4

Fig. 4 is designed as an aid to those who intend to analyse the coloured orientation maps along these lines. The colour which is extra/intrapolated from the periphery into the center of the hypercolumns may not be the same in all hypercolumns.

References

Blasdel GG, Salama G (1986) Voltage-sensitive dyes reveal a modular organization in monkey striate cortex. Nature 321:579-585

Bonhoeffer T, Grinvald A (this volume)

Braitenberg V, Braitenberg C (1979) Geometry of orientation columns in the visual cortex. Biol Cybern 33:179-186

Braitenberg V (1985) Charting the visual cortex In: Peters A, Jones EG (eds) Cerebral cortex vol III: Plenum Publishing Corp, New York London, p 379-414

Braitenberg V, Schüz A (1991) Anatomy of the cortex. Statistics and geometry. Springer-Verlag, New York Berlin

Götz KG (1987) Do "d-blob" and "l-blob" hypercolumns tesselate the monkey visual cortex? Biol Cybern 56:107-109

Götz KG (1988) Cortical templates for the self-organization of orientation-specific *d*- and *l*-hypercolumns in monkey and cats. Biol Cybern 58:213-223

Grinvald A, Lieke E, Frostig RD, Gilbert CD, Wiesel TN (1986) Functional architecture of cortex revealed by optical imaging of intrinsic signals. Nature 324:361-364

Livingstone MS, Hubel DH (1984) Anatomy and physiology of a colour system in the primate visual cortex. J Neurosci 4:309-356

Löwel S (this volume)

Cortical Maps

Hubert Preißl

Max-Planck-Institut für biologische Kybernetik, 7400 Tübingen, Germany

Two long outstanding problems in neuroscience are how cortical maps develop and how they are organized. There were and are a lot of efforts to reveal the underlying principles of their development - leading to a certain organization - both on theoretical and experimental levels. In the case of the visual cortex, two kinds of models can be distinguished. One kind is especially concerned with the problems of development, the other one with structural questions. In this contribution I will focus on the developmental part of this story.

Introduction

During cortical information processing, various stimulus features are evaluated from the signals which are transmitted to the cortical network by fibres from the sensory organs, e.g. the eye or the ear. One basic principle of the cortical network organization is, that in different cortical areas these projections result in a two-dimensional representation of selected stimulus features. A projection is called a map, when certain relations of these features in the sensory space are preserved during this process.

In the case of the visual cortex, several different maps are known. Hubel and Wiesel (1962, 1963) showed in their famous work on cat visual cortex, that cells respond best to a bar stimulus with a certain orientation: the so-called orientation specifity. They also showed that neurons generally get their input not equally strong from both eyes, but that some cells in primary visual cortex are more sensitive for input from the left, others to input from the right eye: the so-called ocular dominance. Furthermore they showed that these features of orientation specifity and ocular dominance are not randomly distributed over the cortex, but that a certain order exist. For example, preferred orientation changes gradually if one records from different cells during a horizontal penetration and does not change during a vertical penetration. For the ocular dominance they determined stripes in which the ocular dominance did not change. These experiments were carried out with adult animals. I regard these kind of results as *organizational information*. There are some theoretical models to describe these results (compare the contribution of Braitenberg, this volume). There are more recent experimental results about the organization of the cortex. It could be shown for example that orientation tuning is not organized in stripes but rather in a patchy distribution (for example see the contributions of Bonhoeffer and Löwel, this Volume).

Hubel and Wiesel (for a review on the monkey see Hubel et al. 1977a, b) also showed that these maps are not genetically fixed, but that they can be changed by environmental changes. For example, in an adult cat one finds nearly the same number of cells responding to the left or right eye. This relation, however, can be shifted by covering one eye during what is called a 'sensitive period'. After this deprivation more cells are sensitive to input from the uncovered eye. This I call the *developmental information*. After the experimental work of Hubel and Wiesel, a number of models for the creation of such maps were developed.

Models of map formation

From the findings of developmental studies of cortical maps one can derive some general principles of the processes taking place in the brain during this formation.

First of all one has to make a very crude picture of what is going on in the primary visual cortex during development. From the retina of the two eyes the visual fibres transmit the information to the LGN (lateral geniculate nucleus) where the input of the two eyes is still separated. From this station the fibres project to layer IV of the primary visual cortex. Here they contact cortical cells, and the input of the one location in the visual field of the two eyes project to one location in the cortex (retinotopic projection).

This leads to three main questions:

1) How do the fibres find their way to the right projection site?
2) How can ocular dominance evolve, when the two eyes project equally to the cortex?
3) How do feature detectors develop, which respond best, for example to certain bar orientations?

These questions were addressed by some models which were developed over the last 20 years, although not all these questions were investigated in a single model. For example, certain models concentrated on the development of retinotopic projections (Willshaw and von der Malsburg 1976, 1979; von der Malsburg and Willshaw 1977), others on the development of ocular dominance (von der Malsburg 1979; Linsker 1986c; Miller et al. 1989). Another class of models is concerned with the development of feature detectors, e.g. orientation specific cells at different levels of cortical stages (von der Malsburg 1973; Linsker 1986a-c).

There are some common features in these models. They all assume that the establishment of the maps is a self-organizing process in a large network of similar elements (compare von der Malsburg and Singer 1988). One of the major principles of self-organizing systems is that the global organization is determined by local rules. In the context of brain research these local rules are mainly learning rules, i.e. learning in the sense of changing synaptical transmission (strengthening or weakening). One of the most famous learning mechanisms was proposed by Donald Hebb (1949), who assumed that the synaptic strength between two cells increases by coincident firing of these cells.

One of the first models trying to resolve the problem of map formation in the cortex is that of von der Malsburg (1973). This model incorporates findings going back to learning systems like Perceptrons as well as anatomical and physiological facts. Two-dimensional representations for the retinal input layer and for the cortical layer were used. In the cortical layer excitatory and inhibitory cells are uniformly distributed. Von der Malsburg was able to show that a learning rule similar to the Hebb rule leads to a cortical map which shows similar orientation tuning as observed in physiological experiments. One important aspect of this model was that only the afferent synapses were able to learn, whereas the intra-cortical connections were predetermined and fixed to certain values, depending on distance.

Models which are strongly related to feed-forward nets were investigated by other researchers, with special emphasis on the influence of different learning rules (modified Hebb rules; see Bienenstock et al. 1982).

Under the influence of a renaissance of artificial neural networks, this kind of models were recently investigated using a different approach. One of the most prominent studies is the series of papers by Linsker (1986a-c). He modelled the map formation process with a feed-forward net of up to 7 layers. Examing the evolution of the synapses under a Hebbian learning rule, he was able to show that orientation selective cells become visible in the seventh layer without a structured input. Incorporating lateral interaction in the different layers he showed that the orientation selective cells are ordered in a structure similar to orientation columns. This work is related to an approach of Oja (1982) for eigenvalue analysis in a neural network system.

Another important point in development is the ocular dominance map. Related to this problem is the retinotopic projection from the retina to the cortex, with neighbouring points on the retina projecting to neighbouring points in the cortex. In this case one has to establish a topographic mapping between two 2-dimensional spaces, e.g. the image on the retina to a image on the cortex. This problem was investigated by von der Malsburg and Willshaw (1977), who used a algorithm from optimisation theory. The retinotopic projection evolves with the help of chemical markers, which codes a pre-synaptic position. This model was extended by von der Malsburg (1979) for the formation of ocular dominance stripes by incorporating additional markers. An alternative model was proposed by Swindale (1980), in which the ocular dominance evolves from reinforcing synapses from the same eye and inhibitory influence from different eyes. This model was worked out further by Miller et al. (1989), who gave a more detailed analysis of the model together with more simulations for the development of ocular dominance. This model also incorporates a Hebb like learning rule for the map formation.

Kohonen (1984) developed a more detailed theory for neighbourhood preserving mappings between spaces of different dimensions. A related approach was adopted for map formation in the cortex by

Durbin and Mitchison (1990). These authors investigated the self organization of a map, when the parameter space is a 4-dimensional feature space (coding retinal position and orientation tuning) which has to be mapped on a 2-dimensional surface. Their model tries to incorporate different mappings in a unified context. Using a Hebbian learning rule and a modified elastic net algorithm they showed that the resulting map is similar to maps found physiologically.

Discussion

As I pointed out, there are many models for the development of cortical maps. As a matter of fact, there are even more models I did not mention at all. One of the basic questions in the different models is the assumed learning rule. Most models contain a learning rule, which is inspired by the idea of Hebb that correlated firing leads to a stronger cooperation of connected elements. This is a strictly local learning rule, in which only pre- and postsynaptic elements are involved. For the development of ordered mappings, however, cooperation alone is not enough. In addition, one needs competition between the elements, otherwise it would not be possible to get different features into a single map.

Future work on cortical mappings will have to investigate questions whether a local learning rule according to Hebb is ideal for such a problem or whether one has to incorporate also non-local effects, such as observed by Bonhoeffer et al. (1989). There is first evidence that such a non-local rule, in this case based on diffusive chemical substances, can modify synaptic strength (Gally et al. 1990). Another important issue is what computational processes actually take place within these maps.

Summarising, although many aspects of map formation have been measured as well as modelled in great detail, many questions, predominantly dealing with the functional aspects remain. Future work can contribute most in this important field.

References

Bienenstock EL, Cooper LN, Munro PW (1982) Theory for the development of neuron selectivity: orientation specifity and binocular interaction in the visual cortex. J Neurosci 2:32-48

Bonhoeffer T, Staiger V, Aertsen A (1989) Synaptic platicity in rat hippocampal slice cultures: Local "Hebbian" conjunction of pre- and postynaptic stimulation leads to distributed synaptic enhancement. PNAS 86:8113-8117

Durbin R, Mitchison G (1990) A dimension reduction framework for understanding cortical maps. Nature 343:644-647

Gally JA, Montague R, Reek GN, Edelman GM (1990) The NO hypothesis: Possible effect of a short-lived, rapidly diffusible signal in the development and function of the nervous system. PNAS 87:3547-35551

Hebb DO (1949) The organization of behaviour. Wiley, New York

Hubel DH, Wiesel TN (1962) Receptive fields, binocular interaction and functional interaction in the cat's visual cortex. J Phys 160:106-154

Hubel DH, Wiesel TN (1963) Receptive fields of cells in striate cortex of very young, visually inexperienced kittens. J Neurophys 26:994-1002

Hubel DH, Wiesel TN (1977a) Functional architecture of macaque monkey visual cortex. Proc R Soc Lond Ser B 198:1-59

Hubel DH, Wiesel TN, LeVay S (1977b) Plasticity of ocular dominance columnes in monkey striate cortex. Phil Trans R Soc Ser B 278:377-409

Kohonen T (1984) Self-organization and associative memory. Springer-Verlag, New-York

Linsker R (1986a) From basic network principles to neural architecture: Emergence of spatial opponent cells. PNAS 83:7508-7512

Linsker R (1986b) From basic network principles to neural architecture: Emergence Of orientation selective cells. PNAS 83:8390-8394

Linsker R (1986c) From basic network principles to neural architecture: Emergence of orientation columns. PNAS 83:8779-8783

Miller KD, Keller JB, Stryker MP (1989) Ocular dominance column development: Analysis and simulation. Science 245:605-615

Oja E (1982) A simplified neuron model as a principle component analyser. J Math Biol 15:267-273

Swindale NV (1980) A model of the formation of ocular dominance stripes. Proc R Soc Lond Ser B 208:243-264

von der Malsburg, C (1973) Self-organization of orientation sensitive cells in the striatal cortex. Kybernetik 14:(1973) 85-100

von der Malsburg, C (1979) Development of ocularity domains and growth behaviour of axon terminals. Biol Cybern 32:49-62

von der Malsburg C, Willshaw DJ (1977) How to label nerve cells so that they can interconnect in an ordered fashion. PNAS 74:5176-5178 von der Malsburg C, Singer W (1988) Principles of cortical network organization. In: von Seelen W, Shaw G, Leinhos UM (eds) Organization of neural networks. VHC-Verlag, Weinheim

Willshaw DJ, von der Malsburg, C (1976) How patterened neural connections can be set up by self-organization. Proc R Soc Lond Ser B 194:431-445

Willshaw DJ, von der Malsburg, C (1979) A marker induction mechanism for establishment of ordered neural mappings: Its application to the retinotectal problem. Phil Trans R Soc B 287:203-243

Part Four
Outlook

Views of a Theoretical Physicist

Gérard Toulouse

Lab. de Physique Statistique, Ecole Normale Supérieure, 24 rue Lhomond, 75231 Paris, France

Introduction

I shall start with an analogy between the present effort to design intelligent machines and another big project, about 150 years ago: to make power machines, able to emulate and replace animal work. Along the text, the analogy will prove to be suggestive in more than one regard.

Next comes the main argument of this contribution, which describes the impact of statistical physics on neural network theory, and also the reciprocal effect, that is not negligible, since neural network theory has now become a new horizon of statistical physics.

These views end with an effort of reflexion on the limitations of this type of theoretical modelling, and also on possible openings. (An enlarged version of this text will appear elsewhere (1991)).

An analogy

I suppose the reader is convinced that the conception of intelligent machines, able to emulate and replace biological brains, is a major scientific goal of our end of century. He is then invited to remember that, about one and a half century ago, there was an equally magnificent project, namely: how to conceive energetic machines, in order to emulate and replace animal work.

To this project, that might be called the science of energetics (see Fig. 1), were to contribute three categories of actors:

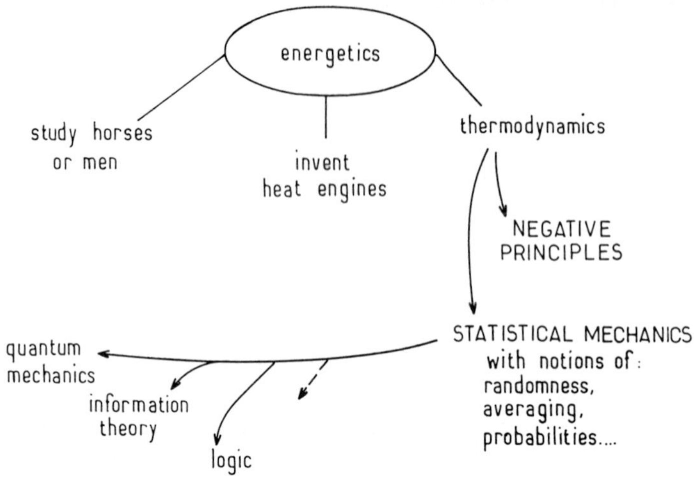

Fig. 1

- biologists, studying the muscles of horses and men,
- inventors, designing heat engines,
- theoreticians also, who created thermodynamics.

Then the theoretical activity followed an unexpected path, one that was not always along the preferences of the biologists or the inventors.

Firstly, thermodynamics essentially produced negative principles; it is well known that one can formulate the three principles of thermodynamics using sentences starting with: 'It is not possible ...'

1. It is not possible to build perpetual machines of the first kind (or, shortly: 'You can't win').
2. It is not possible to build perpetual machines of the second kind (or: 'You can't even break even').
3. It is not possible to reach the absolute zero of temperature.

These principles provide essentially bounds and limitations. Secondly, thermodynamics was 'reduced' to statistical mechanics, along the ideas of Boltzmann, and meanwhile the notions of randomness, of averaging, of probabilities, and also of reproducibility, of universality, entered into physics. This conceptual adventure was already a noticeable deviation from the initial project, but it was only a beginning. There would be a repeated process of sprouting of new ideas, leading to the unfolding of new branches of knowledge: quantum mechanics, information theory, even affecting logic and thus the core of mathematics. At the end of this paper, we shall return to this analogy, underlining the resemblances (three populations, negative principles, new branches) and also the differences with the thematics of neural networks.

Why statistical physics, in the study of neural networks?

This intervention of statistical physics is both natural and surprising. Natural because:

a) statistical physics is traditionally concerned with the study of assemblies made of a large number of elements, and with the emergence of their collective properties, such as phase transitions. Now the question 'Mind from matter?' may be reformulated as: How can intelligent collective behaviour emerge from a large assembly of neurons, each of them being a mindless automaton? True, there are many other problems of biological interest that would qualify within the ballpark of large assemblies, such as: protein folding, cell differentiation, immune system, etc. But moreover,

b) neural networks are devices that manipulate information, and it has been known since the times of John von Neumann and Claude Shannon that a special link exists between thermodynamics and information theory.

All the above being said, this entry of physics is nevertheless surprising because:

c) we shall see that the concepts put to use are those of equilibrium statistical physics; whereas these systems are conspicuously out of equilibrium; and furthermore

d) the interactions (synapses) between elements (neurons) are asymmetric; this is an essential difference with the material systems under usual study, where Newton's third law applies, allowing for the definition of an energy function, that serves as cornerstone for the formalism of statistical mechanics.

Historical steps

For pedagogical reasons, seven steps (seven is a number carefully chosen to fit the capacity of human short term memory ...) are highlighted, as an introduction to our topic (Toulouse 1989). In 1943 W.S. McCulloch and W. Pitts defined a formal neuron as a binary element, 'all-or-none'. The famous psychologist D.O. Hebb (1949) introduced two fundamental ideas (not yet quite demonstrated up to this day) which have shaped the theoretical framework of most neural network studies during the last forty years: the idea that a percept or a concept is represented in the brain by an assembly of simultaneously active neurons (Hebb assembly) and the idea that the mnemic trace, the material modification necessary for any learning process, takes place at the loci of interaction between neurons (Hebb synapses). The first analogy between a net of neurons and an assembly of magnetic moments came with B.G. Cragg and H.V. Temperley (1954) who noted also that, in order to deepen this analogy, it would be helpful to find equivalents for the notions of temperature and energy. As for temperature, it took twenty years (W.A. Little, 1974, uses a temperature to model the stochastic character of the neurodynamics) and roughly ten years longer for energy (J.J. Hopfield, 1982, makes the analogy with spin glasses and proposes a model of content-addressable memory, for which he computes the storage capacity associated with a given learning rule). The next two steps mark the two main successes of statistical physics. In 1985, the Jerusalem trio (D.J. Amit, H. Gutfreund, H. Sompolinsky) reveals that it is possible to obtain exact solutions and, thus, surprising results, for a large class of memory models. In 1988, E. Gardner proposes a new approach to the problem (inverse formulation of statistical mechanics), that yields absolute bounds (for the errorless storage capacity).

The neuron and its nets

It is now timely to introduce the main protagonist: the neuron, stripped to its simplest form. Out of all anatomical and chemical complexity, and of all the natural diversity, there will remain only a binary element (active or inactive) endowed with the dynamics of a probabilistic threshold automaton: algebraic summation of inputs (coming from afferent neurons) weighted by the synaptic efficacies, comparison to a threshold, sigmoid-shaped probability for the triggering of an action potential (Amit 1989). The spatial structure of dendrites, as well as the diversity of temporal delays, are neglected. This simplification is purposeful, and part of a strategy (sometimes called 'connectionist'), viz.: to explore the consequences of the synaptic variability hypothesis on the nets' processing and learning capacities, everything else being simplified as much as possible (Abbott 1990). Such a strategy is familiar to the physicist; it is remindful of the theory of perfect gases, where the terribly reductive hypothesis of ignoring altogether the atomic interactions, bearing only attention to their motions, is adopted. Nevertheless this hypothesis (that one does not care to call 'kineticist', dressing it up with a word in -ism) turns out to be greatly instructive, and a kind of passage obligé toward more refined theories. It is a bit of the same bet that is made here.

Two network structures have been mainly studied, because of their simplicity, and because they represent conveniently opposite limit cases:

- feedforward layered structure, named perceptron or multi-perceptron (according to the number of layers), without any feedback;
- self-coupled structure, with complete feedback, each neuron being coupled to every other neuron.

Layered structures will be said to perform computation by dynamic flux. Nothing could be simpler than this mode of computation: inputs come in at the first layer, outputs come out at the last layer. The computation mode of self-coupled nets is more original: the inputs are supposed to clamp the initial state of the network, that subsequently evolves freely under its own internal dynamics and converges toward an attractor (this may be, in all generality, a persistent state, or an oscillating one, or more complex), that contains the result of the computation. Self-coupled nets are said to perform computation with attractors.

Associated with any of these two net types, a historical line of antecedent works can be traced back: a well known line for layered structures (including the books of F. Rosenblatt, 1961, of M.L. Minsky and S. Papert, 1969, and the backpropagation algorithm, as e.g. in Rumelhart et al. 1986, etc.), a less notorious one (at least in the pre-

Hopfield era) for self-coupled nets (allusions to 'reverberating states' in Hebb and precursors; Kohonen maps; etc.). To this day, computation with attractors has been essentially used for memory purposes, or for optimisation in problem solving tasks.

Two successes

Starting in 1985, exact solutions have been obtained for self-coupled nets, where the memory storage is made according to some given learning prescription. The results have yielded very rich phase diagrams, quantitative estimates for memory storage capacities and retrieval qualities, etc. Along with a good tradition in theoretical physics, solvable models have a precious advantage over ad hoc models: they afford to get surprises, i.e. more than what was put inside in the first place. Since these works are now classics, and well analyzed in textbooks (Amit 1989; Geszti 1990), I jump without further ado from praise to criticism, that contains two quite serious charges.

In order to apply the formalism of statistical mechanics, it was necessary to use an 'energy' function that governs the couplings between neurons. (The quotation marks are placed here to warn that this is a formal energy, unconvertible into normal chemical or electrical energy). So doing, one had to assume that the coupling (i,j) of neuron i on neuron j was equal to the coupling (j,i) of neuron j on neuron i, a biologically very unrealistic hypothesis. If neuron i has a synapse on neuron j, nothing impels neuron j to have a synapse on neuron i, and even if it happens to be so, nothing impels both synapses to be of the same sign, and even if it happens to be so, it would be pure chance if those two efficacies turned out to be equal. Thus the hypothesis of symmetric interactions is a step backwards, as far as biological plausibility is concerned, and this did not fail to make a bad impression (and a longlived one) on some people.

The second criticism bears on the arbitrariness in the choice of the learning prescription that is adopted. In the absence of absolute bounds (i.e. learning rule independent), it is difficult to pronounce a judgment on whether some particular rule is good or bad. This situation led to deafs' debates between rival schools adept of such or such rule.

The approach proposed by Elizabeth Gardner has allowed one to go beyond these two drawbacks, and to attack the problem from a reverse side. The question becomes: Given a set of patterns to be stored, find the couplings which stabilize them. In other terms, instead of working in activity space, with given interactions (as is customary in statistical physics), one works in interaction space, under the constraints provided by the stabilisation of the given memory patterns. Within this huge space of interactions, corresponding to all possible values of the couplings, interest will be focused on the subspace of solutions (those values of the couplings that define nets satisfying the constraints), whose volume will permit the definition of an "entropy" (with *double* quotation marks now, since this is at a higher degree of abstraction than the Hopfield level), and then an "energy", etc.

First advantage: one obtains in this way absolute results, independent of any particular learning rule (cf. the optimal yield of Carnot, in thermodynamics). As the learning session goes on, the maximal capacity is reached when the volume of the subspace of solutions vanishes. It becomes also possible (Virasoro 1990) to ask 'generic' questions such as: do neural nets tend to categorize? The term categorisation is taken here in the precise following sense: suppose a net has learnt a fair number of variants of a given prototype, will it tend to store the prototype itself (to which it has never been exposed), and if so, will the prototype be stored with larger stability than the explicitly learnt variants? The answer is: yes, for almost all learning rules (it is thus a property of the hardware, arising from the neural infrastructure). One of the most popular rules (the projection rule), though, does not possess this property, thus betraying its oddity. Finally, it is also possible to extend the analysis, and to study the effect of biological constraints, such as the restriction to neurons which are either excitatory or inhibitory (all efferent synapses of one neuron having the same sign) (Amit 1989).

Second advantage: in this new formulation, there is no longer any restriction to symmetric synapses (it would even appear now as a nuisance to impose such a constraint). Thus a reunification occurs in the analysis of monolayer perceptrons and self-coupled nets (at least as far as errorless storage is concerned).

Thus the model introduced by Hopfield in 1982 appears in retrospect as a clever step backwards. The deviation via the hypothesis of symmetric couplings has turned out to be profitable (both for neural network theory and for statistical physics) since it has directed the efforts in a way that has allowed to bypass the initial obstacles and to move ahead.

All biologists know full well that the idea of turning around obstacles in order to reach a desirable goal, instead of knocking endlessly against the obstacle (as does the fly on the window pane), is a proof of intelligence (which for instance distinguishes superior monkeys from inferior ones). However some biologists, when it comes to scientific research, lose sight of this fact; they would want that theoretical models always move in a direction of greater biological plausibility, and they are still irritated against Hopfield who, admittedly, never defended his model as a step backwards ...

Biological relevance

Grosso modo, feedforward layered nets are now being mainly used as models to interpret the neurobiological data obtained on input systems, following Fodor's famous terminology. Thus it is hypothesized that, in such areas, the data processing occurs according to a mode of computation by dynamic flux, and then the theoretical effort is mainly directed toward understanding the function of intermediate units (those neurons sitting in layers intermediate between the input and output layers).

For higher areas, in contrast, the observation of states of persistent activity, specially during tasks involving a working memory (delayed matching tasks), suggests interpretations in terms of computing with attractors. And this is doubtless the main conceptual progress with regard to past analyses. It seems that some features of central cognitive systems can be simulated by such simple models, thereby opening a new path for meaningful dialogue between theory and experiment.

Thus one important question is already raised: Is there unicity or multiplicity of computation modes in the neocortex? In view of the remarkable anatomical homogeneity of this sheet-like structure, it is tempting to assume that local functional specialisations are only induced by the differences in the inputs (different data being processed here and there, but according to a similar computation mode). However the suggestion that primary areas function on a mode of computation with attractors, invites considering the possibility of deeper differentiations.

How can one see the evolution of this science of intelligent machines, sometimes called neuro-informatics, in the light of our analogy of Section 1 and Figure 1? To this project (see Fig. 2), contribute three categories of actors:

- biologists, studying the brains of monkeys and men,
- inventors, designing computer devices,
- theoreticians also, not within one unique framework, but rather with a mixture of logic (one may mention the names of Gödel, Turing, Chaitin, ...), of algorithmics (notions of algorithmic complexity, of algorithmic information), and last but not least the statistical physics of neural networks, that is the topic of this paper.

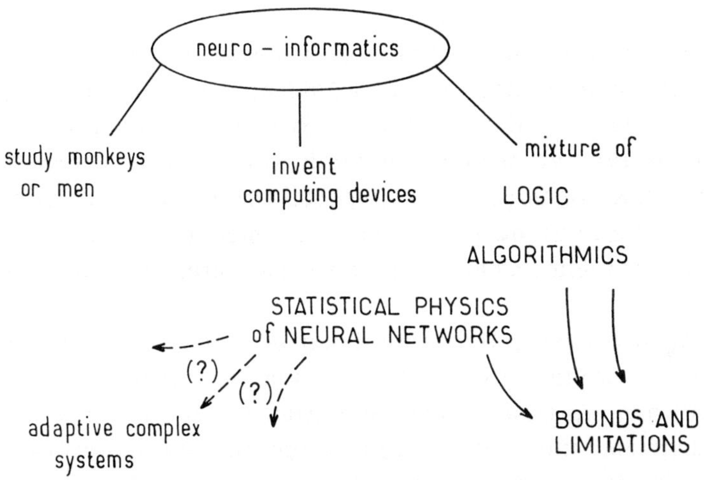

Fig. 2

As a common feature, these various theories have been conspicuously producing bounds and limitations (suffice it to recall the incompleteness theorem of Gödel, the book of Minsky and Papert, and Gardner's bounds).

One may also notice a tendency to move away from the initial motivations and to explore new domains. And perhaps should be confessed the secret hope, sheltered by many theoreticians, that these research efforts to understand intelligence, instead of proceeding straight towards their target (that would be a little dull), will experience a process of sprouting, with the unfolding of new and superb branches of knowledge. It seems that the outlines of a science of complex adaptive systems (wherein neural networks would find place aside with immune systems, evolution processes, etc.) are emerging, but this still belongs to prophecy.

Limitations and openings

Let me finish this chapter with mentioning some limitations of this type of theoretizing, as well as some possible openings

a) The strength of statistical physics lies upon the legitimacy to perform a statistical averaging over some disorder. Thus the importance of the controversy between the two opposite views of the brain, seen as 'maximally amorphous' or 'maximally ordered'. In the latter case, there would be little or no disorder to be averaged over; in the former case, the tools of statistical physics would appear well suited. It is not too risky to suggest that the truth might lie between the two extremes, and that the relative proportions might differ from species to species, and vary from one to another part of the same brain. The biological paradox is that the disorder seems to be more prevalent in higher animals and in higher centers, that exhibit greater ability to learn.

But anyway, statistical physics cannot hope for similar success in the study of brains as in the study of gases (where thermodynamics triumph): never will one equation abolish evolution.

b) As far as artificial intelligence applications of neural networks are concerned, we are in a phase of inventive fascination. In contrast with standard expert systems, neural networks seem to open a possibility of solving hard problems, without a need for the human programmer to understand the solution process: the burden of comprehension is left to the network, that must search its way alone to extract the rule from examples. But how far can one go solving without understanding? A divergence shows up here between the inventor who cares for solutions (nevermind, and even so much the better, if the net works better than it should), and the research scientist who insists on understanding (at the risk of disenchanting the miracles).

c) Biological experimentation on living beings raises moral problems, that I wish to evoke here, because physicists are often ill prepared for them. A good part of the pleasure of research in physics stems from the fast exchange between theory and experiment, and from the possibility to test ideas, even if they are slightly 'crazy', on matter or on a computer. In neurobiology, when it means to hurt or to sacrifice living beings, the imagination gets a little stifled. Thus the interest of physicists for developing methods of observation or visualisation that are non invasive, or soft, like nuclear resonance, magnetoencephalography, optical methods (rather than electrode recordings), tissue cultures in vitro, or also for the top-down approaches of psychophysics.

d) One of the appeals of biology is that this science studies objects which have meaning; those objects are present because they have been kept by evolution, because they fulfill some function; they have been sorted out and selected. Whereas the materials of physics and chemistry are often out there from mere inertia, when they are not the product and artefact of the scientist's fancy.

If furthermore some biological objects subserve thought and other higher brain functions, their interest is further increased. However one experiences rather rapidly some limitations in the satisfactions that may be gained in explaining the mind from the brain. Indeed, we have an intuitive, immediate, knowledge of our consciousness, compared to which neuropsychological explanations appear often as tangled and cumbersome as the jargon of Molière's doctors. A neuronal theory of humour would probably be the summum of ridicule. Let us end this paragraph with a sentence from a contemporary mathematician: 'It happens that nature lacks wit, this is the ground that physics exploits'.

In manner of conclusion

Albert Einstein said: 'The most incomprehensible thing in the world is that we can understand it'. I submit the following addendum: 'The most incomprehensible of the incomprehensible would be if we could understand how we understand'.

References

Abbott LF (1990) Learning in neural network memories. Network 1:105

Amit DJ (1989) Modelling brain function. Cambridge University Press, Cambridge

Amit DJ, Gutfreund H, Sompolinsky H (1985) Spin glass models of neural networks. Phys Rev A 32:1007-1018

Cragg BG, Temperley HNV (1954) The organization of neurones: a co-operative analogy. EEG Clinical Neurophysiol 6:85-92

Gardner E (1988) The space of interactions in neural network models. J Phys A: Math Gen 21:257-270

Geszti T (1990) Physical models of neural networks. World Scientific Publishing, Singapore

Hebb DO (1949) Organization of behavior. A neuropsychological theory, 2nd edn (1961) Wiley & Sons, New York

Hopfield JJ (1982) Neural networks and physical systems with emergent collective computational abilities. Proc Natl Acad Sci USA 79:2554-2558

Little WA (1974) The existence of persistent states in the brain. Math Biosciences 19:101-120

McCulloch WS, Pitts W (1943) A logical calculus of the ideas immanent in nervous activity. Bull Math Biophys 5:115-133

Minsky ML, Papert S (1969) Perceptrons. MIT Press, Cambridge Mass.

Rosenblatt F (1961) Principles of neurodynamics: Perceptrons and the theory of brain mechanism. Spartan Books, Washington, DC

Rumelhart DE, Hinton GE, Williams RJ (1986) Learning internal representations by error propagation. In: Rumelhart DE, McClelland JL (eds) Parallel distributed processing: explorations in the microstructures of cognition, vol I, MIT Press, Cambridge Mass. pp 318-362

Toulouse G (1989) Perspectives on neural network models and their relevance to neurobiology. J Phys A 22

Toulouse G (1991) The contribution of statistical physics to neural network theory. In: Proc. of the 8th European Physical Society Meeting, Amsterdam 1990, in press

Virasoro MA (1990) Maximum entropy principle and brain models. In: Theumann W, Köberle R (eds) Neural networks and spin glasses. World Scientific Publishing, Singapore

Manifesto of Brain Science*

Valentino Braitenberg

Max-Planck-Institut für biologische Kybernetik, Spemannstrasse 38, 7400 Tübingen, Germany

1. We believe that there are questions of such philosophical import that they deserve being pursued without any consideration of utility. One of them refers to the nature of thought processes, or more generally, of complex behaviour.

2. We are convinced that ultimately a satisfactory explanation of thought and behaviour will be given in a language akin to that of physics, i.e. in mathematical terms.

3. The physics of living organisms, with its specialized branches of physiology and biochemistry will undoubtedly underlie such an explanation, but it will not be sufficient by itself as a theory of behaviour. In fact, when boiled down to physical fundamentals, a mouse or even a worm is not very different from man. But we are ultimately interested in thought and behaviour of people, not of worms.

4. The difference in behaviour in different species reflect different ways of coping with the environment, or with distinct niches of the environment. These different behaviours have their material counterpart in different brains. Therefore the peculiar nature of any animal brain cannot be explained from the physical components alone, the explanation necessarily involving causes residing outside the animal, i.e. information derived from the environment.

5. Concepts such as (Shannonian) information, coding, computation, are outside of physics (even if the formulas look like physics) but are

---

* This was prepared for a meeting in Brussels where the European Commission considered the future of Neurobiology in Europe.

central to brain science. They are also fundamental concepts in electronics and computer science. This is the basis for a lively discourse between certain branches of engineering and brain science. Another common aspect is that both deal with functions directed to a goal, which physics does not.

6. Our object being the discovery of computer-like operations in brains, the hypotheses we test in our experiments are really inventions of computing schemes, and are therefore necessarily more complex than hypotheses in other branches of science. Thus we are inventors of computing devices much as our colleagues in Artificial Intelligence are and we can learn from them as much as they learn from us. Some ideas in brain science (e.g. neural networks) have already turned into eminently practical applications.

7. Computation in brains is a fine-grain operation, requiring a spatial resolution of about one to ten micrometers. The functional elements are fibers and neurons, and in most cases many neurons are involved in a significant functional pattern. This requires special techniques of observation which are being developed: multiple electrode recording, optical recording by means of voltage sensitive dyes. In most cases the vast amount of information produced by these recording techniques can only be stored and digested by means of large computers. Their theoretical analysis also requires sophisticated computing techniques, and often computer simulation.

8. We believe that the distribution of electrical signals observed at a spatial resolution of 1 μm and a temporal resolution of about 1 ms is all we need to know as the material counterpart of behaviour. Behaviour may be modified by hormones, or by pharmaca, or by pathological unbalance of some transmitter substance, but the actual effect of these is always expressed in terms of the occurrence or not occurrence of action potentials in neurons.

A more fine-grain analysis, say at the molecular level, is relevant for the understanding of the individual cell, but probably unnecessary for the understanding of behaviour, or may even obscure the picture there.

9. Developmental neurobiology is a branch of general biology, not of brain science as defined here. "How do the fibers from the eye find

their way into the optic tectum?" The answer to this question will tell us much about how the arteries find their way into the kidney, or the roots of a tree into the earth, but very little about the problem of the analysis of visual information in the optic tectum.

10. Efficient research groups in brain science are small. Everybody is groping for experimental techniques and for conceptual models. If someone draws up a gigantic project in order to solve the problem by brute force, he is likely to have missed the complexity of the situation and is sure to produce much waste.

To illustrate my points, I want to mention some successes of modern brain science in its interaction with information engineering.

(a) The paper by McCulloch and Pitts (1943) proposed an equivalence between nets of neurons connected by synapses and propositions of Boolean logics. The terminology and the diagrams of this paper were immediately taken over by the designers of calculating machines (e.g. J. v. Neumann) and the basic ideas became the starting point for more than one theoretical development, e.g. Automata Theory and Chomskian linguistics (via the formalization proposed by Kleene, 1956).

(b) Some ideas were exchanged repeatedly to and fro between brain science and engineering. The idea of the Perceptron (Rosenblatt 1962), a randomly connected image processor, was inspired by neuroanatomy and neurophysiology. It has admirable technological consequences even today (Sejnowski 1987). It received criticism on theoretical grounds by Minsky and Selfridge, who thought that a machine equipped with preset form detectors ("Pandemonium") would be much more efficient. The Pandemonium inspired neurophysiological work by Lettvin and others which turned into the seminal paper "What the frog's eye tells the frog's brain" (1959). Parallel to it, in the same intellectual environment, work on the cat (and monkey) visual cortex in the hands of Hubel and Wiesel produced splendid, Nobel prize winning results. The Hubel and Wiesel "feature detectors" in turn gave the engineers ideas, who produced several efficient image processing devices along the same theoretical lines.

(c) Filter theory, auto- and crosscorrelation, generalized Fourier analysis are theoretical concepts developed in electronics. Reichardt (1970) described the results of his (and Hassenstein's) experiments on optomotor reactions in insects in those terms. This was the first model of animal behaviour which made detailed predictions on the neurological wiring underlying the behaviour, and the predictions were in part confirmed anatomically (Braitenberg 1977). The technological fallout was a patent for a device designed to measure the direction and velocity of a moving panorama.

(d) Associative memory was postulated by psychologists (Hebb) as a principle underlying cognition and behaviour. This idea turned into a variety of mathematical models, one of which, the neural net of the Hopfield kind, is hailed now as the cornerstone of a new age of computing technology. It was shown that the statistics of connections within the cerebral cortex (Braitenberg and Schüz 1991) can best be explained as being specialized for associative memory. The global states of activity which the Hopfield theory postulates, a sort of resonant modes or "eigen-states" of the cortex, have been shown with computer analysis of multiple electrode recordings (e.g. Aertsen and Gerstein 1991; Vaadia and Aertsen, this volume).

References

Aertsen A, Gerstein GL (1991) Dynamic aspects of neuronal cooperativity: fast stimulus-locked modulations of effective connectivity. In: Krüger J (ed) Neuronal Cooperativity, Springer Series in Synergetics. Springer, Berlin Heidelberg

Braitenberg V (1977) On the texture of brains. Neuroanatomy for the cybernetically minded. Springer, Berlin Heidelberg New York

Braitenberg V, Schüz A (1991) Anatomy of the Cortex. Statistics and Geometry. Springer, Berlin Heidelberg New York

Hebb DO (1949) The organization of behavior. Wiley, New York

Kleene SC (1956) Representation of events in nerve nets and finite automata. In: Shannon CE, McCarthy J (eds) Automata Studies, Princeton University Press

Lettvin JY, Maturana HR, McCulloch WS, Pitts WH (1959) What the frog's eye tells the frog's brain. Proc Inst rad Engrs 47:1940-1951

McCulloch WS, Pitts WH (1943) A logical calculus of ideas immanent in nervous activity. Bull Math Biophys 5:115-133

Reichardt (1970) The insect eye as a model for analysis of uptake, transduction and processing of visual data in the nervous system. 34. Physikertagung 1969, Salzburg, Plenarvorträge. BG Teubner, Stuttgart

Rosenblatt F (1962) A comparison of several perceptron models. In: Yovits MC, Jacobi GT, Goldstein GD (eds) Self-organizing systems. Spartan Books, Washington

Sejnowski TJ, Rosenberg CR (1987) Parallel networks that learn to pronounce English text. Complex systems 1: 145-168

Vaadia E, Aertsen A (this volume)

von Neumann, J (1956) Probabilistic logics and the synthesis of reliable organisms from unreliable components. In: Shannon CE, McCarthy J (eds) Automata Studies, Princeton University Press

Druck: Mercedesdruck, Berlin
Verarbeitung: Buchbinderei Lüderitz & Bauer, Berlin